POSITIVE HEALTH:
FLOURISHING LIVES, WELL-BEING IN DOCTORS

MARSHA W. SNYDER, MD., MAPP.

BALBOA.
PRESS
A DIVISION OF HAY HOUSE

Balboa Press books may be ordered through booksellers or by contacting:

Balboa Press
A Division of Hay House
1663 Liberty Drive
Bloomington, IN 47403
www.balboapress.com
1 (877) 407-4847

Because of the dynamic nature of the Internet, any web addresses or links contained in this book may have changed since publication and may no longer be valid. The views expressed in this work are solely those of the author and do not necessarily reflect the views of the publisher, and the publisher hereby disclaims any responsibility for them.

The author of this book does not dispense medical advice or prescribe the use of any technique as a form of treatment for physical, emotional, or medical problems without the advice of a physician, either directly or indirectly. The intent of the author is only to offer information of a general nature to help you in your quest for emotional and spiritual well-being. In the event you use any of the information in this book for yourself, which is your constitutional right, the author and the publisher assume no responsibility for your actions.

Any people depicted in stock imagery provided by Thinkstock are models, and such images are being used for illustrative purposes only.
Certain stock imagery © Thinkstock.

ISBN: 978-1-4525-9830-7 (sc)
ISBN: 978-1-4525-9831-4 (e)

Library of Congress Control Number: 2014919870

Print information available on the last page.

Balboa Press rev. date: 09/17/2016

Contents

Foreword

In this unprecedented book, Marsha W. Snyder, MD, MAPP, applies the latest wisdom and science of positive psychology to the widespread problem of medical-student and clinician burnout as she presents a vision for "positive health" and educational transformation. She draws on a wealth of experience in psychiatry, health-care administration, and graduate studies in the innovative Masters of Applied Positive Psychology program at the University of Pennsylvania with the distinguished "father" of positive psychology, Professor Martin E. P. Seligman.

Those of us in medical education know how serious the "distress of ill-being" (to use the author's phrase) is among clinicians and students. There are so many reasons for it, including overwork and fatigue, decline in clinician compensation and astronomical indebtedness, increasing malpractice suits, patient load and time-restricted patient care, the complex paperwork required for processing patients, adversarial and cold interprofessional relationships, the loss of professional autonomy, and the assumption that each clinician or clinician-in-training has to have solutions at hand for every patient despite human and medical limits. Dr. Snyder refers to the latter as the attitudes that prevent clinicians from acknowledging their emotional and physical limits and from being able to entrust their patients to their peers.

The reasons are complex, but the realities of physician depression, disability, anxiety, dissatisfaction, and burnout are everywhere. Many physicians these days, even a slight majority of them, report thinking about leaving practice. When doctors do experience burnout, the results for patients are suboptimal care, sloppy diagnosis, decreased patient satisfaction, medical error, and poor patient adherence to treatment.

Dr. Snyder is well-steeped in medical education and takes note that as many as 25 percent of medical students experience depression in their first two years of medical school. This problem, the author reminds us, starts to surface about halfway through the first year due to factors such as the stress of exams, long hours, and sleeplessness; and in the clinical settings, other factors arise, such as humiliation, maltreatment, and feeling incompetent.

The author's Rx is the integration of positive psychology and positive health into the medical-school curriculum and into curricula for clinicians. She focuses on resiliency skills, the uplifting strength of moral integrity, emotional intelligence, empathy and self-awareness, balance, authentic professional community, and the various other virtues or character strengths that positive psychology has come to offer, with conceptual clarity, scientific evidence, and practical how-to guidance. Dr. Snyder writes of "positive health," which requires us to think not just about illness and disease in ourselves and in others, but flourishing in the form of optimal well-being. Her approach is evidence-based throughout, as well as eminently practical in laying out various exercises, both somatic and cognitive, that can both protect students and clinicians and allow them to experience emotion and professional growth despite immense challenges.

As one who has been involved in medical-school education for thirty years and counting at the University of Chicago, Case Western Reserve University, and Stony Brook University, I endorse Dr. Snyder's diagnosis and prescription. Our students and clinicians are struggling to maintain their mental and physical health. Many physicians I know are advising their children not to go into medicine due to innumerable stresses and relatively low pay levels outside of the very competitive specialties. These residents today, burdened by immense debt, low-paying residencies, and overwork almost all at some point throw up their hands in desperation. Dr. Snyder prescribes her integrative curricula not just for medical students, but for residents, house staff, and all those who are part of the culture of health care and its delivery.

Being a doctor is harder now than it was a few decades ago, and the wounded healers are everywhere. Dr. Snyder, who has suffered with burnout firsthand, is offering an innovative and beneficial vision for healthier students and physicians, and ultimately, for the better care and treatment of patients. I endorse her visionary integration of positive psychology, positive health, and clinician well-being into medical curricula and across medical educational venues of all types.

Stephen G. Post, PhD
Professor of Preventive Medicine
Head, Division of Medicine in Society
Director, Center for Medical Humanities, Compassionate Care, and Bioethics
Stony Brook University School of Medicine

Preface

Although research tells us that distress and ill-being in the physician population has reached epidemic proportions worldwide, precious few in the medical field actually focus on, and specialize in, exploring this phenomenon, including its impact on patients and health-care economics. Hence, a solution to the problem remains beyond our understanding.

The health and well-being of physicians has been a topic of great interest and concern to me since I first entered medical school. As a graduate of an outstanding Ivy-League baccalaureate nursing program and a dedicated professional nurse, I was dismayed and discouraged in medical school by the cold, impersonal, disrespectful, and competitive attitude of professors and instructors toward students, patients, staff, and one another (a major contrast to the positive attitude of faculty in my nursing-training experience). It was obvious to me that this culture of coldness could not result in a happy, healthy professional with the key skills necessary for relating to patients, families, and their own life challenges.

It is, therefore, not surprising that in my role as chair of psychiatry for a four-hospital health-care network, I took on the management and advising of the system's physician-health policies and committee, and the clinical management of distressed physicians became an increasingly large percentage of my practice.

With increasing success in my career and my ability to help physicians, no one was more surprised than I was when I fell victim to the same process of physical burnout, leading to a sudden and severe physical illness that totally disrupted every aspect of my life for two years.

My experience as a patient with an undiagnosed and gradually worsening illness, the concomitant losses of physical and role function, and my journey to find my true self and my purpose on my road back to healing were the motivating wisdom and knowledge behind this book.

An important part of my broadening included an intense and comprehensive fourteen months of education in the masters program in applied positive psychology at the University of Pennsylvania with Dr. Martin Seligman, the "father" of positive psychology. It was he who introduced me to the body of research in positive health. I instantly realized how important this body of knowledge could be when applied to physician well-being, health of the population, and health-care economics.

Step one for me is to introduce physicians and medical students to this vitally important body of knowledge. Research shows that physicians only teach to their patients that which they themselves actively practice. This book was, therefore, written in order to: (1) Provide research-based evidence of the epidemic of physician ill-being and associated problems in current medical-school curricula; (2) Introduce critical additions to medical-student and physician education based on the science of positive health (positive emotions, engagement, positive relationships, meaning, accomplishment, etc.), resilience, and professionalism; and, (3) Review topics that should be included in that curriculum through the chapters of the book, including group discussion questions and individual assignments for those who would like to use the book as a self-teaching tool.

Once physicians are actively practicing positive health, research shows that they will then teach this to their patients. This will lead to a healthy and flourishing population, decreased morbidity and mortality, and decreased health-care costs.

My hope and motivation is for positive compassionate change in medicine and in physician well-being. I hope no other physician or patient suffers as I did for the reasons that I did. I hope for flourishing lives and health and well-being for all humans. In order to accomplish this, the "business" of health care (in which large corporations financially benefit from treating illness) and the cold competitive culture of medicine must become things of the past. They must be replaced by doctors and medical leaders who understand, model, and teach positive health, loving-kindness, and thriving to the entire population. This book introduces the materials to help build that reality.

I would like to acknowledge and give special thanks to Kathryn Britton, who selflessly gave of her time and editing expertise, in my labor of love to give birth to this book.

Marsha W. Snyder, MD, MAPP, 2014

Note from the Author

Each of us as human beings will face challenges and difficulties in our lives. Throughout this book, you will learn about positive health and read of many people who exemplify these ideals.

The illustrations contained in this book were all drawn by Sabine R. Snyder, my daughter, who has always been a role model of positivity for me. Born with a severe form of autism and limited in her verbal communication, Sabine has always communicated through her drawings. With a creative imagination and a wonderful sense of humor, she tells stories filled with love and laughter involving her favorite characters.

The characters in these drawings are based on singer Klaus Nomi (with permission from his estate) and Sabine herself.

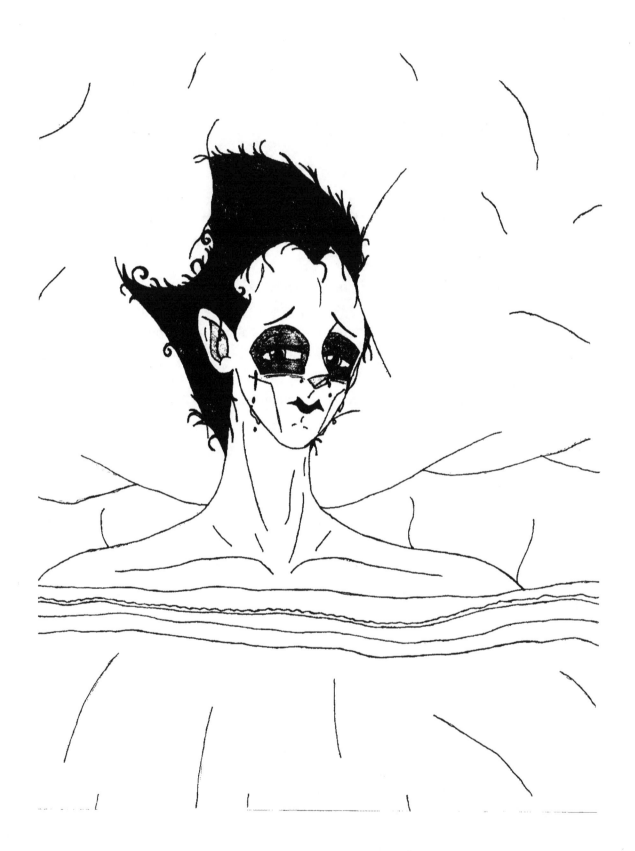

Chapter 1

Why Positive Health and this Curriculum?

This book documents the distress of the medical profession and proposes an innovative curriculum, based firmly in positive health, resilience, professionalism, compassion, and purpose. This is an important first step in effecting a significant positive change. Neither physician ill-being nor attempts at correcting it are unique, as researchers and practitioners began offering solutions a generation ago. This book, however, highlights three unique aspects that have been absent from the literature: the extent and complexity of ill-being in medical students and physicians; the importance of psychological and physiological resilience in the well-being of physicians; and the unique opportunity that positive health represents both to physician well-being and the thriving of their patients.

This curriculum is innovative in two ways. It is the first curriculum for doctors based on the scientific principles of positive health, resilience, and positive psychology. It is also the first medical curriculum that provides tools for improving the health and well-being of doctors, their patients, the population, and the health-care economy.

To document the needs and current state of doctors and medical students, this chapter begins by exploring why the medical profession is at risk. It highlights the issues of distress and burnout in doctors and medical students, while identifying their sources of origin to provide the context for interventions regarding physician well-being.

Next, the chapter takes an in-depth look at the construct of resilience in the context of psychological science. Although many physicians' health advocates emphasize the importance of resilience in doctors, there remains no consensus of what is meant by *resilience*. As a result, ineffective solutions and conjecture dominate.

The next section in this chapter introduces the construct and science of *positive health*, as an outgrowth of positive psychology. The section includes a review of the teaching and practice of behaviors that build positive health and how these can benefit medical students, physicians, and their patients.

Finally, the chapter synthesizes the key themes of this inquiry, and establishes it as a unique and pioneering work in physicians' health, medical education, and positive psychology. These themes will be clearly explained throughout this chapter.

Theme one is that the cause of ill-being in medical students extends beyond the students, into issues with faculty and administration.

Theme two suggests that many physicians who are troubled or burned out relate some of their difficulties to ethical issues in the system. This reflects a complex system-wide problem that cannot be fixed by a single intervention or curriculum. Evidence regarding resilience training's effects in other domains positions this curriculum as a high-leverage, low-resource opportunity that can produce positive outcomes.

Theme three points to the understanding, defining, and teaching of resilience skills to physicians. These skills have not been clearly defined in physician-health literature or taught formally in medical-education settings. Teaching resilience skills will promote flexible and accurate thinking for student and faculty excellence.

Theme four involves the creation of well-being in doctors and the rest of society by incorporating the science of positive health. This is the first documented training for medical students or faculty using this body of science. In addition, this is the first documented application of positive health applied directly to the medical profession.

Theme five states that medical training and practice must move from an outdated pathology-based model to a health-based/prevention-based model. Health care is fundamentally a human activity involving multiple interactions that must be guided by professionalism, ethics, and complex interpersonal skills. These skills must be taught and cultivated early in the professional life of physicians, preferably as students. The relevant values and skills fall under the umbrella of professionalism, and require sophisticated competencies, such as emotional intelligence, communication skills, integrity, and high moral and ethical standards. This theme, coupled with the other four, suggests a strong need for change in medical-school curricula. The information presented in this book is a small step toward effecting that change.

MEDICINE: A WORKFORCE AT RISK

The medical profession has long been known as one filled with potential risks to the health and well-being of its members. Issues such as low physician satisfaction, fatigue, anxiety, depression, suicide, substance abuse, disability, divorce, and burnout are well-documented in the profession (Rosenthal & Okie, 2005). Changes in the health-care environment have created multiple additional stressors for today's practicing physicians. These include time-constrained patient care, a lack of resources, a decline in compensation, an increased threat of malpractice litigation, and an erosion of professional autonomy. They have contributed to a further deterioration of dignity, spirit, and will (Hu, et al., 2012; Dunn, Arnetz, Christensen, & Homer, 2007).

Additional factors cause more anxiety and ill health. Medicine is filled with uncertainty owing to the issues involved in daily practice. These include death, helplessness, the limitations and challenges of accurate prognoses, intense human emotion, and the inevitable human capacity for error. The fact that these can lead to personal anxiety in the physician is not the major resulting problem.

Optimism, activism, and heroic attitudes are endemic in physicians. As a result, physicians feel they must exert superhuman capabilities, fix everything, and even snatch patients from the jaws of death. This never-give-up attitude is part of medical training, part of the professional identity, and part of the public's expectation of their doctors. Uncertainties, such as death and unpredictable patient outcomes, conflict with this superhuman belief and result in anxieties that interfere with physicians' ability to effectively and empathetically negotiate their professional role among patients and society. Every patient death is viewed as a physician mistake by the public, and becomes a devastating professional and personal failure to the physician (Christakis, 2003).

This gap between expectations and reality has consequences. Forty percent of American surgeons in one 2009 study met criteria for burnout, and in most cases, a poor quality of life, with younger surgeons exhibiting the highest risk. However, the problem is neither limited to the United States nor to surgeons. Forty-six percent of New Zealand general practitioners felt work had affected their physical health, and 57 percent indicated they often thought about leaving general practice. In a recent study of young surgeons from Australia and New Zealand, 27 percent of the participants reported burnout (Henning, Hawken, & Hill, 2009).

A study exploring Canadian physicians' personal coping strategies for dealing with stress while at work revealed that the three most frequently used strategies were all significantly correlated with emotional exhaustion. They included keeping stress to one's self, concentrating on what to do next, and going on as if nothing had happened. While the coping strategies physicians used at home tended to rely more on family and supportive relationships (which is therapeutic), this does not compensate for maladaptive strategies used in the workplace. An overall lack of resilience and an absence of knowledge regarding effective coping strategies seems to pervade the medical profession, along with a lack of workplace support for effective coping (Lemaire & Wallace, 2010).

In addition to the negative consequences of burnout and stress suffered by physicians, the resultant feelings of depersonalization and loss of empathy lead to decreased patient satisfaction and prolonged recovery time for patients, along with an increase in medical errors (Halbesleben & Rathert, 2008). Additional studies have noted the negative effects on patient care associated with physician distress (McCray, Cronholm, Bogner, Gallo, & Neill, 2008; West, Tan, Habermann, Sloan, & Shanafelt, 2009). West and associates, looking at 16,394 US internal medicine residents, noted a clear association between burnout and lower scores on the Medicine In-Training Exam (a knowledge-based examination taken by all residents) in all postgraduate years (West, Shanafelt, & Kolars, 2011). Measured depersonalization also was associated with how frequently physicians report delivering suboptimal care to patients (Shanafelt, Sloan, & Habermann, 2003). The higher the degree of burnout, the more the number of reports of suboptimal care reported by physicians. Burnout is also associated with decreased career satisfaction, decreased physician and patient satisfaction, and poor patient compliance (Dimatteo, et al., 1993; Linn, et al., 1985).

What is the source of physician ill-being?

Many experts have tried unsuccessfully to solve the puzzle of the source of ill-being in physicians and correct it. However, some detective work as to its origin may be helpful.

Numerous studies have found a high prevalence of psychological distress among medical students in the United States and abroad. Much of the distress encountered by students in medical schools surfaces about halfway through the first year and manifests as burnout, stress, depression, anxiety, poor mental and physical quality of life, and fatigue (Dyrbye & Shanafelt, 2011). A recent survey of first-year and second-year students at a West Coast medical school found that approximately one quarter of the students were depressed (Rosenthal & Okie, 2005).

As with physician ill-being, medical student ill-being is an international phenomenon. In a study of medical students in Australia, it was found that 16–25 percent of students reported some degree of suicidal ideation before examinations. A study of medical students in Turkey demonstrated that students transitioning from year one to year two had significantly higher scores for depression, anxiety, and ill health than comparable students studying physical education or economics (Henning, Hawken, & Hill, 2009).

As is the case with physicians, the usual suspects, such as long work hours, lack of sleep, and academic problems and pressures, have been explored, but without a satisfactory explanation for the widespread student ill-being (Dyrbye & Shanafelt, 2011). A look at less commonly explored factors may be helpful.

Medical student maltreatment is a troubling reality in medical education and has been since the early 1980s. Unfortunately, it is rarely discussed openly as a causal factor for medical student or physician ill-being. From the early 1980s (Rosenberg & Silver, 1984) through the early 1990s (Baldwin, Daugherty, & Eckenfels, 1991), researchers have reported its occurrence, severity, and consequences (including verbal, physical, and sexual abuse). Further, investigators typically reported a rate of occurrence near 20 percent for abuse incurred by medical students (Baldwin, Daugherty, Eckenfels, & Leksas, 1988; Haviland, et al., 2012). In 1992, the Association of American Medical Colleges (AAMC) issued a memorandum establishing standards of behavior regarding medical student treatment and procedures that deal with behaviors not conforming to the standards. In 1999, the Liaison Committee on Medical Education established a follow-on standard requiring each allopathic medical school to define standards of conduct in the teacher-learner relationship, as well as standards for preventing and reporting abuses. These standards are now part of the medical-school accreditation process. Although rates of reported abuse dropped as low as 14 percent from 2002 to 2006, more recent reports from 2007 to 2010 indicate the rates of abuse incidence rising to 17 percent, close to the pre-guideline levels (Haviland, et al., 2012). A key point to consider is that these are merely reported rates. Establishing guidelines and consequences may have actually decreased the rate of reporting by institutions monitored to avoid negative consequences.

In a longitudinal survey involving sixteen nationally representative US medical schools, with an 80 percent response rate of 2,316 students, 42 percent of seniors reported experiencing harassment and 84 percent reported experiences of belittlement during medical school. Sources of harassment and belittlement were primarily from residents (27% and 71% of med students experienced harassment / belittlement from residents) and clinical professors (21% and 63% of med students experienced harassment/belittlement from clinical professors) (Frank, Carrera, Stratton, Bickel, & Nora, 2006). Those who reported being harassed or belittled were more likely to experience stress, depression, suicidal behavior, alcohol abuse, and discontent for their chosen specialty than those who were not affected by this abuse. They also indicated lower overall satisfaction with life and a lower locus of control. In addition, researchers of these findings also made a sad discovery, finding that 11 percent of harassment and 32 percent of belittling actually came from other medical students. This negative behavior among medical students has not been documented in the earlier literature (Frank, Carrera, Stratton, Bickel, & Nora, 2006). The severe and damaging psychological and behavioral effects of sexual abuse, racial/sexual identity discrimination, and public humiliation and belittlement are well-studied and well-known (Mattke, Schmitz, & Zink, 2009; Witte, Stratton, & Nora, 2006).

With careful and clear guidelines in place, particularly among medical schools, where enforcement is linked to accreditation, it seems unlikely that the incidence of medical student abuse could once again be approaching pre-guideline levels. However, this begins to make sense when considering the widespread unwillingness by students to report such abuse, due to fear of reprisal, receiving poor grades, and making a spectacle of themselves. In addition, the long-standing culture of abuse tolerance in medicine is well-known—for example, "That's just the way Dr. X is, but he's a great doctor," (Mattke, Schmitz, & Zink, 2009)·

The following example, reported by a physician, represents her experience as a senior medical student and illustrates some of these issues.

> I was on my surgery rotation as a medical student at a well-respected medical school. After work, the residents and students often went to the restaurant across the street to get a bite to eat or have a beer. About two weeks into the rotation, the chief resident left the restaurant the same time I did and started to walk home with me. I was confused at first, uncertain if he lived nearby. When we got to my building, a high-rise with a doorman, I said good-bye, but he kept following.
>
> When we reached the door, he grabbed my hand and said, "I'm coming up." I said, "No." Then he said, "Don't forget that I'm the chief resident, and I have power." He proceeded to rape me in my own apartment, forcing me to have sex with him three times over what was an eight-hour nightmare.
>
> The next day, I made an emergency appointment with my gynecologist, who was also a faculty member at the medical school, but I refused to identify the perpetrator for fear of the repercussions. I had to continue the last two weeks of the rotation working directly with my perpetrator, pretending as if nothing had happened.
>
> This was my first clinical rotation as a medical student. It damaged my trust and my spirit. This is the first time I have ever told anyone about it (Name Withheld, personal communication).

A second infrequently discussed factor, though equally compelling, is the prevalence of burnout in faculty who teach the medical students. Dyrbye, Shanafelt, Thomas, and Durning conducted a cross-sectional, multi-institutional study to evaluate the presence of burnout in internal medicine clerkship directors (2009). With a 75 percent response rate from all 110 institutional members of the Clerkship Directors in Internal Medicine (82 responses), 62 percent met criteria for burnout. Responders with burnout were two to four times more likely to report attitudes of lack of empathy toward students and of students being burdensome. Of note, burnout was more prevalent among internal medicine clerkship directors who were allotted ten or fewer hours per week for their primary educational role (Dyrbye, Shanafelt, Thomas, & Durning, 2009).

Several additional studies corroborate these findings, suggesting that faculty at academic medical centers are dissatisfied and are considering leaving academia as a result (Shanafelt, et al., 2009). In a stratified random sample of 4,578 full-time faculty members from 26 US medical schools, with a response rate of 52 percent, 14 percent had seriously considered leaving their institution during the prior year, and 21 percent had considered leaving academic medicine altogether during the prior year owing to dissatisfaction (Pololi, Krupat, Civian, Ash, & Brennan, 2012). Of particular significance was the primary nature of faculty's dissatisfaction: **There are negative perceptions and distress about the nonrelational and ethical culture of the workplace. Significant predictors of intention to leave include feeling vulnerable and unconnected with colleagues, moral distress, perceptions of the culture as being unethical at times, and feelings of being adversely changed by the culture. Low sense of engagement and lack of alignment of faculty's personal values with perceived institutional values also predicted intention to leave** (Pololi, Krupat, Civian, Ash, & Brennan, 2012).

Once again, exploring the origins of medical student burnout and ill-being from the standpoint of faculty as mentors and role models, two new issues of concern stand out: feelings of disconnection, and ethical/moral distress. Research on social learning theory from Bandura suggests that people learn by observing others' behavior, attitudes, and outcomes of those behaviors. When observing the actions of others, we form an idea of how behaviors, particularly new behaviors in new situations, are performed. In future situations, this coded information serves as a guide for action. Particularly when role models or people of admired status exhibit behaviors, they are more likely to have the greatest effect. Because internal medicine clerkship directors serve in an important mentorship capacity, their own burnout could greatly influence the attitude and behavior of medical students (Bandura, 2001).

According to self-determination theory, the social contexts in which individuals are embedded must be responsive to basic psychological needs to provide an appropriate atmosphere in which an active, well-integrated learner can develop. Excessive control, suboptimal challenges, and lack of connectedness disrupt the inherently positive natural tendencies, resulting in distress and even psychopathology. Feelings of lack of connection and exclusion in faculty lead to alienation (as opposed to engagement) and ill-being (as opposed to high intrinsic motivation and high achievement) (Ryan & Deci, 2000b). If we regularly observe this problem in faculty, we also are likely to see it in their students.

Regarding faculty issues of ethical/moral distress, the 21 percent of faculty who entertained thoughts of leaving academic medicine answered positively to statements: (a) must be a self-promoter to get ahead, (b) working here is dehumanizing, (c) culture discourages altruism, (d) felt pressure to behave unethically, (e) people need to be deceitful to succeed, (f) others have taken credit for my work, (g) must compromise values to work here, and (h) must be more aggressive than I like (Pololi, Krupat, Civian, Ash, & Brennan, 2012).

Adding to the obvious distress this causes faculty and the loss of valued, principled faculty members, this creates for medical students a third issue, that is, the apparent medical-school curriculum versus the hidden agendas and covert realities faced by students. It has long been noted that medical students become less altruistic and more cynical through their years of medical training (Feudtner, Christakis, & Christakis, 1994). **If the ethical, professional, and moral values of the formal medical-school curriculum are not reinforced through the medical school's and hospital's institutional values (including their fair and ethical treatment of faculty, students, employees, and patients), the institution will undermine its own teaching.**

The training of humane and empathetic physicians should be a concern to medical educators. There is a growing public perception that physicians have become too impersonal and detached, lacking empathy (Verrees, 1996). A 2007 multi-institutional cross-sectional survey involving 1,098 medical students in Minnesota found that burnout inversely correlated with feelings of empathy in the students. In contrast, students' sense of personal accomplishment demonstrated a positive correlation with empathy, independent of gender (Thomas, et al., 2007). Therefore, student distress and burnout, coupled with a distressed faculty and an unspoken negative agenda of parent institutions, help grow this negative trend rapidly. The medical student who enters school with a noble purpose and a desire to be a healer finds it waning by the middle of year one.

What solutions have been attempted?

Despite the state of ill health among medical doctors, residents, interns, and medical students and multiple attempts at effective interventions, little substantive positive change has occurred in the fight against physician ill-being. The high prevalence of distress and its serious personal and professional ramifications remains. Although the Liaison Committee on Medical Education requires medical schools to have a student wellness program (Accreditation Standard MS-26), there are no clear guidelines on content and structure for such a program (Haviland, et al., 2012).

Most programs that have been empirically studied use a series of short-term activities or interventions, followed by a comparison of physician data immediately before and after the intervention. Krasner and coworkers designed a continuing medical education course, taken by seventy primary care physicians, that focused on mindfulness meditation and self-awareness exercises (2009). The course involved an eight-week intensive phase of two and a half hours per week, plus one seven-hour retreat, followed by a ten-month maintenance phase of two and a half hours per month. Results at the end of the program (12 months) and three months later (15 months) demonstrated increased mindfulness and empathy, along with decreases in burnout and depersonalization scores during the program. However, no further measures were obtained beyond fifteen months, and outcomes such as physician quality of life, physical well-being, and career satisfaction were not measured.

In 2008, the Northwestern University Feinberg School of Medicine introduced a required six-week healthy living unit into the second-year medical-school curriculum. This unit addressed the competency of personal awareness and self-care in medical students (Kushner, Kessler, & McGaghie, 2011). The theme of student self-care was addressed via a behavior change plan, in which students attempted to change one of their own self-selected health behaviors. The most frequently selected target behaviors were exercise, nutrition, and sleep. Each student kept a journal throughout the process. Results revealed that 40 percent of students reported positive goal achievement. However, 49.6 percent reported that their goal was not achieved, and 9.9 percent were uncertain. The authors suggested that the lack of success, as reflected in student feedback, was due to highly competitive demands placed on students and their own disproportionately high expectations.

The American Medical Student Association developed a Web-based tool for medical students to encourage self-reflection, promote positive lifestyle habits, and educate students about their own health (Rakel & Hedgecock, 2008). Between August 2005 and August 2006, there were 10,683 hits on the Web site. Survey results of the first five hundred medical students and residents who completed the survey revealed that only 38.5 percent agreed that the module would change their behavior toward improved health and 50.6 percent felt that what they learned would help them communicate health concepts to future patients.

At one medical school in Australia, teachers taught a required mindfulness-based health enhancement program to 270 second-semester first-year medical students (Hassed, De Lisle, Sullivan, & Pier, 2009). Measurements taken at the end of the program demonstrated significantly less depression and hostility scores, with no significant change in anxiety or physical health scores, compared with preprogram scores. No further follow-up was performed, and no conclusions could be drawn regarding the possible long-term benefits of this program.

The challenging culture of medicine

In 2009, Henning and colleagues passionately and rigorously pursued the mystery and causes of poor quality of life and ill-being in New Zealand doctors. The authors suggest a need to address issues of quality of life for doctors at all levels, starting with medical-student selection and training, through faculty modeling and self-care, including promoting quality-of-life programs and networks of support for doctors in practice, and scrutiny and change respecting the medical culture. Additionally, health-care organizations must respect and care for physicians and employees in the same way they require their employees to care for patients. Finally, these organizations must eliminate the culture of secrecy and shame in health care (Henning, Hawken, & Hill, 2009). Although the authors made no specific programmatic suggestions, simply identifying these issues is a significant first step for the medical culture if substantive changes are to occur.

The following examples of these issues faced by two different physicians help to highlight the above.

> I was part of a group practice that was bought by the local hospital. My patient satisfaction scores were very high, and I had never had an error or a malpractice suit. My patients loved me and I loved what I did. Suddenly, the hospital decided that we had to see twice the number of patients in an hour than we currently scheduled (which we felt was the safe number) because the practice was not bringing in enough income. They sent a nonphysician administrator to enforce this policy, who treated my colleagues and me disrespectfully. I spoke to the administrator and said that seeing any more patients would be unsafe for the patients. He ordered the secretaries to comply with his orders in spite of what I told him. I left the practice shortly thereafter (Anonymous Source, personal communication).

And the second:

> I am a physician who has worked in a group practice that has tried to stay independent from hospitals. Hospitals are buying up most of the practices in the area, but we heard that most of the employed physicians felt mistreated. At one of the two hospitals where we are on staff and do our surgery, we heard they were trying to get rid of any physicians at their hospital who competed with the practices that they owned. However, I had not encountered any problems. Then one day, during a critical case, while I had the patient's chest open on the table, some nurse came into my room from another operating room demanding that I had an instrument that was needed in the other room. In a firm, but not loud or unprofessional tone, I told her that I could not help her and went back to my patient. The next day, having been charged with harassment, I was instructed to take a leave of absence from the hospital and to seek treatment (Anonymous source, personal communication).

An opportunity: rethinking medical education

The goal of medical education has been to train knowledgeable, competent, and professional physicians equipped to care for the nation's sick, advance the science of medicine, and promote public health (Dyrbye, Thomas, & Shanafelt, 2006). The highly competitive selection process to enter medical school in the United States involves required undergraduate training in biology, chemistry, and physics, and taking the Medical College Admission Test examination. Although some schools recommend undergraduate humanities courses, they are not required. For many medical students, the severe competition with fellow students for grades, and an overemphasis on the sciences, begins as an undergraduate.

Skills taught in the first year of medical school uniformly focus on basic sciences of medical pathology, such as pathology, pathophysiology, histology, pharmacology, and microbiology. The competitive climate continues, with the focus now being the need to be the best to earn the best residency slot at the time of the post-medical school residency match.

While this definition and model may have served us well in earlier decades, perhaps this model has outlived its usefulness. Scientific research has moved medicine ahead from a primarily illness-based and pathology-based focus, to the possibility of a focus on prevention and the development of health assets (M. E. P. Seligman, C. Peterson, A. J. Barsky, J. K. Boehm, L. D. Kubzansky, and N. Park, unpublished data, 2010). Secondly, although the specialized knowledge of medical and human pathology and pathophysiology those medical students learn in their first year is based in the science of disease, health care is fundamentally a human activity involving a focus on wellness and multiple complex human interactions. These complex interactions require attaining specific values and skills that must be taught and cultivated (Lesser, et al., 2010). These values and skills fall under the umbrella of professionalism and require medical students to master sophisticated competencies such as resilience, self-awareness, self-control, emotional intelligence, communication skills, integrity, empathy, and the highest moral and ethical standards and behavior. A story shared by a fellow physician about when he was an intern illustrates:

> It is really important for a physician to be open-minded, nonjudgmental, and compassionate with each and every patient. One night as an intern, I was on call in the emergency room, and we got what I thought was our typical "dump": a young, unconscious man, dirty and smelling of alcohol. I figured he was our typical homeless guy living on the street who gets drunk and passes out from alcohol intoxication and has pneumonia from living on the street. I started him on antibiotics and alcohol detox. About an hour later, he had a seizure, but again, I figured it was the alcohol withdrawal. It was the end of my shift and I \went home.
>
> The next day when I returned to work, one of the nurses asked me, "Did you hear about the hospital CEO's son? Last night he had gone out to have a beer with his friends after working for a few hours in his toolshed. After drinking only half of his beer, he left because he felt ill. While walking to his car, he

lost consciousness, was picked up by the police and brought to our ER without identification. They thought he was a drunk and treated him for detox, until he had multiple seizures and a cardiac arrest. After the multiple seizures, someone ordered a CT scan of his brain and found a 3-cm brain tumor, probably malignant, based on location and configuration. About an hour later, the family reported him missing, and the police put two and two together and directed the family to the hospital. The CEO is in the ICU with the son and the rest of the family right now."

Because of my own moral judgments, my lack of insight and professionalism, I nearly killed a young man with a wife and young children (Name Withheld, personal communication)!

I suggest a new goal for medical education: **to train outstanding medical professionals whose goal is to educate and support a healthy, thriving population (including self and colleagues) in a life filled with flourishing, and to advance the science of medicine and well-being, including the ability to lead and support a team of harmonious multidisciplinary health professionals.** Based on that goal, a radical change in the first-year curriculum is appropriate and essential.

In studies involving American medical students (Frank, Carrera, Elon, & Hertzberg, 2007; Frank, Segura, Shen, & Oberg, 2010), a strong, consistent, and positive relation is demonstrated between the health practices that doctors actually teach patients and the practices that they personally perform. An important corollary of this conclusion is that *doctors will not teach self-care and preventive health skills to their patients if doctors themselves do not practice them.* Therefore, a primary focus of the first-year curriculum for medical students must become the teaching and practice of self-care and prevention, along with the other professional competencies of professionalism and human behavior.

Resilience: a necessary asset for an effective medical professional

Resilience seems to be the popular term among those specializing in physicians' health. For every national and international conference on doctors' health in the last twenty years, one has heard the word used time and again. The repeated theme is "Doctors must learn to be resilient to cure their ills." However, no one is able to define the term *resilience* or outline the specific skills that doctors must learn to possess it.

Actually, there are multiple theories of resilience and related concepts that are reviewed in depth in chapter 7, "Identifying, Defining, and Building Resilience." Resilience skills are crucial for a successful life. Importantly, resilience can be taught and developed. Several studies demonstrate that individuals taught specific psychological resilience skills subsequently engage in behavioral changes allowing them to become more resistant to pathology such as anxiety and depression (Reivich & Shatté, 2002).

So why aren't doctors resilient?

Why are physicians so susceptible to developing emotional distress, burnout, career dissatisfaction, and depression? Because physicians tend to use maladaptive coping mechanisms, such as withdrawal, denial, and substance abuse. It is countercultural for physicians to admit emotional vulnerability. Perhaps most importantly, coping strategies have never been a regular part of the medical-school curriculum (Hu, et al., 2012), nor has resilience training.

In a study of orthopedic surgery residents in which 33 percent demonstrated significant psychiatric morbidity, stress levels were rated as moderately high, and scores were in the upper third for emotional exhaustion and depersonalization. Residents reported faculty mentors as providing little or no help (Sargent, Sotile, Sotile, Rubash, & Barrack, 2004). A survey of 108 physicians from a different institution is revealing. In this study, 53 percent of the physicians had been involved in at least one serious adverse patient event, 57 percent of the physicians had experienced a significant personal stressor within the last year, and 94 percent indicated they would anticipate wanting support for one or more of these stressors. Unfortunately, the vast majority of doctors (89%) indicated a lack of time as the primary barrier to seeking such support. Most also indicated other concerns that prevented them from accessing care, including a lack of confidentiality (68%), a negative effect on their career (68%), fear of documentation on their record (63%), stigma of accessing mental health care (62%), uncertainty where to go for help (61%), and difficulty accessing services (52%) (Hu, et al., 2012). Consequently, physicians are not simply unaware of or lacking in coping skills; their professional environment discourages the use of adaptive coping mechanisms or even acknowledging the need for help. The implicit messages they receive, coupled with the responses role-modeled by physician peers and mentors, create a reinforcing cycle of ill health.

Nearly 40 percent indicated that using services means that they are weak, and more than 20 percent indicated the feeling that nobody would understand their problems or that their problems were not important. All of these barriers to obtaining support are driven by a lack of knowledge, falsely negative beliefs, and fear; the aforementioned conspire to produce an absence of resilient thinking and mature coping behaviors (Hu, et al., 2012).

Marsha W. Snyder, MD., MAPP.

Evidence-based methods for teaching resilience

Resilience skills are critical for leading a successful life. Reivich and Shatté note that humans have four fundamental uses of resilience: (1) to overcome the obstacles of childhood, (2) to steer through everyday adversities, (3) to help us deal with major setbacks or life-altering events so that we can regroup and continue to move forward, and (4) to reach out to others so that we can find renewed meaning and purpose in life and achieve optimal performance (2002).

Resilience can be taught. Various studies demonstrate that individuals taught specific psychological resilience skills subsequently engage in behavioral changes that allow them to become more resistant to psychopathologies such as anxiety and depression (Reivich & Shatté, 2002; Brunwasser, Gillham, & Kim, 2009). To accomplish this goal requires a refocusing on a strengths-based, rather than a deficit-based, approach. Using an individual's emotional and psychological strengths allows a proactive response that builds on an individual's self-efficacy, rather than a reactive approach that is ineffective and reinforces weakness (Reivich & Shatté, 2002).

As noted by the studies above as well as many others, resilience is an ability and a skill set that can be taught and developed, along with accurate thinking, empathy and connection, self-efficacy, impulse control, self-regulation, and emotional intelligence. These constitute critical resilience skills that must be learned by future competent, skillful, and compassionate physicians.

Resilience for Physicians and Physicians-in-Training

The literature points to a disappointing trend: physicians demonstrate a surprising propensity toward maladaptive or immature psychological resilience skills, and subsequently experience negative outcomes such as poor self-care, burnout, anxiety, depression, substance abuse, and other deleterious functional outcomes. Resilience is a critical need in the curriculum of medical students, faculty, house staff, and practicing physicians. A new curriculum should highlight and teach essential individual skills and create an environment where positive coping skills are seen as an asset, not a weakness. A curriculum that teaches resilience skills to first-year medical students can set a firm foundation that will pay dividends throughout the individual's career as a student and as a physician. It is one of the most important solutions to implement now, especially because other solutions can take longer to implement. Students must have the skills to deal effectively with their own challenges and withstand the burdens of a system needing reform and change.

A new construct in medicine and health: positive health

Positive health refers to health assets that exist above and beyond the mere absence of disease. These "assets" are attributes that enable flourishing and longevity. Health *assets* are distinguished from health *risks*, which are factors that predict or enable disease and mortality. The positive-health initiative is an outgrowth of the field of positive psychology (Seligman, 2011).

Positive psychology is an umbrella term for the scientific study of those factors that allow humans to flourish (Seligman, 2011). The field of study has been evolving for decades; it was formally labeled "positive psychology" in 1999, when the then-president of the American Psychological Association, Dr. Martin Seligman, declared a need to broaden the field of psychological research beyond the current concept of psychopathology. Much of the philosophical stance that drives the field is based on the observation that people want to lead meaningful and fulfilling lives, to cultivate what is best within themselves, and to enhance their experiences of love, work, and play (Seligman & Csikszentmihalyi, 2000).

Before Seligman's declaration of positive psychology, most psychological and psychiatric research was oriented toward a disease model that emphasized mitigating pathology and correcting weaknesses. While helpful in treating certain illnesses, the practical outcomes of this research did little to prevent disease, which is an important focus of positive psychology. While bolstering the positive aspects of life and cultivating flourishing, some positive-psychology interventions also have been shown to prevent prevalent pathologies, such as anxiety and depression (Seligman, 2008). This requires not only building individual competencies and strengths, but also cultivating environments and institutions that foster them.

Positive psychology has three central areas of concern: positive emotions, positive individual traits, and positive institutions. *Positive emotions* entail the study of the array of emotional states that contribute to contentment with the past, happiness in the present, and hope for the future (Seligman & Csikszentmihalyi, 2000). *Positive individual traits* consist of the study of strengths and virtues, such as the capacity for love and work, courage, resilience, compassion, creativity, curiosity, integrity, self-knowledge, moderation, self-control, and wisdom. *Positive institutions* entail the study of the strengths that foster better communities and organizations, such as justice, responsibility, civility, parenting, nurturance, work ethic, leadership, teamwork, purpose, and tolerance. *Positive interventions* are the intentional and evidence-based tools that create these desired positive outcomes. Methodologically, they represent the enhancers of human flourishing. Specifically, a positive intervention is an activity that targets a given system or function through an active ingredient and produces a desired outcome (J. Pawelski, personal communication, 2011).

Positive health is the study of health assets—individual factors that produce longer life, lower morbidity, lower health-care costs, and better prognosis and quality of life when illness does strike (Seligman, 2011). *Positive health* describes a state beyond the mere absence of disease that is measurable (Seligman, 2008). The emerging concept of positive health takes an innovative approach to health and well-being that focuses on promoting behaviors that can lead ultimately to a longer, healthier life. Positive health is predicated on identifying potential health assets from the research literature. Then, looking longitudinally at these candidate health assets while holding risk factors constant, those with empirical legitimacy can be identified (M. E. P. Seligman, C. Peterson, A. J. Barsky, J. K. Boehm, L. D. Kubzansky, and N. Park, unpublished data, 2010).

The second stage is to develop interventions that amass these health assets. The third stage measures the results and cost-effectiveness of these interventions (M. E. P. Seligman, C. Peterson, A. J. Barsky, J. K. Boehm, L. D. Kubzansky, and N. Park, unpublished data, 2010). The knowledge base presented in this book is a proposed intervention intended to bolster health assets; research evaluation has already determined its effectiveness in accomplishing this goal.

In 1948, the World Health Organization defined health as *a state of complete physical, mental and social well-being, and not merely the absence of disease or infirmity* (World Health Organization, 1948). Our health-care system is oriented toward the treatment of disease (Martin, Lassman, Washington, & Catlin, 2012). Despite this, people desire well-being, that is, more than a mere relief of suffering. They want well-being that embodies a true sense of thriving. Well-being—manifested in positive affect, engagement, positive relationships, meaning, and accomplishment (PERMA)—may be one of our biggest weapons against developing common mental disorders. Multiple studies have shown that interventions that build positive states alleviate depression and anxiety (Seligman, 2008).

Positive health is not the treatment of disease. The concept of positive health is to build an individual's health assets that are desirable in their own right and that also may protect the individual from future illness. Positive health is also distinct from disease prevention, which focuses on eliminating or mitigating risk factors, leading to *avoidance of disease*. The target of disease prevention is avoiding or delaying illness, and its main focus in health is solely those factors that are useful in preventing illness (Heymann, 2008). Positive health overlaps with disease prevention in its use of interventions to prevent disease and its focus on early intervention strategies. However, the targets of positive health are broader than simply illness, and include such items of importance as subjective well-being, emotional well-being, positive relationships, and other life factors. Positive health focuses on building up positive health assets and strengths, as opposed to risk factors, leading to *better health and thriving* (see table 1-1).

Table 1-1: Positive Health Versus Disease Prevention

	Goal	Method	Focus
Positive Health	Better health, longer life, thriving	Building or enhancing specific positive health assets	Subjective, biological, and functional health assets; subjective and emotional well-being; positive life factors and positive relationships
Disease Prevention	Avoiding disease	Eliminating or mitigating risk factors	Only factors useful in preventing illness

Positive health changes how we think about health and health care. It reframes the goal of our care and education of medical students specifically, and the overall population, in general, from treating and preventing disease to building more robust health and thriving. Therefore, when we teach positive health and resilience to medical students, and when they master the knowledge base and begin to build their own health assets, they will begin to exhibit greater physical and emotional well-being and thriving. As they build their resilience skills, they can better deal with the stresses of their environment, creatively manage others, and teach (and role-model) positive health to their patients when they reach their clinical rotations.

CONCLUSIONS AND NEXT STEPS

The data presented in this chapter demonstrate that physicians at all levels, from students to house staff to practitioners, need a significant change.

When medical-school curriculum focuses exclusively on hard sciences related to disease—to the exclusion of social sciences that allow for human thriving and professionalism—coupled with an atmosphere of competition that is fostered by a faculty with a high rate of burnout (Pololi, Krupat, Civian, Ash, & Brennan, 2012), one can see how students entering medicine schools with altruistic motives can easily become disillusioned.

If we view the medical profession as an individual, with its various levels as organ systems, it might look something like this. The heart of the medical profession is clearly ill.

Studies have shown high rates of burnout and exhaustion among all levels of practitioners (Henning, Hawken, & Hill, 2009; Lemaire & Wallace, 2010). Students, interns, and residents are the circulation, or the supply line of new talent once their training is complete. This chapter has clearly described the problems with depression and burnout in this population. The brain controls the rest of the body. Therefore, the brain represents the hospital/medical school/university administrative entity. Although this entity has not been directly addressed in this chapter, disease in this organ system is implied from the high rates of dissatisfaction of faculty members at academic medical centers (Shanafelt, et al., 2009) and the high rate of concern regarding the ethical culture of the workplace (Pololi, Krupat, Civian, Ash, & Brennan, 2012), and many of these concerns have prompted a complete exit of young talent from academia.

We have a hypothetical individual with multisystem failure, a weak heart and brain, and inadequate circulation. If we looked at this from the basic science and disease point of view currently taught by most medical schools, we might put the individual (system) on life support.

We know from resilience theory that improving individual functioning is possible, and by refocusing on strengths, those improvements can be permanent (Reivich & Shatté, 2002). We also know from positive health that despite the risk factors for any disease, if we begin to build positive health assets, we fortify the individual with factors that lead to longer life and better prognosis and quality of life. As the metaphor applies to medicine represented by an individual, it carries equal weight and validity to medicine as a system.

While research has moved modern medicine ahead from a primarily illness- and pathology-based focus to a focus on prevention and developing health assets, and despite the fact that health care is a fundamentally human activity involving multiple interactions that must be guided by positive health, professionalism, resilience, and meaning and purpose, and their implicit skill sets, the basic science-focused curriculum structure has not changed in more than forty years. Particularly during the first year of medical school, when students are most vulnerable, the absence of a solid foundation in health asset-building skills, including resilience, emotional intelligence, self-awareness, self-control, optimism, communication, meaning and purpose, and ethics, is alarming and problematic.

This book is not proposing a major change to the goals and structure of medical education overall, However, a logical and achievable first step is the integration of a curriculum for medical students and house staff, the clinical faculty and physicians who will provide supervision for their clinical activities and mentoring, and CME activities for physicians, in positive health, resilience, and professionalism. The learning experience is highly interactive and relational. Major goals include the ability to understand, build, and teach positive health assets, the development of professional competencies, including resiliency skills, and enhancing skills of human understanding, including emotional intelligence, communication skills, self-awareness, empathy, optimism, meaning and purpose, and flourishing.

The recommended second tier of the curriculum for students and house staff involves training of clinical faculty in similar skill sets and competencies as those taught to the students. The goal is to prepare the clinical faculty to reinforce the professional competencies, skills, and human understanding taught in the student curriculum, while encouraging the continued building and teaching of positive health assets, professionalism, and resilience skills. Further, it prepares the faculty for the important role of a mentor. As part of a positive health curriculum, each student should be assigned to a faculty mentor who has been trained in this body of knowledge. This important relationship will optimally continue throughout medical school or training.

In conclusion, it is doubtful that one curriculum change will heal an entire distressed system. However, endowing our medical students and physicians—the future of our profession—with the appropriate skills to meet the needs of themselves, their patients, and their colleagues is certainly a good place to start.

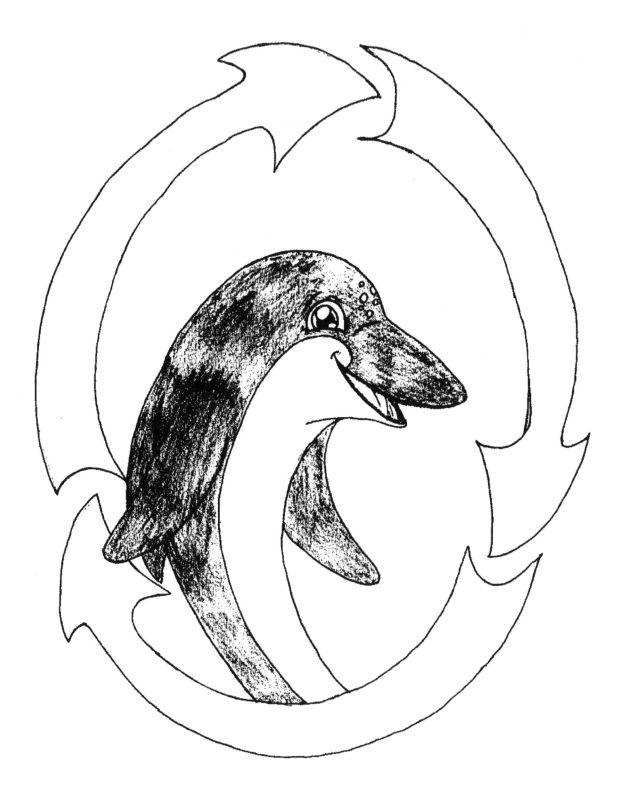

Chapter 2

Health Assets:
The Building Blocks of Positive Health

People are desirous of well-being in its own right, and they desire it beyond relief of their suffering (Seligman, 2008). As the preamble to the Constitution of the World Health Organization states (1948), "Health is a state of complete positive physical, mental, and social well-being and not merely the absence of disease or infirmity."

Positive health describes well-being that exists beyond the absence of disease and beyond risk factors for disease. The positive-health initiative is more clearly understood by examining its roots in positive psychology. Positive psychology, as a discipline and body of research, challenged the assumption that mental health was merely the absence of mental illness. Instead, mental health consists of positive emotions, positive relationships, engagement, meaning and purpose, and other positive states that lead to a sense of well-being. These states are not guaranteed to be present, nor are they achieved, merely by avoidance or removal of mental illness. At the same time, the presence of mental illness does not prevent them from existing (M. E. P. Seligman, C. Peterson, A. J. Barsky, J. K. Boehm, L. D. Kubzansky, and N. Park, unpublished data, 2010). Positive psychology does not deny the reality of ill-being or suffering. Rather, it suggests that one of the best ways to address psychological problems is by leveraging positive psychological strengths.

With this model of positive psychology in mind, defining what is meant by positive physical health is critical to the positive-health initiative. Positive health is definable and measurable by excellent status on biological, subjective, and functional measures (referred to as health assets). Further, it predicts increased longevity, decreased health-care costs, improved well-being in aging, and better prognosis when illness does strike (Seligman, 2008).

Research findings have linked positive interventions and well-being to positive health assets. For example, in a study conducted by Fredrickson in 2001, physicians with positive scores on measures of mood could reach a diagnosis with greater accuracy and in less time than those with lower mood scores (Fredrickson, The role of positive emotions in positive psychology: The broaden-and-build theory of positive emotions, 2001).

Positive health research, then, includes the empirical study of candidate health assets. A health asset is an individual factor that produces longer life, lower morbidity, lower health-care expenditure, better prognosis when illness does strike, and higher quality of life. To date, three categories of health assets have been identified: biological, subjective, and functional. The assets within each category are independent, quantifiable, and therefore, measurable. This is essential in establishing each one's validity with regard to the target goals of positive health, such as decreased morbidity and mortality and increased quality of life. For example, seven studies have examined the relationship between optimism (a subjective health asset) and cardiovascular mortality (M.E.P. Seligman, C. Peterson, A.J. Barsky, J.K. Boehm, L.D. Kubzansky, and N. Park, unpublished data, 2010). These studies have consistently demonstrated that optimism is associated with reduced risk of developing cardiovascular disease or with decreased cardiovascular disease-related mortality.

In this chapter, we will first review and examine the three major categories of health assets that contribute to positive health. Once this general conceptual understanding is established, we will look at specific candidate asset examples from each category in greater depth for purposes of clarity and greater specificity of knowledge.

POSITIVE HEALTH ASSETS

Because it is a relatively new and evolving field, positive health seeks to determine which factors will qualify as true health assets, leading to longer life, lower morbidity, decreased health-care costs, and thriving. This is done through longitudinal studies of candidate assets while holding risk factors constant. Numerous studies have been completed to date by the University of Pennsylvania Positive Psychology Center Group in conjunction with the Robert Wood Johnson Foundation Frontier Grant on positive health (M. E. P. Seligman, C. Peterson, A. J. Barsky, J. K. Boehm, L. D. Kubzansky, and N. Park, unpublished data, 2010).

The first task in the development of positive health is to identify these likely candidate health assets, whose ability to produce positive health outcomes can then be empirically assessed. Candidate assets, derived from extensive literature reviews, fall into three categories: biological, subjective, and functional.

Biological health assets

The human body, from birth and throughout life, consistently faces varied challenges. These challenges come from environmental sources, internal and external sources, and emotional and physical sources. It is each individual's biological characteristics, anatomical and physiological, that are determinants of positive adaptation to challenges and stresses, thereby increasing disease resistance and retarding aging. These biological characteristics must, by definition, be positive and specific attributes. The absence of a disease or of a negative potential laboratory abnormality (such as the absence of diabetes or the absence of elevated LDL cholesterol) would not be a positive health asset.

Biological health assets often involve objective measurements of biological substances or states in the body, thereby facilitating objective comparison over time or across conditions.

Candidate biological health assets

An obvious indicator of good health is the rate of wound healing. A foot wound is likely to heal much faster in a healthy twenty-one-year-old than in an elderly individual with type 2 diabetes mellitus. Of note, age difference alone, or the presence or absence of a disease state alone, does not determine rapidity of wound healing. A host of factors are involved in rapid wound healing, such as good nutritional status, intact immune system function to ward off infection, and even personal hygiene to keep the wound clean and dry. Rapid wound healing is, therefore, an example of a candidate biological health asset.

High heart-rate variability (high parasympathetic nervous system tone) is also a candidate biological health asset, and one that has been well-studied. High heart-rate variability refers to the variation in the time interval between successive ventricular contractions. In the presence of environmental or physiologic stressors and under the influence of sympathetic nervous system control, the heart rate increases and variability between contractions decreases. While this might be helpful in the short run to facilitate fighting or fleeing, in the long run a persistently increased heart rate can cause undue stress and strain on the heart muscle, with potentially life-threatening consequences.

However, an intact parasympathetic nervous system, mediated through the vagus nerve to the heart, prevents this potential disaster from occurring, by counteracting heart-rate arousal on a beat-to-beat basis, thereby resulting in high heart-rate variability (Tsuji, et al., 1996). Thus, high heart-rate variability is an indicator of the presence of high vagal tone, which protectively slows and modulates the heart rate and protects the heart muscle. This is considered another positive biological health asset.

Oxytocin is yet another well-researched candidate biological health asset. Oxytocin is a nine-amino acid peptide, synthesized primarily in the brain, in the supraoptic and paraventricular nuclei of the hypothalamus. Neurons from both of these nuclei project to the posterior pituitary gland, where oxytocin is released into the bloodstream in response to various physiological and psychological stimuli. Oxytocin surges during labor in a pregnant female and is also involved in lactation, in both cases to facilitate maternal-infant bonding. In fact, oxytocin is stimulated by any physical touch in both females and males. The behaviors associated with high levels of oxytocin include increased interpersonal trust, attachment, marital fidelity, and other prosocial behaviors. Given the association of positive relationships with thriving and well-being, oxytocin can well be considered a candidate positive biological health asset (M. E. P. Seligman, C. Peterson, A. J. Barsky, J. K. Boehm, L. D. Kubzansky, and N. Park, unpublished data, 2010).

Low body mass index (BMI) is another potential positive health asset, of which both professionals and the public have growing awareness. Body mass index is a ratio derived from an individual's height and weight that is widely used as an index of healthy body size versus obesity. High body mass index is a known risk factor for multiple unhealthy conditions, such as cardiovascular disease and diabetes mellitus. Research has yet to clarify if an exceptionally low body mass index is a health asset or if the relationship between BMI and health is a U-shaped curve, with either end leading to poor health, and only an ideal midrange value serving as a health asset.

Another interesting candidate biologic health asset is greater-than-average telomere length for one's age. Telomeres are attached to the ends of all of our chromosomes in all of our cells. Their purpose is to facilitate the replication of DNA and cells. Once telomeres become too short, cells can no longer replicate to replenish body tissues. Studies show that individuals with long telomeres are more likely to live longer and have more years of healthy living. The progressive shortening of telomeres, on the other hand, is predictive of chronic disease, such as cardiovascular disease, diabetes, some cancers, depression, osteoarthritis, and vascular dementia (Calado & Young, 2009). Telomerase, an enzyme that helps to lengthen telomeres, prevents the shortening of the chromosome ends in cells that are rapidly dividing, and can promote the health of certain types of cells and tissues.

Telomeres and telomerase are a focus of research in the scientific understanding of aging, stress, and chronic disease. Research has shown a consistent association between chronic stress and both shorter telomere length and lower telomerase activity. Fortunately, this condition is reversible. Comprehensive lifestyle changes, such as a healthy diet, regular exercise, and stress management, resulted in increased telomerase activity and increased telomere length.

There are many other positive candidate biological health assets, such as a high HDL/LDL cholesterol ratio, low levels of interleukin 6 (an inflammatory hormone), maximal uptake rate for oxygen in the blood (VO_2 max), low serum fibrinogen, and rapid recovery from illness. It is important for us, as doctors and as healthy individuals, to understand the circumstances and interventions that will lead to the increased accumulation of these valuable assets in ourselves and in our patients.

Subjective health assets

It is well-established in the literature that individuals with high psychological well-being are significantly less likely to die of any cause than those with low psychological well-being (Seligman, 2011). Psychological well-being includes a variety of positive states and experiences, such as positive emotions, optimism, emotional vitality, and meaning in life.

Research has shown that, beyond being an important outcome in its own right, high psychological well-being may have even greater consequences for overall health. For example, at least seven scientific studies have linked optimism to reduced risk of cardiovascular disease (M. E. P. Seligman, C. Peterson, A. J. Barsky, J. K. Boehm, L. D. Kubzansky, and N. Park, unpublished data, 2010).

The psychological traits or characteristics that are components of psychological well-being are usually assessed by self-reports using validated research instruments. They become subjective positive health assets when they are linked by research to lower rates of morbidity and mortality, lower health-care costs, or higher levels of thriving. However, careful and ongoing investigation of these relations is critical to determine whether the relation between the psychological characteristic and the physical change is a direct physiological one, or simply mediated through changes in health- or illness-related behaviors. Only those with direct relations qualify as subjective health assets.

Although the positive states and experiences that comprise subjective health assets are, generally, not as objectively measured as many biologic health assets, such as body mass index, many validated research instruments exist to consistently measure these levels across time and populations.

Candidate subjective health assets

As mentioned above, optimism is a frequently studied subjective health asset. Optimism is the expectation of an abundance of positivity and good events in the future, with an accompanying minimum of negative events. It can be measured in a variety of ways, including self-report surveys, content analyses of open-ended material, or reconfigured personality inventories. Multiple studies have demonstrated a consistent relation between optimism and both longevity and better health (Peterson, 2000).

What specifically are the mechanisms by which optimism causes good health? Research has not been clear as to a single mechanism, but points to the suggestion of multiple pathways (Peterson, Park,, & Kim, 2012). For example, optimism has been associated with improved immune-system function, slower progression of carotid intima thickening, more rapid wound healing, and healthier blood pressure and cortisol regulation. Behaviorally, optimists demonstrate better health habits due to their expectation of positive outcomes and their perception that their actions can have a significant impact on their health. Socially, optimists tend to have better social connections and social support, both of which have proven health benefits.

A study done on dispositional optimism, looking at 6,044 adults over the age of fifty years who were stroke-free at baseline, revealed that higher optimism was associated with a lower risk of stroke. On an optimism measure ranging from 3 to 18, each unit increase in optimism was associated with an age-adjusted odds ratio of 0.90 for stroke ($P < .01$). The effect of optimism remained significant even after adjustment for a comprehensive set of sociodemographic, behavioral, biological, and psychological risk factors (Kim, Park, & Peterson, 2011).

The experience of frequent positive feelings and emotions, along with the extent to which an individual experiences more prolonged positive moods (positive affectivity), represents another candidate positive subjective health asset. Positive emotions and moods can be measured using a self-report questionnaire such as the Positive and Negative Affect Schedule (PANAS) (Watson, Clark, & Tellegen, Development and validation of brief measures of positive and negative affect: The PANAS scales, 1988). In this particular scale, positive and negative mood-associated terms are rated separately, resulting in a calculation for positive emotion that is independent of negative emotion. The scores obtained using the PANAS tend to show stability across years of repeated administration to individuals.

Positive affectivity is more commonly seen in extroverted and more socially active individuals with more friends and a greater investment in their social community. Men and women are represented equally among those with positive affectivity. In addition, those with higher positive affectivity are more likely to be happily married and to like their jobs than are those with lower positive affectivity.

Research has consistently linked the presence of meaning (and purpose) to health and well-being, thereby making meaning another well-documented subjective health asset. A meaningful life is one in which people feel connected to, and motivated by, something larger than themselves. Research demonstrates that a life filled with meaning is more satisfying than a life centered solely on pleasure, a fact that surprises many Americans.

Meaning is usually assessed by interviews or self-report surveys. Individuals with high levels of meaning and purpose report greater life satisfaction, more positive affect, higher optimism, and increased self-esteem. They are less likely to have psychological problems, and they tend to have greater longevity, living longer than those whose lives lack meaning (Sone, et al., 2008).

Meaning and purpose play a very special role in the life of a physician (see chapter 8). Those physicians who have an abundance of meaning in their lives tend to demonstrate greater career satisfaction and lower levels of burnout, in addition to the health advantages this asset provides. Because of the key role that meaning and purpose play in both the professional life and health of a medical doctor, an entire chapter of this book will be devoted to an in-depth exploration of this topic, including exercises to help doctors build the deep self-knowledge needed to discover their true purpose in life and work.

Vitality is yet another candidate subjective health asset. Vitality can be defined as a composite of positive emotions that provide energy for effective problem solving and emotional regulation. This relation is reciprocal in that effective emotional regulatory processes and coping skills also, in turn, help to preserve vitality and avoid energy-depleting negative emotions (Rozanski & Kubzansky, 2005).

Various self-report measures exist to indicate levels of vitality, from those that focus primarily on physical energy to those focused more on the psychological aspect of feeling energized and engaged in life. Physicians should be aware of the fact that specific measures of vitality have been associated with cardiovascular outcomes (Kubzansky & Thurston, 2007).

Additional candidate subjective health assets include zest, internal health locus of control, engagement, curiosity, mastery, and sense of coherence (this concept will be covered in the chapter on resilience), among many others yet to be discovered.

Functional health assets

The concept of positive health involves optimal physical functioning and optimal role functioning. The assets that allow for and indicate this high level of physical and role function are included in the functional health assets.

To further clarify, this state of optimal functioning is that which exists beyond physical disability or the absence of role impairment. Therefore, the true indicator of positive health in this domain is one's ability to function effectively in the physical activities and role functions one chooses as ideal for oneself and one's life. This is an extremely important concept as it allows for adaptation and return to optimal functioning in those who experience unforeseen physical and role losses. For example, an able-bodied soldier goes to war and loses a leg in battle, resulting in an unforeseen physical loss; a young mother of a one-year-old child endures an unforeseen loss of role function when her young child is accidentally killed in an auto accident. With the ability to heal and adapt their physical and role functions to what is optimal for themselves at the time, they once again achieve a state high in positive functional health assets.

There are two overall categories of functional health assets. The first, positive physical function, refers to an individual's physical capacities and abilities. Physical functioning can refer to anything from sensory acuity, to motor performance and musculoskeletal function (strength, endurance, flexibility), to central nervous system functioning (such as balance, coordination, and memory).

The second category of functional assets is positive role function. This refers to one's ability to carry out occupational, social, and family roles successfully, along with one's ability to integrate in a social community and receive support from others. Positive role function requires matching of an individual's physical, emotional, and intellectual abilities and the requirements of, and support offered by, his environment and chosen lifestyle. An individual's ability to successfully adapt to and meet the demands of his or her lifestyle is an indicator of positive health. This includes one's ability to flexibly adapt and change as situations might demand. For example, as one's visual acuity weakens with age, the use of reading glasses, driving only during the day, and using brighter light to make reading easier allow one to optimize visual functioning, and therefore, the ongoing ability to drive and see friends, read and pay bills, and continue to remain employed until an age of desired retirement.

A particular emphasis will be given to that aspect of role functioning that falls within the social domain. As you will see in chapter 9, numerous studies have linked positive social relationships with good health (Cohen, 2004). The quality of one's marriage, social relationships, and the perception that one has friends and a social network with social support from others are associated with longer life and lower mortality rates from a variety of causes (Cohen & Janicki-Deverts, 2009).

However, predicting outcomes solely on the basis of functional health assets can be a tricky business. Consider the following scenario: both a father and a son, involved in a motor vehicle accident, sustained spinal cord trauma that resulted in paralysis from the waist level down. The father, a fifty-eight-year-old banker with gout and mild hypertension controlled by medication was able to recover, undergo rehabilitation, and quickly return to his job as a bank executive, with some appropriate accommodations to both his home and office. His son, on the other hand, was a twenty-nine-year-old Major League Baseball player in excellent physical condition with no health problems. Although he, too, made a quick initial recovery in the hospital, his progress slowed in rehab. With the realization of the many losses he had sustained—loss of career, livelihood, direction in life, so much of what he loved and for which he had worked so hard—he felt lost and sad. Therefore, although the son appeared initially to be higher in functional health assets than his father, the circumstances of the accident and the ability of each to adapt to it soon revealed the father to be more adaptable under the initial circumstances and, therefore, higher in functional health assets.

Now let's look at the son a year later. He has a job as a play-by-play announcer on a major television network for Major League Baseball games. What happened? When his rehab started to slow, it was suggested that he talk to one of the psychologists on the rehab center staff about his loss and his future. The opportunity to therapeutically deal with his losses and, once again, recognize his strengths and possibilities for a positive future allowed him to find new meaning in his life and creatively adapt his life direction to match his abilities and strengths. He was, once again, flourishing and high in positive functional health assets.

Candidate functional health assets

As highlighted above, candidate functional health assets fall into two overall categories. In the category of positive physical functioning, candidate assets include: sensory acuity (such as vision, taste, and hearing), motor performance and musculoskeletal function (such as strength, endurance, flexibility, and fine motor skills), central nervous system functioning (such as balance, coordination, cognition, and memory), and adaptability to states of change or ill health.

In the category of positive role function, candidate assets include an enjoyable and steady job or occupation, a stable happy marriage, supportive friends and family, a positive peer group or social community from whom one derives social support, and avocations and recreational activities of interest.

Most of the measures of positive physical functioning can be easily obtained by physical examination and health history. Positive role function can be obtained through various self-report measures and surveys.

THE ONGOING STUDY OF HEALTH ASSETS

In this chapter, an introduction to health assets has been provided, including a review of biological, subjective, and functional health assets. Because these assets are the building blocks of positive health, it is essential that any student of positive health have a clear understanding of health assets, what they are, and the function they serve. As stated at the outset of this chapter, because this is a young science and research to develop and identify candidate health assets is ongoing, it is neither necessary nor possible to develop a comprehensive list of these health assets. It is for this reason that only several well-researched assets in each category were reviewed in depth in this chapter. With ongoing research in positive health, these lists, as well as our knowledge of the assets that lead to human thriving, will grow far beyond what we know today. In the chapters that follow, we will be exploring a variety of positive health assets and states and how they can be built and embraced in the life of a busy professional physician as well as in the lives of the patients we serve.

What is essential for physicians and physicians-in-training to recognize is that those of us who have burnout, ill-being, stress, depression, and ill health also have a significant loss or absence of positive health assets. When these assets are lovingly rebuilt, as the chapters of this book hope to do, physicians can flourish both personally and professionally. Doctors actively practicing positive health in their own lives can then lovingly teach this same practice to their patients. These are the ultimate goals of this curriculum: to end the epidemic of physician ill-being worldwide; to create a compassionate positive practice of medicine that is patient-centered; to have physicians teach positive health to their patients, which will result in longer life, decreased morbidity and mortality, lower health-care costs, and faster recovery when illness does strike; and to have a thriving population.

MiNomiSADolphin.

by Sabine "Bean" Rebecca Snyder.

Chapter 3

Introduction to Positive Psychology, Emotions, and Flourishing

Guest Author: Tom Heffner, MAPP

A QUICK GLANCE AT THE RECENT HISTORY OF PSYCHOLOGY

What does it mean to live life? What can we expect? Sigmund Freud and Arthur Schopenhauer, two of the most influential thinkers in the past two hundred years, thought that the best humans can hope for in life is not to suffer (Seligman, personal communication, September 7, 2012). By the time you finish reading this chapter, you will realize that this idea is both empirically and morally wrong. Unfortunately, those in the field of psychology have believed this view to be true for the past seventy years and have spent that time supporting it with research, practice, and application. Worse yet, this mind-set has pervaded nearly every domain of life—from parenting and education to relationships, sports, and the workplace.

This decades-long focus on disease and pathology was triggered by the events of World War II (Peterson C., 2006). Soon after the United States joined the war, a flood of injured soldiers returned home with horrific physical and psychological wounds. Consequently, Veteran Affairs Hospital psychologists focused almost exclusively on disease diagnosis and treatment. This approach was for good reason, because these soldiers returned with unclear diagnoses, such as battle fatigue or shell shock. Since then, the United States engaged in several wars, producing a steady stream of physically and psychologically wounded soldiers. The result was that areas of research and application such as performance excellence, well-being, purpose, and meaning—to name a few—went untouched until recently.

During this long period of traditional psychological research, academic and practicing psychologists continued to respond by examining and identifying an exponentially growing number of psychological diseases. The first edition of the *Diagnostic and Statistical Manual of Mental Disorders* (DSM-I), published in 1952, listed 106 mental disorders within its 130 pages (Grob, 1991). Fast-forward to the current edition of the DSM (DSM-5), published in 2013, and the list balloons to approximately 297 disorders described within 991 pages. The number of disorders has almost tripled, while the page count has multiplied by ten compared with the original edition. It becomes apparent that psychologists have been busy researching and identifying everything that is wrong with mankind.

According to Seligman, fixing the bad in our lives does not necessarily lead to a life of well-being or flourishing (2011). Although resolving issues, whether mild or severe, is important, it is only one piece of the puzzle. To live a good, fulfilling life requires more. This belief is encompassed by the domain of positive psychology. Christopher Peterson, noted author, researcher, and expert in psychology, defined positive psychology as *the study of what makes life worth living* (2006). Positive psychology is the study of how we thrive and succeed in our lives. It is the study of how communities, organizations, and institutions flourish.

This chapter will now introduce five key characteristics of positive psychology and how they can contribute to increasing one's well-being and ability to live a good life: positive emotions, engagement (flow), positive relationships, meaning, and accomplishment. (Note: Several of these concepts will be explored in greater depth in subsequent chapters of this book.)

POSITIVE EMOTIONS

The foundation of a good life—and one of the central tenets of positive psychology—is the study and cultivation of positive emotions. Positive emotions play a crucial role by affecting practically every element of a good life (e.g., engagement, positive relationships, meaning, achievement, etc.). Barbara Fredrickson, one of the world's leading experts on positive emotions, lists the ten most important positive emotions as joy, gratitude, serenity, interest, hope, pride, amusement, inspiration, awe, and love (2009).

Why are positive emotions so important? Most people will intuitively grasp the potential of these emotions, but there is more behind the science of positive emotions. According to Fredrickson, when we experience positive emotions, they open us up in a variety of important ways (2001; 2003; 2009). They expand our visual acuity, our emotional capacity, and—perhaps most importantly for medical practitioners—our cognitive abilities. Scores of research studies support this claim, and one research experiment in particular is pertinent to the medical field.

In the experiment noted above (Fredrickson, 2003), researchers presented physicians with a complex liver diagnosis case. They asked the physicians to think and talk out loud throughout their diagnostic process and clinical reasoning. The participants were divided into three groups. The researchers induced one group with positive emotion, another group with negative emotion, and the control group with neutral emotion (i.e., no affective change). The group induced with positive emotions were given a small bag of candy. Through careful observation and analysis, the researchers confirmed they could reliably produce a degree of positive emotion in the physicians by using this intervention. In a similar manner, they produced negative and neutral emotions in the other two physician groups.

The big payoff for the researchers was that the physicians who were induced with positive emotions were quicker and more skillful at assimilating case information and they did not become attached to their initial ideas (Fredrickson, 2003). Positive emotions deterred the physicians from making a premature diagnosis.

So, how exactly does a process as simple as experiencing positive emotions trigger such beneficial changes in a person's cognitive abilities? According to Barbara Fredrickson (2001; 2004; 2009), when we experience positive emotions, we broaden our awareness, which in turn encourages new exploratory behaviors and ideas. This process allows us to build new skills, resources, and assets. For most persons, positive emotions help people to cultivate the psychological, physical, and social skills and the resources that increase individual well-being. In medicine, positive emotions can help practitioners cultivate their case-integration skills and clinical reasoning over time.

Although the immediate outcome of positive emotions can be dramatic and swift, their enduring and transformative effects can be even more dramatic. For example, experiencing a preponderance of positive emotions allows you to experience and cultivate stronger and more rewarding relationships. In addition, you will be more productive and successful at work. Perhaps most relevant to positive health is that positive emotions can change our internal biochemistry and immunity for the better. Sheldon Cohen and his experiments investigating positive emotions and the rhinovirus illustrate this concept (Cohen, Alper, Doyle, Treanor, & Turner, 2006).

In his experiment, Cohen purposely infected three groups of participants with the rhinovirus (Cohen, Alper, Doyle, Treanor, & Turner, 2006). After administering the rhinovirus, he kept the subjects in quarantine for six days, collecting both subjective data (e.g., self-report of symptoms) and objective data (e.g., measuring the amount of mucus in the tissues by weight and the congestion level using the length of time required by dye injected into the nose to reach the back of the throat). By design, Cohen divided the participants into groups based on the level of their positive emotion (i.e., low, middle, and high). The results of the experiment were nothing short of astounding. Those persons with the highest levels of positive emotion at the time of the experiment were less likely to contract a cold, and when they did, they experienced symptoms from the cold for a shorter time compared with persons in the middle emotions group. In contrast, those persons in the low-level group who experienced the fewest positive emotions were most likely to contract a cold and showed the longest-lasting symptoms.

When designing his experiment, Cohen made several decisions that helped validate the study's results. He chose to quarantine all subjects for six days while waiting for the colds and symptoms to develop. This method ensured that other environmental factors did not contribute to the results (Cohen, Alper, Doyle, Treanor, & Turner, 2006). For instance, the participants did not return to their homes, where exposure to sick persons may have varied among participants (e.g., participants who worked in child care versus those who did not). In addition, because participants were kept in quarantine, variations in sleep, diet, stress (cortisol), zinc intake, and exercise could be ruled out. As a result, the study clearly showed that positive emotions affect the human biology and immune system in a helpful manner.

Application and practical exercises

Awareness of positive emotions is among the first steps to a good life, but they are not enough. We must apply the knowledge that we have gained in a way that helps us every day, and positive-psychology experts have designed various exercises to achieve this goal. One real-world application is an intervention known as the "What-Went-Well Exercise" or "Three Blessings." At the end of your day, you write down three things that went well for you (Seligman, Steen, Park, & Peterson, 2005). Whether you use a traditional journal, a computer, or a smartphone is up to you. The most important aspect of this intervention is keeping a physical record of what you wrote (Seligman, 2011). The three things that you list can range from an activity of little importance in your life (e.g., my wife made my favorite dinner) to a life-changing event (e.g., my son was just accepted into college). For each good thing that happens, you should also write down why this experience was a good thing for you or what caused it to happen.

Researchers tested this exercise against several other positive interventions by using the rigorous standard of a random-assignment, placebo-controlled experimental design (Seligman, Steen, Park, & Peterson, 2005). Remarkably, they found that two of the positive interventions, "What-Went-Well" and "Using Signature Strengths in a New Way," significantly increased happiness levels and decreased depressive symptoms for six months. Signature strengths are those strengths that people use effortlessly and effectively every day and in almost every domain of life (Peterson C., 2006). (Note: Signature strengths will be covered in greater depth in chapter 6.)

One reason this exercise works so well is because it uses the pathway of positive emotions. It trains people to focus on the good things that happen in life on a daily basis, thus making it a habit. Considering the beneficial effects of positive emotions, cultivating them into a habit is the best way to increase your well-being. The practice allows you to build those skills, resources, and assets that you have gained day after day. This benefit is important because many people have an inherent negativity bias or a tendency to focus on the things that go wrong. We all engage in negative thinking and for good reason; historically, it has allowed humans to thrive when everyday life was filled with ever-present danger. The challenge is to counteract this innate tendency by focusing on positive emotions.

As discussed earlier, positive emotions form the foundation of the good life and support almost all of the elements of a flourishing life. The model of this flourishing life is known as PERMA (Seligman, 2011), which stands for *p*ositive emotions, *e*ngagement (flow), positive *r*elationships, *m*eaning, and *a*ccomplishment. Although various well-being models exist, PERMA stands strong as one of the most recognizable, and it is supported by many studies performed by the leading well-being and illness researchers (e.g., Martin Seligman, one of the most cited and well-known psychologists). In his book *Flourish, A Visionary New Understanding of Happiness and Well-Being*, Seligman (2011) outlines and describes his model, stating that when we experience success in each of these elements, we can be described as *flourishing* in our lives. As such a model, PERMA acts as an indicator of well-being and is descriptive, not prescriptive.

Group discussion questions

- How might you cultivate more positive emotions in your life?
- How can your medical school or hospital administrators cultivate an atmosphere that allows for more positive emotions?
- What causes the most negative emotions in your life? Of these, what are changeable or controllable, and how might you change them for the better?

ENGAGEMENT (FLOW)

Engagement or *flow*, the second key element of living the good life, is a state of mind in which a person is completely absorbed in an activity (Csikszentmihalyi, 1997). When you are in this state, it is as if time stands still, taking up your focus, energy, and attention. Anyone can experience flow, and in any domain (e.g., work, games, sports, etc.). For example, superstar basketball player and Hall of Famer Michael Jordan unwittingly described this mental state perfectly when asked how it feels to dominate (as he did so often when taking the lead during games). When asked how it felt, Jordan described the feeling as being *in the zone*. For many, flow is just that. It is being in the zone. Mihaly Csikszentmihalyi, an expert on flow, describes the act of skiing down a mountain to illustrate this concept:

> Imagine that you are skiing down a slope and your full attention is focused on the movements of your body, the position of the skis, the air whistling past your face, and the snow-shrouded trees running by. There is no room in your awareness for conflicts or contradictions; you know that a distracting thought or emotion might get you buried face down in the snow. The run is so perfect that you want it to last forever (Csikszentmihalyi, 1997, pp. 28-29).

Unlike the other elements of PERMA, the act of flow does not involve positive emotions. In fact, Seligman argues that flow is the opposite of positive emotions (Seligman, 2011). That is because there is no conscious thought or feeling during flow. It is only after the state of flow ends that a person experiences its benefits, such as a feeling of accomplishment (i.e., a positive emotion). For instance, if a person described his black diamond skiing experience as Csikszentmihalyi did above, he or she might feel elated and prideful.

Flow is important to well-being. To achieve a state of flow, a person must use some of his or her signature strengths in the service of flow-inducing activity. Furthermore, the activity must have clearly set goals that are challenging yet still attainable. In the medical profession, for example, think about the physician engaging in a difficult surgery. Almost always, the surgeon has clear goals in mind, which can pose a significant challenge. For example, a cardiovascular surgeon who performs bypass surgery knows the surgical goals and requirements very well. He also knows that his performance will not be easy and will require his full attention.

As stated above, one of the main benefits of flow is that it requires the full use and service of signature strengths. Through the process of flow, a person can cultivate his or her signature strengths, as well as experience the benefits of positive emotions after the fact. Cultivating signature strengths helps to improve overall human performance and to increase well-being (Niemiec, 2012b). Supporting this theory and explaining the power of flow, researchers found that flow can lead to improved performance in a range of areas (e.g., sports, learning, teaching, and artistic creativity). Finally, flow can lead to advanced learning and skill development.

Group discussion questions

- What activities induce flow in your life? Try to be specific. The activities can encompass any domain of your life (e.g., medical school, work, family, athletics, etc.).
- What character strengths help you to find and sustain flow? (See list in Chapter 6, Fig. 6-1, for a complete listing of the twenty-four VIA Character Strengths).

You can use these strengths or identify your own strengths or skills that help you to find and sustain flow.

- How are flow and engagement connected to your well-being?
- Brainstorm ways to increase engagement in your daily life.

POSITIVE RELATIONSHIPS

Although positive emotions form the foundation of positive psychology and a flourishing life, perhaps no concept, skill, or resource is as important to the good life as relationships. When asked to summarize positive psychology and how to live a good life, Dr. Christopher Peterson replied: "Other people matter." (2006, p. 249). A simple phrase, it summarizes much of the research on well-being into one easily digestible piece of advice. This notion does not mean that solitary endeavors (e.g., achievements and activities) do not matter; however, much of what is positive in life involves other people.

Take a moment to reflect on your own life and the times or events that gave you great happiness. For example, think about when you were accepted into medical school. Think of a time that you laughed so hard and for so long that you cried, or a time that you sensed great meaning in your work as a physician (e.g., helping to ease someone's pain through palliative care). Most likely, those events involved other people.

It is important to highlight the powerful effect that entry into the medical profession has on relationships. The incredibly competitive nature of gaining entrance to medical school, residencies, fellowships, and internships can lead to a significant lack of trust among many physicians and, as a result, isolation. Furthermore, the formal educational philosophy in medical school emphasizes that good physicians are tough, detached, and unemotional. Combined with the competitive nature of medical professionals, these behaviors lead to chronic isolation in physicians, which greatly contributes to ill-being and burnout.

Application and practical exercises

One can become apt at promoting positive relationships by practicing kindness with friends, classmates, or any other person. Recent research shows that practicing kindness benefits life satisfaction and overall happiness (Lyubomirsky, Sheldon, & Schkade, 2005). This process works by building positive emotions in both the giver and the recipient. In doing so, positive emotions strengthen the relationship quality among those that practice kindness. You should keep in mind three points when practicing kindness:

First, diversity of the activity is important (Lyubomirsky, Sheldon, & Schkade, 2005). Studies have shown that it is beneficial to vary the types of kind acts that you perform because doing the same activity over and over can become tedious and ritualized. One day, you can offer to host a meal and roundtable discussion on tough medical cases that each guest is treating. The next day, you could bring bagels for the morning meeting. Another day, you could propose a lunch outing for a doctor who is known to be struggling to give him a break from work.

Second, frequency of the kind acts performed is also essential (Lyubomirsky, Sheldon, & Schkade, 2005). Research suggests that stacking kind acts all in one day (e.g., five acts in one day) produces greater benefit compared with spreading out the five acts over five days.

Finally, counting kindness is imperative. Research shows that simply counting the number of times that one has engaged in a kind act each day can boost happiness. This activity of counting works by bringing important practices related to social activity to the top of a person's awareness. And if one develops more humanity and propensity toward socializing, one is more likely to strengthen relationships with other people.

Another exercise originates from Dr. Christopher Peterson's latest book, *Pursuing the Good Life, 100 Reflections in Positive Psychology* (2013), and is called the "But-Free Day." Peterson describes the exercise as follows:

"When someone relates good news, respond without using the word *but*. The generalized version of this intervention is to go through an entire day without using the word *but* or any of its close cousins like *however, whereas, yet, then again*, and *on the other hand*." (Peterson, 2013, p. 309)

Here too, the idea is to learn to strengthen relationships with other people. Affirming someone's good news instead of negating it or qualifying it is a great way to do so. To go even further, work on elaborating the good news of the person sharing it. Use phrases like "Tell me more," "How did that feel?" or "What did the other person say or do?" to help the person who is sharing the news relive the positive event.

Group discussion questions

- List five ways to increase the number of times that you see and positively interact with your closest friends or family members during the week.
- How would practicing acts of kindness strengthen relationships in your life?
- What does a life in medicine look like with meaningful relationships with your coworkers included?

MEANING

Meaning is the next building block of well-being in the PERMA model. Seligman describes meaning as *belonging to and servicing something that you believe is bigger than the self* (2011, p. 13). This idea of belonging to something bigger than oneself is common. One needs only to look at spirituality and faith. People seek out faith as a way of making sense of their place in this world and finding meaning in their lives. They often find happiness and well-being in the process. Meaning, however, is not limited to the providence of a higher being. For example, men and women join the military every day in search of meaning and purpose in life. For many, this purpose becomes joining a fraternity of soldiers who fight to protect their country.

The nature of meaning—this desire to belong to and service something bigger than the self—suggests that a person might find himself, at times, relegating other elements of well-being to the back burner while pursuing meaning. In fact, this is a common error of medical professionals, who sacrifice close relationships and suffer from an excess of negative emotions by devoting an overabundance of energy and time to their professional pursuits at the expense of having a life balance. While the search for meaning and purpose involves giving of oneself and the pursuit of important goals, it is only valuable and positive in the context of a well-lived, well-balanced life.

It is for this reason that the physician who chose a career in medicine solely to make money tends to suffer. He crams in as many appointments as possible in a day to push through as many patients as he can. He runs his patients through numerous diagnostic tests allowed under legal and medical guidance, not in the interest of helping to heal his patients, but rather, to protect himself legally. He is the physician who is frustrated by the always-changing and complex medical insurance system, as well as the Medicare and Medicaid cuts. He wakes up every morning planning his retirement because he cannot wait to leave behind the problems of his complex practice and fixing his patients.

Compensation is important to everyone, including those who are not medical professionals; however, physicians, like all professionals, must make sure that compensation is not the most important factor in their career. Otherwise, the search for meaning and purpose might take a backseat and significantly affect their well-being.

Application and practical exercises

Often a sense of purpose is wrapped up inextricably with meaning. Purpose is the vehicle that helps us to find meaning in our lives. Chapter 8 in this book will explore meaning and purpose in great depth, including relevant theories and exercises in formulating one's meaning and purpose in life. However, the following brief exercise might give you a peek at what lies ahead. The exercise is called "Creating Your Purpose Statement" and is taken from one of Dr. James Pawelski's classes in the University of Pennsylvania's Master of Applied Positive Psychology (MAPP) program. For this exercise, consider your purpose or mission in life (Rockind, personal communication, November 12, 2011). Which unique strengths, values, passions, and talents do you offer to influence others in a positive way? How do you and will you make your impact? Once you have thought this through, consider on whom you will have an effect and how you can affect the lives of others.

To put your mission into words, take a look at the three criteria for sense of purpose, as put forth by Damon, Menon, and Bronk (2003):

- A purpose provides an ultimate aim toward which one can make progress
- Your purpose is meaningful to you; in other words, you are the driving force behind your purpose—not your friends or your parents or your teachers.
- Your purpose is also meaningful to others; it is different from other kinds of meaning in that it seeks to benefit not just you but others as well.

Now, write a short personal purpose or mission statement by using no more than ten words. This exercise is more difficult than it may seem at first. A helpful way to tackle the assignment is to start by describing your sense of purpose in one paragraph, then distilling it into one sentence, and finally, articulating it in ten words or less. Make sure to keep your purpose statement close by. Stick it on the bathroom mirror. Tape it to your computer screen at work. Whatever you do, just make sure that you come back and read it regularly and whenever you feel as if your life's direction is at odds with your purpose.

A note for the reader: This exercise is a variation on a classic creative writing assignment. Legend has it that a Nobel prize-winning novelist was once challenged to write a story in just six words. He promptly offered up the following tale: "For sale: baby shoes, never worn." *SMITH Magazine* has since made a niche publishing *Six-Word Memoirs*®. Remember not to get bogged down by the format when writing your individual purpose—this is meant to be a fun and creative assignment.

Group discussion questions

- What is meaning, and why is it important to well-being?
- How do you cultivate meaning in your life?
- Is your search for, and cultivation of, well-being helping or harming your well-being? How so?

- Do your character strengths help you to cultivate meaning in your life?
- What role do relationships play in cultivating meaning in your life?
- Are positive emotions necessary to find meaning?

ACCOMPLISHMENT

The fifth and final element in the well-being model of PERMA is accomplishment or achievement. The element of accomplishment is multifunctional; the drive to achieve can be used, for instance, to find flow. Look back to Csikszentmihalyi's example of finding flow while skiing (1997). To find flow, a person must develop and cultivate a set of skills to be used in service of an activity. To achieve your mastery level of skills and strengths is to take a giant step toward finding flow.

The will to achieve has also fueled many meaningful and purpose-filled endeavors throughout history. Consider Dr. Martin Luther King Jr. and his fight for civil rights. A life already pregnant with meaning gave birth to a new era of civil and racial equality in the United States when King delivered his famous "I Have a Dream" speech on August 28, 1963. In that moment, driven by his will to achieve racial equality, Dr. King achieved what no one else had been able to do before him: he moved most Americans to fight for racial equality and end racial discrimination.

And he did it at a time when most people thought it was impossible.

In addition to multifunctionality, accomplishment is often pursued for its own sake (Seligman, 2011). People will exhaust their mental and physical limits; they will fight and do whatever it takes—just for the sake of winning, achieving, and mastering the task. Former tennis player and coach Brad Gilbert exemplifies this characteristic of accomplishment. By his own admission, he did not possess preternatural physical gifts or tennis skills (Gilbert & Jamison, 1993), yet he became a fixture in the top ten ranking for nine of his first ten years on the Association of Tennis Professionals men's tennis tour. He also went on to beat the top three players: Boris Becker, Jim Courier, and Stefan Edberg.

How did Brad Gilbert accomplish such a feat for someone so poorly equipped with physical attributes and tennis skills? In his own words, he did it by "winning ugly." For Gilbert, it did not matter how he won the match. He did not care if he was as elegant and graceful as Stefan Edberg when executing a serve and volley—so long as the ball landed inside the line and he won the point. He did not possess a beautiful arcing one-handed backhand. Instead, he used an unsightly two-handed backhand that won him the point effectively. In the end, all that mattered to him was winning and accomplishing as much as he could in his career. Accomplishment leads to increased self-esteem, the satisfaction of goal achievement, and the positive emotions that it produces, including the joy of pursuing meaningful goals.

Application and practical exercises

The best exercise involving the well-being element of accomplishment is arguably writing about your life achievements. Dr. Christopher Peterson popularized this intervention called "Writing Your Own Legacy" in his book *A Primer in Positive Psychology* (2006, pp. 22-23). Think about this exercise as writing your own eulogy. For this exercise, you are still alive (obviously) and experiencing the luxury of crafting your own eulogy.

To help kick-start your creativity, think ahead toward the end of your life. How might you evaluate your life? What would be your life's greatest accomplishments? What do you want to be remembered for? What would be your life purpose and meaning? What were your signature strengths, and how did they help you to accomplish your life goals or achievements? Whom did you love? Who loved you?

As you write down your life goals, dreams, and hopes, take a moment to reflect on your life as you see it now. Take stock of the direction in which your life is going. Are you making progress toward these goals? Do you have a plan for short-term dreams and long-term aspirations? Most individuals, particularly young physicians, struggle with this question and these issues. These are some of the key issues that will be addressed throughout this curriculum to enhance your ability to sustain well-being and positive direction in your life and career.

Group discussion questions

- Can accomplishment harm our well-being? If so, explain how.
- Can we prioritize both accomplishment and other well-being elements at the same time (e.g., positive relationships, positive emotions, etc.)? Or do you think they are incompatible?
- Does flow (engagement) help us achieve more in our life? Less? And can we use the concepts of flow and achievement to improve our well-being?

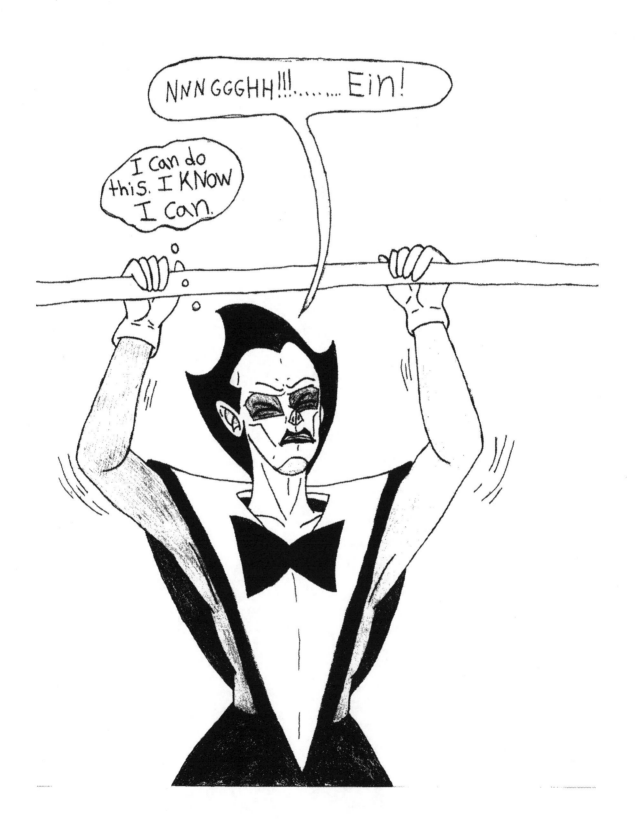

Chapter 4

Positive Fitness, Movement, and Mindful Breathing

Guest Author: Elaine O'Brien, MAPP

"Lack of activity destroys the good condition of every human being, while movement and methodical exercise save it and preserve it." —Plato

"Movement is life." —R. Tait McKenzie, MD, physician, surgeon, physical therapist, physical educator, scholar-athlete, soldier, and sculptor. Inspired by Dr. McKenzie's example, the aim of this chapter is to advance the idea of connecting positive exercise practices (PEP) to medical training and to desired health outcomes.

This chapter's focus is on how positive fitness, movement, and mindful breathing can benefit you, whether you are a medical student, instructor, physician, health practitioner, fitness leader, patient, or family member. I hope to encourage you to embrace and harness the growing body of empirical wisdom of "joy in movement," here described as positive exercise practices (PEP). This chapter will give you the rationale and many benefits of promoting individual and group fitness training in your practice. It will also introduce a wide variety of physical activity practices for you to enjoy. When we become more connected to our body and movement, we heighten our feelings of awe and wellness. Raising kinesthetic awareness and experiencing greater vitality are important positive health goals.

Research shows that physicians can have far-reaching influence on people's lives: doctors help shape habits, decisions, behaviors, choices, and outcomes of their patients. A recent survey by the American Council on Sports Medicine (ACSM) found that nearly two-thirds of patients (65%) would be more interested in exercising to stay healthy if advised by their doctor and given additional resources (Jonas & Phillips, 2009). Your patients look to you, particularly when you lead by example. This chapter includes a variety of information and resources to help boost exercise literacy and offers some innovative, positive movement strategies, including tactics, tips, and an experiential component to help you "walk the talk" in advancing physical activity training as a positive intervention.

Promoting and prescribing PEP to patients of all ages and fitness levels will help put more life into their years. Individual and group exercise, along with basic lifestyle fitness programming, is a cost-effective, life-enhancing recommendation.

There is an exciting emerging global initiative called Exercise is Medicine.Ô Exercise-is-medicine visionaries are fighting what epidemiologist Dr. Steve Blair calls, "the epidemic of inactivity." Your voice, involvement, and action matter! Your action and example as a physician are vital in helping reduce the growing risks of "diseases of inactivity"— cardiovascular disease, cancer, diabetes, and pulmonary lung disease. Exercise has been shown to have a positive effect in reducing these, as well as in lowering the risks of depression and even Alzheimer's disease.

HISTORIC VIEW OF FUSING PHYSICAL EDUCATION AND MEDICAL TRAINING

An early adopter of physical activity for whole health, R. Tait McKenzie, was a pioneer in physical education and medical-school training. McKenzie entered McGill University at age eighteen, graduated, and worked there for nearly twenty years as a medical doctor and as the university's medical director of physical training. After his tenure at McGill, Dr. McKenzie charted new ground at the University of Pennsylvania (Penn) from 1904 until 1931, where he was a professor of medicine and also Penn's first director and professor of physical education. McKenzie was attracted to University of Pennsylvania in no small part by the newly constructed gymnasium at Franklin Field. He viewed this move to Philadelphia as an opportunity to test his understanding of physical education as a vehicle of preventive medicine.

At Penn McKenzie taught undergraduates and medical students about the beneficial relationship between physical education and health. Dr. R. Tait McKenzie was in the vanguard of advancing the value of physical activity as a necessary and beneficial preventive measure for restoring health and vitality.

McKenzie taught how exercise keeps human beings well and how physical activity helps the student academically (McGill, 1980). He demonstrated how exercise improves efficiency and learning. Dr. McKenzie began this uniting of physical education and medical training in the United States over a hundred years ago via his teachings, practices, and his iconic book *Exercise in Education and Medicine* (McKenzie, 1909).

An exemplar and visionary, McKenzie lived his whole life with harmonious passion. McKenzie is known as a pioneer of *The Joy of Effort*, the title of his biography. McKenzie was a renowned sculptor who continued working until his death in 1938. In keeping with his belief that the heart was the seat of the soul, McKenzie's heart was buried in Edinburgh at the base of his sculpture *The Call 1914*, which he considered his best work. Inspired by Dr. McKenzie's example, the aim of this chapter is to advance the idea of connecting PEP to medical training and to desired health outcomes. Ultimately, our hope is to help, heal, and empower medical students, instructors, doctors, and our patients by reframing notions of physical activity training more positively and encouraging proper energy management (proper eating, rest, and exercise). The goal is to build healthy habits in the context of a positive, sustainable balanced life.

PHYSICAL ACTIVITY: A HEALTHY, HEALING, AND PREVENTIVE MEASURE

The importance of physical activity in helping to extend longevity, decrease morbidity, lower health-care costs, and thus, contribute to a more robust health economy is of high importance. Physical inactivity, on the other hand, leads to a steady growth in chronic diseases and their attendant costs. Renowned epidemiologist Dr. Steven Blair discussed how physical inactivity is THE biggest public health problem of the 21st century after measuring the effects of cardiorespiratory fitness on mortality in a sample of over 53,000 male and female subjects (2009).

Arguably, the scientific community first took notice of the relations among physical activity, fitness, and cardiovascular disease in a 1953 study by Dr. Jeremy Morris. Morris observed that active bus conductors (who walked the aisles of double-decker buses) in the United Kingdom presented with about one-half of the coronary heart disease rate compared to their counterparts, the sedentary, seated bus drivers. Morris identified a lower risk of myocardial infarction in the physically active bus conductors (those who climbed up and down steps all day checking tickets) (Morris, Heady, Raffle, Roberts, & Parks, 1953). Paffenbarger in 1971 reported an inverse relation between the risk of cardiovascular death and the work-related caloric expenditure in longshoremen. This provided further evidence that work-related physical activity was associated with a lower rate of cardiovascular death (Paffenbarger, Gima, Laughlin, & Black, 1971).

Walking is one of the easiest ways to keep in shape, manage weight, and improve your quality of life. Walking as little as thirty minutes a day has been shown to maintain health and weight. The experience increases in positivity if, in addition to walking, you reconnect with your inner spirit, spend time with your favorite friends, explore new places, revel in the beauty of nature, or engage in other forms of positive thinking. Along with health benefits, regular walking reduces the risk of heart disease by as much as 40 percent.

Practice: Dorsiflexion or toe raises (lifting and dropping your toes with your heels on the ground) is a great way to strengthen your shins and stretch your calves for walking.

Toe raises help improve walking balance and heel strike, prevent shin pain, and promote ankle flexibility. You can tap your toes in sets of eight, twelve, and twenty repetitions, working up to three sets daily. You can do toe raises almost anywhere.

PEP AND SOMATIC MOVEMENT AS AN INTERVENTION

"Physical activity interventions can provide a constructive synchronicity between positive psychology, health, and education." —Dr. Ray Fowler, valued past president of the American Psychological Association and pioneer in positive health and movement

Creating appropriate somatic interventions and applying the tenets of positive psychology and physical training are relatively new ideas. The intersection of positive psychology and physical activity is the realm of PEP. Positive exercise practices have been newly developed through years of observing best exercise practices and recognizing the value of appreciative movement. These mindful interventions allow us to be more fit and vibrant, and promote health and well-being. There is no "one size fits all" measure for how much activity is required; ideally the promotion of physical activity and PEP follows the guidelines of the American College of Sports Medicine: for adults, 150 minutes of moderate-intensity exercise a week; for children, ninety minutes a week, especially with time spent in free play. These recommended exercise practices include aerobics exercise, strength training, flexibility training. and balance training. We encourage you to lead by example, moving well and often, daily, and ultimately to prescribe moderate exercise to yourself and every patient.

Standing cat curl stretch: This exercise helps maintain a flexible and supple back and helps reduce the risk of low-back pain. Here's how it's done:

- Stand tall, with your feet hip-width apart. Place your hands on the top of your thighs above your knees.
- Put your weight slightly back into your heels, bend your knees, and squat slightly, as if you are going to sit.
- As you inhale, look forward and lengthen your spine, stretching from the crown of the head to the base of your tailbone.
- As you exhale, look downward and round your back, drawing your belly button into your spine, tucking your tailbone under, and spreading the shoulder blades wide.
- Repeat five or six times as you breathe rhythmically, easily, and freely.

"The world experienced, comes at all times with our body as its center, center of vision, center of action, center of interest." —William James cited by Shusterman, creator of the pragmatic discipline of somaesthetics (Shusterman, 2006, p. 7)

Shusterman explores the body in aesthetic experience and ultimately demonstrates how greater body awareness (embracing proprioception and kinesiology) can lead to the attainment of fulfilling experiences (2006). Shusterman, a professional Feldencrais "Awareness Through Movement" practitioner, teaches people how to improve the way they move, feel, and think. This method of neurologic retraining is based on small, gentle movements done with focus and concentration.

In *Thinking through the Body,* Shusterman (2006) offers a rich understanding of a "new" burgeoning interdisciplinary field. His essays discuss somaesthics and how they impact depression, self-knowledge, meditation, pragmatism, teaching styles, and the art of living. Shusterman argues that we need better somatic knowledge to improve our understanding and performance in the arts and human sciences, and to help us perfect our humanity and living better lives. Shusterman discusses how Socrates recognized the importance of the cultivation of the body as an "indispensable tool" for all human achievement.

As Dr. Marsha Snyder has pointed out, positive health interventions are innovative tools that practitioners apply to help people thrive, prevent disease, and live longer and healthier lives through positive psychology. Today we can develop and apply positive movement and fitness interventions that will offer health professionals and patients beneficial insights about our behaviors. These positive movements will ultimately enrich the lives of ourselves, others, and society for the better.

In the PERMA theory (see chapter 3), the focus is on developing overall well-being, with the goal of increasing the amount of flourishing both in one's own life and for others on the planet. The five-prong strategy—positive emotions, engagement, positive relationships, meaning, and (5) achievement—called PERMA can be adapted into a fitness program model for people at every life stage, and can especially help aging adults move toward greater health and independence. Exercise programs with PERMA in mind can serve our patients well, and especially those who are growing older.

THE AGE WAVE AND ACTIVE SENIOR FITNESS

"If you had to pick one thing that came closest to the fountain of youth, it would be exercise." —Dr. James Fries, MD, Stanford University (Greider, 2011, p. 1)

Seniors are the fastest-growing segment of the population. Experts estimate that by 2030, 20 percent of Americans will be sixty-five or older. Because of this, designing positive health and fitness programs for seniors is more important than ever. Here are some innovative thoughts for combining quality exercise (PEP) and positive psychology or PERMA to foster active, happy, and independent older adulthood.

1. To build and encourage positive emotions through motion:

    *   Move to uplifting music you love. Listen to music that reminds you of peak moments in life (Langer, 2009).
    *   Be active in your community. Our "Trendsetters" class in Spring Lake Heights, New Jersey, supports local events such as Race for the Arts 5K, Komen Race for the Cure®, and Walk to Cure Diabetes. We have food drives. During the winter holidays, we gather goodies and treats, and make up gift boxes for families and children in need.
    *   Have a laugh while exercising with friends.

2. We create engagement when we are fully present, mindful, and creating opportunities for flow that lead us and our patients to achieve greater levels of well-being. Flow happens when the entire body is involved in the activity at hand and we "become one" with it (Csikszentmihalyi, 1990). The following exercises give examples of how to build engagement.

    *   Develop skill levels by varying movements and activities. Go outside and enjoy "green exercise."
    *   Encourage mindfulness and appreciation for being in the present moment.
    *   Close your eyes to fully experience your senses. What does it feel like to be in your body?

3. Create positive relationships: positive social connections, promoting social integration and social support, have been linked to positive health behaviors (McGonigal, 2007).

    Relationships can offer a powerful positive influence on our overall health and happiness, particularly for older adults (Peterson C., 2006).

    How to build positive relationships into exercise:

    *   Learn to partner dance or learn the benefits of ballroom dancing for children.
    *   Get in touch with people you miss; show you care; make plans to meet and exercise together.
    *   Take a dance or fitness class with friends. Go for a hike and connect with nature and each other. Join an athletic team. Train for a group event.

4. Meaning can be found in a variety of situations. Consider how different cultures celebrate, honor, and give tribute. Are there dances, processions, or movements around sacred times or that have special significance? Using these dance exercises can build meaning to physical rituals.

5. Achievement is about accomplishing goals. The following are ideas on how to build achievement in yourself and others:

    •   Promote SMART (*s*ystematic, *m*easurable, *a*ction-oriented, *r*ealistic, *t*imed) goals.
    •   Catch yourself and others doing something right and celebrate it!
    •   Recommend a positive exercise prescription. Write it down. "A goal is an idea until you write it down." —Anonymous

THE GO4LIFE INITIATIVE

The National Institute on Aging (NIA) has activated a campaign, Go4Life, with a goal of promoting lifelong physical activity. The Go4Life literature emphasizes how anyone at any age, particularly older adults, can benefit from some type of physical activity. This NIA campaign is encouraging physicians to prescribe physical activity to patients (both young and elderly). The NIA wants you to know that they and your patients are looking to you, as physicians, to take the lead. They suggest as part of your ongoing conversations with patients, including a discussion about exercise and physical activity. Here are a few suggestions the NIA has for you to consider when talking to your patients about exercise. This valuable information is for you and your patient, whether just starting out, or if you would like to significantly increase your activity level.

Encourage and promote cross-training and include the following components of fitness:

1. Aerobic activity, the key to cardiovascular fitness
2. Strength training
3. Flexibility training
4. Balance training
5. Work together with patients to determine the best activities for them.
6. Create a safe activity plan that provides the most benefits.
7. Exercise is critical to maintaining health and managing many chronic illnesses.

Experience: Do your part. Recommend your patients lower their risk for "diseases of inactivity" via positive exercise practices (Joy, Blair, McBride, & Sallis, 2013).

Work together to determine the best activities for your patients. Join forces with your patient to boost his or her self-determination (autonomy, competence, relatedness).

1. Cocreate a safe activity plan that provides the most whole health benefits and incorporates the elements of cardiovascular, strengths, flexibility, and balance training.

2. Discuss warning signs. Encourage your patients to talk with you if they experience any of the following symptoms now or in the future:

   - unplanned weight loss
   - dizziness
   - foot or ankle sores that won't heal
   - shortness of breath
   - chest pain or pressure
   - joint swelling
   - feelings that their heart is fluttering, skipping, or racing
   - blood clots
   - infection
   - fever
   - muscle aches

3. Encourage continuing progress. Many people start out enthusiastically but find it hard to stay motivated. Group exercise can be helpful in boosting adherence and in building motivation and accountability.

4. Help patients stay safe and attracted to being mindfully active with this advice:

   - Start out exercising at a comfortable level and progress slowly.
   - Make physical activity part of a daily routine.
   - Try different activities to keep things fun and interesting.
   - Choose to move more via daily activities, as well as planned exercises.

EIGHT THOUGHTS ABOUT KEEPING A TRAINING JOURNAL

Creating a "Positive Health Habits Journal" is a great place to get started. This powerful practice can boost a more mindful awareness, self-regulation, and greater clarity around your own daily approaches, actions, and choices. Here are eight things to keep in mind about keeping a training journal:

1. Create an intention and focus on what you hope to accomplish (in a training session, for the day, week, month, season, year).
2. Boost your accountability and savor your eating, exercising, and resting/relaxation times.

3. Gain momentum as you reach mini-goals, gaining strength, tone, flexibility, balance, and greater aerobic capacity. Research shows that writing down goals increases the likelihood of achieving them from 20 percent to more than 90 percent.

4. It feels great to keep challenging yourself, so make note of your progress and successes. Build your self-awareness by tracking your mood before and after exercising.

5. Write down key numbers, for example, resting heart rate, waist circumference, and percentage of body fat (if you have an electronic scale). You can also compute your body mass index (BMI).

6. Notice your body clock and circadian rhythms. Notice if your performance is better at certain times of the day.

7. Notice patterns and habits unfolding. Can you be proactive and plan ahead for successes in your training, health, and healing? Plan for times of anticipatory savoring as you look forward to more positive health and fitness.

8. Over time, marvel at your improvements. Write down what you appreciate about your health. Write down three blessings each day.

GAVIN'S INNOVATIVE PERSONALITY AND EXERCISE STRATEGY

In an article in *The Physician and Sportsmedicine*, Gavin suggests building a better understanding about what "moves you" and how introspection in this regard may be a key to success (2004). Gavin recommends that before actively embarking on a fitness program, it is most helpful if you (and your patients) consider what activities will best suit their temperament. In a research study of seven hundred new gym or health club members, Gavin looked at personality dimensions in relation to fitness activities. Gavin found that assessing people according to seven aspects of character—competitiveness, sociability, motivation, sense of adventure, spontaneity, aggressiveness and ability to focus—before recommending a type of exercise that matched their disposition significantly improved the likelihood of their sticking to a fitness program. Gavin explains that people have personalities and so do sports and fitness activities. Someone will feel better about attempting an exercise type within his or her comfort zone or which matches his or her style. The shy, solitary type, for example, who is encouraged to attempt a gregarious aerobics class could be too uncomfortable to attend class a second time.

A change to another fitness program could make all the difference. A sociable person who becomes bored with running could be encouraged to try a Zumba class that would provide similar cardiovascular benefits. Gavin believes the overarching goal is to get people moving in the first place. He points out that only 20 percent of adults in the West currently exercise regularly. He believes that the strategy of matching personality to exercise activity will help to promote activity for the sedentary. We know exercise can reduce anxiety and improve mood, but choosing the proper activity depending on the person's mental makeup can help the person stick to something, enjoy it more, and learn some important lessons for life (Gavin, 2004).

Gavin hopes his model will help people to think beyond the stereotypes of fitness, and think of new forms of movement with a greater potential to influence personal development. Considering your personality in beginning an exercise program can inspire you to get moving and keep moving.

Experience: What personality type(s) resonate with you?

- Social (typified by "I don't enjoy doing things by myself"). Try group classes such as spinning, circuit training, aqua aerobics, or working out with a personal trainer.
- Spontaneous ("I like doing things on the spur of the moment"). Try kickboxing, karate, or salsa classes.
- Self-motivated ("I have strong willpower and don't rely on others for support"). Try jogging or trail-running, circuit sessions at which you can chart your progression, in-line or ice-skating, indoor climbing, or swimming.
- Competitive ("I perform better when I compete"). Try any team sport or activity, spinning or other class in which you can compete against yourself, or a mini indoor triathlon class (these are held in many gyms).
- Aggressive ("I am assertive and won't let things get in my way. I make sure my needs are met"). Try cross-country or competitive running, boxing, or martial arts.
- Focused ("I enjoy getting absorbed in what I am doing"). Try tae kwon do, yoga, or Pilates. Take swimming lessons because they require learning and concentration.
- Risk-seeking ("I am willing to take big risks in order to do things that appeal to me"). Try any new, stimulating workouts. Every month have a go at something different, such as outdoor circuits around parks. Work with a personal trainer to set new goals, like running a marathon, and to help you work toward achieving these.

PHYSICAL ACTIVITY FOR PEOPLE WITH DISABILITIES

The landmark July 2012 issue of *The Lancet* presented an overview of important cross-cultural contexts and adaptive considerations to promote physical activity training for all, and for the greater good (Barnet, et al., 2012). This issue discussed how there are more than a billion people with disabilities worldwide. Engaging in a healthy lifestyle while having a disability can be a daunting task. People with disabilities often are at greater risk of serious health problems associated with physical inactivity. This raises important questions and challenges us as a society to take greater care and consideration in creating and building programs and environments that can serve people with disabilities.

There is a call to action to promote epidemiologic research and practices that offer physical activity for all. Research demonstrates that adults and children with disabilities thrive with access to recreational, leisure, and sporting activities in both inclusive and disability-specific settings. The outcome of inclusive physical activity communities is a society that respects and values the rights of all to have equal access to physical activity.

WATER EXERCISE FOR HEALTH, HEALING, AND PERFORMANCE

Throughout history, water has been used to restore one's health. Water soothes and protects us in a sensual, graceful medium. Water is an exercise medium appropriate for anyone, be they novice exercisers, professional athletes, or people with disabilities.

Beyond horizontal swimming, people can benefit from vertical water-fitness training. Vertical water-fitness training is best performed in waist-high to chest-deep water. A floatation device like a vest or noodle may be used in deep water. Water should be approximately 80 to 84 °F.

Exercising in water is made easier for novice or overweight exercisers because the target heart rate is approximately 10 percent lower in water than on land, and because individual apparent body weight in water is only 10 percent of one's real body weight (because of buoyancy). Water exercises employ variations of buoyancy, pressure, and drag forces to promote safe and effective training.

Water density is about 25,000 times greater than that of air. Changing the effective area of body parts moving through water and changing velocity of movement can vary drag forces.

Some tips to increase the benefits of exercising in water include the following:

- Increase the speed of movement.
- Increase the length of the lever.
- Increase the range of motion of a specific joint.
- Flex extremities to implement resistance or drag forces.
- Increase the width of the frontal plane.
- Change directions often (law of action/reaction).
- Combine muscle groups—striding to work the hamstrings and quadriceps, while doing bicep curls to work biceps and triceps.

Experience: Try these vertical water-fitness moves in shallow or deep water:

- Walking/jogging lifting knees high and in front can vary to side, externally rotating, or bring heels to back for hamstring curls.
- Soccer-kicking legs front and back.
- Power striding, like cross-country skiing in water—the best!
- Jumping Jacks with front-knee raises
- Lunges with side raises
- Pendulum legs and arms

HIGH-INTENSITY INTERVAL TRAINING AND CONSIDERATIONS FOR "CHOICE" INTENSITY INTERVAL TRAINING

High-intensity interval training (HIIT) consists of alternating short periods of intense exercise with recovery periods of passive or mild-intensity movement. The work intervals last from fifteen seconds to four minutes and approach a high-intensity level of 80 to 95 percent of an individual's maximum heart rate. High-intensity interval training helps boost aerobic and anaerobic fitness, reduces body fat, and improves insulin sensitivity, glucose tolerance, and lipid profiles (among other benefits). High-intensity interval training is geared toward experienced exercisers; HIIT may risk injury, especially in novices, because it is so demanding. Another interval strategy that works well for beginners is to apply a strategy of intervals at a "choice" level of intensity. Choice intensity promotes variance within the heart rate training zone, providing many of the benefits of HIIT, while allowing progression in movement and intensity that may lead to greater exercise adherence. Choice intensity interval training gives beginning or moderate exercisers a chance to experience the benefits of HIIT, with lower risk of injury. Choice intensity interval training sessions can promote feelings of exhilaration.

The President's Council on Physical Fitness debuted a new adult fitness test at http://www.adultfitnesstest.org/. Here you can learn the key dimensions of fitness and determine what type of exercise intensity can work for you. Log in and get inspired by your results!

AEROBICS: THE KEY TO FITNESS

Esteemed cardiologist and founder of the Cooper Clinic, Dr. Kenneth Cooper, coined the phrase and wrote the book *Aerobics* (1968). The term *aerobic* means with, or in the presence of, oxygen. Aerobic exercise involves moving the major muscle groups of our body rhythmically for a minimum of fifteen minutes. Aerobic exercise strengthens virtually all the systems of the body. The American Council on Sports Medicine recommends doing aerobic exercise for at least thirty minutes per day, or for a minimum of three ten-minute bouts. Begin by warming up your body for five to ten minutes and prepare for the exercise that is about to follow by starting to exercise at a gentle pace. This will gradually increase circulation and boost psychological readiness. This also reduces the risk of injury. At the end of your exercise period, gradually decrease the intensity of your pace to lower your heart rate. Following this cooldown (recovery) period, your target heart rate aim is less than 120 beats per minute (Cooper, 1968). Stretching is particularly beneficial after exercise (or after a warm bath or shower) as your muscles are warm and more flexible.

Aerobic, strength, flexibility, and balance training are important parts of a balanced fitness program. Aerobics training is the key to fitness. Examples of aerobic activities include brisk walking, running, dancing, swimming, tennis, cycling, skating, basketball, fencing, jumping rope, skiing, snowboarding, volleyball, badminton, racquetball, water aerobics, table tennis, and step training. Ideally you will pursue training that you enjoy.

WALKING FOR FITNESS AND WELL-BEING

"Don't sit if you can stand. Don't stand if you can walk. Don't walk if you can run (or walk briskly)." —Dr. George Sheehan, MD

As we have discussed, walking is one of the easiest, enjoyable, and most functional ways to keep in shape, improve health, and increase quality and length of life. Research shows that moderate walking (maintaining 55 to 75% of your maximum heart rate) reduces the risk of heart disease by 40 percent. Along with the physiological benefits of improved cardiovascular function, improved bone density, and reduced blood cholesterol, walking has many psychological benefits. Walking can reduce feelings of depression, improve creativity, increase self-confidence, improve concentration and mental performance, and generate feelings of well-being (Archer, 2005).

Fenton discusses walking 10,000 steps per day (2008). He believes that this is the amount of exertion your body needs to reduce the risk of chronic disease. Fenton says that it takes less than a minute to reach one hundred steps, and it is not necessary to get up to 10,000 steps all at once, especially if you are sedentary. Fenton recommends working toward this gradually by increasing your step total each week up to 20 percent over the previous week's total.

Martin Seligman, MD, recommends using a pedometer to measure one's steps. Using a pedometer with the posting of the steps taken offers an opportunity for assessment and reinforcement (Bravata, et al., 2007). An article in *The Journal of the American Medical Association* sought to determine whether pedometers really do trigger greater energy expenditure. The authors found that the average user saw an increase of more than 2,100 steps per day. In analyzing twenty-six studies involving 2,767 participants, the researchers also determined that pedometer wearers were more successful at increasing their daily walking if they had a goal of reaching 10,000 steps per day.

MONITORING AEROBIC INTENSITY

Moderate-intensity aerobic exercise is considered to occur when the heart rate is maintained between 55 and 75 percent of one's maximum heart rate. This range is considered the target heart-range zone for moderate-intensity aerobic exercise. To find an individual's maximum heart rate, you subtract his or her age from 220.

Let's take the example of a forty-year-old. His or her maximum heart rate is 180 beats per minute (220 − 40). The low end of this is ninety-nine beats per minute (55% of 180). The high end is 135 beats per minute (75% of 180). Thus, the moderate-intensity target heart-rate range for a forty-year-old beginning exerciser is between ninety-nine and 135 beats per minute.

The Talk Test: The talk test is another means of measuring your training relative to your exertion level. Archer (2005) explained the Talk Test as follows:

- At low to moderate pace, you can talk easily and carry on a conversation. Breathing is easy.
- At a moderate to high pace, you can still talk, but you cannot easily carry on a conversation. Breathing is harder.
- At a high pace, you can say a few words, but you cannot carry on a conversation. Breathing is labored.

Experience: The average resting heart rate for healthy adults is sixty to eighty beats per minute. Measure your heart rate weekly, and post the number in your journal.

As you and your patients become more fit, your resting heart rate will become lower. You can do more work with less effort. The most accurate way of estimating your resting heart rate is to count your pulse for one full minute before you get out of bed in the morning. Alternately, you can relax for ten to twenty minutes, mindfully slowing your breathing and pulse, and then take your pulse. See if you can mindfully lower your resting heart rate over the next twelve weeks. Take steps to improve your cardiovascular health and general vitality.

MINDFUL BREATHING PRACTICES: RELAXATION AND ENERGIZING TECHNIQUES FOR THE REGULATION OF AROUSAL

Mindful breathing focuses attention on the present moment. We become one in the moment: our breath can link our body and mind. The yogis of ancient India considered fresh oxygen and calmness the key to physical stamina, so breathing in tune with the rhythms of nature has always been an integral part of yoga. You do not have to be a yogi to experience positive benefits from breathing mindfully. Breathing mindfully for even a few moments can boost your mood and clarity and adjust your energy levels. Similar to the benefit of aerobics, rhythmic breathing infuses the body with oxygen and helps rid it of toxins and stress. For the ancients, the goal of mindful breathing was to help people reduce stress and become "better people."

Mindfulness in breathing and in action

Breathing interventions are effective in helping us to direct our conscious attention. By controlling our attention, we are able to reach more optimal states of living and being, and thrive at the peak of our abilities. Attention and happiness are closely related. Improving attention by concentrating on the task at hand allows us to reach a state of inner experience where there is order in consciousness. Our breath, linked with our attention, yields many positive benefits.

The mind in medical practice is often filled with an internal dialogue unrelated to what we are doing. This "chatter" can cloud our concentration, possibly cause unrealistic thinking traps, and cause a sense of anxiety. Zen Buddhism asserts that there is value in mindfulness. Mindfulness is the practice of absorbing yourself completely in each moment, with complete concentration on the task, thought, or conversation at hand. Mindfulness is single-pointed concentration on what we are doing in this moment.[18] What is your breathing like? What does your body feel like in space? Are you lifting up your posture, head, and heart?

The word *respiration* comes from the Latin root *spirare*. Spiritus, a derivative, means "breath of a god." Breathing links our body and mind. It is an unconscious process that can be practiced and made more conscious (Archer, 2005).

Experience: Posture check. Try the following strategy for better standing and seated posture, as well as priming more mindful breathing: Begin with a neutral spine (crown of the head to the sky, ears over your shoulders, shoulders down and over your hips, tall neck, rib cage lifted, abdominals pulled in and up, knees slightly flexed, and the feet grounded into the earth).

Experience: Tadasana-Mountain Pose. Tadasana is a standing pose aimed at relaxing, strengthening, and stretching the body. It is geared toward improving posture and alignment. It encourages elongation of the spine and vertebral alignment.

Here's how to do Tadasana:

- Stand with your feet together, arms relaxed by your sides, and your weight evenly balanced over the feet. Keep your shoulders and chest open. Look straight ahead, and soften your gaze.
- Gently "lift" the knee and thigh muscles, tuck your tailbone under and abdomen in. Feel your spine lengthen from the tailbone to the crown of your head. Allow the back of your head to lift slightly and tuck your chin in.
- Continue to "lift" and stand tall. Hold this pose for up to five breaths.

Experience: Be a better breather.

- Be mindful of your breath as it goes in and out of your nostrils. Try not to breathe through your mouth.
- Be mindful of your belly as it expands and contracts with the breath. You can put your hand on the belly to be more conscious of it.
- Be mindful of the other parts of your body. This is an in-the-body rather than out-of-body experience. It is designed to make you aware of all bodily sensations.
- Be mindful of the sights and sounds around you.
- Have a favorite mantra or word pair to utter to yourself silently as you inhale and exhale. Say one word to yourself slowly as you inhale. Say the second word to yourself slowly as you exhale. (For example, when you inhale say *here*; when you exhale, say *now*).

Practicing present-moment awareness

Mindful breathing focuses attention on the present moment. The present is the most important time in your life. Rhythmic breathing infuses the body with oxygen and helps rid it of toxins and stress. The yogis of ancient India considered fresh oxygen and calmness key to physical stamina, so breathing in tune with the rhythms of nature has always been an integral part of yoga.

Breathing is an important part of meditation. Practicing meditation has been shown to increase positive emotions and lower negative affect (personal communications: Seligman in 2002 and Valliant in 2007). Optimism and subjective well-being have been shown to increase after adding the Loving-Kindness meditation as a positive intervention. The Loving-Kindness meditation, adapted from *The Meditation Year*, teaches selfless or altruistic love (Hope, 2001).

Experience: Muscle-to-mind relaxation skills and strategies.

Exercise: Explore these ways of breathing well (Williams J. M., 2006).

Cultivate and savor these five ways of breath expression:

1. Complete breath/diaphragmatic breathing: Place one hand on your abdomen, and the other on your upper chest. Slowly, and while visualizing the lungs as three chambers, breathe in, filling first your belly, then your chest cavity, and last the top of your lungs (by your collarbone, expanding the shoulders) with air. Exhale and repeat.
2. Rhythmic breathing and sigh of exhalation: Breathe in for a count of four, hold the breath for a count of seven, and exhale audibly for a count of eight. Relax and repeat.
3. One-to-two ratio: Breathe in and out fully. Then breathe in for a count of four, out for a count of eight. With practice you can change the count to 5:10 or 6:12.
4. Five-to-one count: Say and visualize the number five as you take in a full deep breath in and out. Mentally count and visualize the number four, saying to yourself, "I am more relaxed than I was at five." Continue the countdown until you get to one and are totally relaxed.
5. Concentration breathing: breath of thanks: Breathe in for seven counts, hold for seven counts, and exhale out for seven counts. Relax and repeat.

Experience: Breathing and trauma

Experience these six steps to boost and encourage resilience :

Assess levels of posttraumatic stress.

- Encourage expressions of feelings.
- Offer empathy and validation.
- Encourage discovery and expression of meaning.
- Provide didactic information.
- Provide breathing and movement exercises.

Breath is used as a natural medicine and a healing tool. Since no one can control nature, others, and what happens outside of one's self, survivors are assisted in controlling how they respond to the disaster. It is helpful for the medical training, practices, patients, and survivors to know how to move well, breathe, and release fear, uncertainty and resentments.

Experience: Momentary relaxation helps us enjoy controlled, balanced states. Here are some energy management tips:

- Mindful awareness of tension and activation levels helps us make any necessary physical adjustments.
- Relaxation builds skills and strategies to enhance learning. Relaxation should be a priority and taught to improve well-being.
- Momentary relaxation can facilitate imagery and concentration.
- Single-minded focus reduces other thoughts and stimulation, which interfere with what we need in the moment.

Qigong: Moving Meditation

Qigong is the practice of aligning breath, movement, and awareness for exercise, healing, and meditation. With roots in Chinese medicine, martial arts, and philosophy, qigong is traditionally viewed as a practice to cultivate and balance chi, which can be translated as intrinsic life energy. Typically, a qigong practice involves rhythmic breathing coordinated with slow, stylized repetition of fluid movement. The goal is a calm state, with visualization of guiding chi through the body.

Qigong, as an ancient form of healing, meditative movement, offers energy cultivation. Qigong can be regarded as a mindfulness practice combining concentration and present-centered awareness. A mindful approach to movement helps us lower stress, increase energy, improve concentration, raise body awareness, promote relaxation, and decrease the incidence of injury. A mindful approach to qigong practice cultivates a refined awareness of energy flow, along with the ability to direct energy to various parts of the body to heal emotional and physical traumas, reduce stress and pain, and rejuvenate the mind, body, and spirit.

There are many forms and systems of qigong practice. Cammarata discusses the relaxation and energy-enhancing benefits experienced via the Eight Pieces of Brocade, a classic and popular form of qigong (Cammarata, personal communication, 2008). The eight simple movements are designed to relax the body, mind, and emotions, promote calm, enhance stability, and promote the free flow of qi (energy). Cammarata recommends mindfully breathing, relaxing, and enjoying the present moment when practicing.

Experience: The Eight Pieces of Brocade Movements

Practice guidelines are as follow: Relax deeply while standing with your feet firmly rooted to the floor, knees slightly bent. Breathe using slow, continuous breaths. Place your tongue lightly at the roof of your mouth, behind your teeth. Move your body with the lightest of effort, as if you were "swimming in air." Let go of distractions and focus the mind on each movement of the body. With practice, you can naturally coordinate your breath with the exercises by exhaling during expanding movements and inhaling during contracting movements. Learn each individual "piece of brocade" movement and practice eight times each to achieve the greatest benefit.

The 8 pieces are:

- pushing up the heavens
- pulling the bow to shoot the arrow
- separating heaven and earth
- the wise owl gazes backward
- swaying the head and swinging the tail
- two hands hold the feet to strengthen the kidneys
- punching with angry eyes
- bouncing on heels to shake off stress and illness

ANIMATING ENERGY, MINDFULNESS, ACCEPTANCE, AND COMPASSION

Almost every culture of the world has a word to express the concept of an activating energy in the universe. These words include chi, ki, qu, life force, and spiritual energy. This energy exists to sustain life and is the animating force in all living beings. As the animating factor, chi bridges our body and our consciousness and is enhanced by movement (Fritzke and Voogt, personal communication, 2008). "Proper body-mind harmony, proper demeanor, and superior skill for proper action" promotes wisdom and virtue. The positive integration of the mind and body and the incorporation of self-reflection into our movement can empower us and those we serve in our medical practice and training.

Gavin, Seguin, and McBrearty (2006) discussed the many benefits of mindfulness. Interestingly, they suggested that activities like weight training can be as much of a mind-body experience as tai chi, depending on how each is practiced. Gavin, Seguin, and McBrearty also found that an exercise participant's inclination to direct his or her mental activities in a nonevaluative and connected way while training has many additional advantages. The benefits include greater body understanding and awareness, greater body acceptance and satisfaction, greater transfer of training principles to daily life, and the development of deeper compassion for others. These are invaluable perceptions. Movement with intention has the ability to enhance every aspect of performance, including:

- concentration—balance,
- attentional focus—proprioception,
- awareness—efficacy,

- confidence—postural alignment, and
- speed—homeostasis.

Harmonious movement

"There is a force within that gives you life. Seek that." —Rumi

In *Flow: The Psychology of Optimal Experience*, Csikszentmihalyi (1990) revealed that what makes experience genuinely satisfying is the state of consciousness called flow. In this optimum experience, people feel periods of concentration and deep enjoyment. One of the best ways to enjoy more opportunities for flow in life is through movement and music. Csikszentmihalyi discusses physical experience that uses the body as a source of enjoyment, for in fact, a broad range of activities rely on rhythmic or harmonious movements to generate flow (1990).

Experience: Move, dance, or relax to music

Man is music (Seligman, personal communication). In discussing the flow of music, Csikszentmihalyi states that music helps organize the mind, thereby reducing psychic entropy (1990). Because listening to music decreases the probability of anxiety and boredom, focusing on music can induce flow experiences. Music is a fantastic motivator. It can push you to do more and to exercise longer, even longer than you originally planned. Langer discusses the importance of music in her experiments in creating the feeling of "peak years" in her senior adults (2009). When the older adults listened to music from their youth, they responded more youthfully, vigorously, and vibrantly.

Music with a slow beat has been shown to regulate our brain waves and promote relaxation or activation (Fried, 1990). Try to immerse yourself in the sounds you enjoy, and visualize the notes flowing over your body until they envelop, calm, and soothe you.

THE PARADOX OF LEISURE: BASIC NEEDS ASSESSMENT CALLS FOR POSITIVE EXERCISE PRACTICES AND PRESCRIPTIONS

The Greeks believed that free time was the source of the most rewarding experiences in life. Unfortunately, this has not been the case in the United States of the twentieth and twenty-first centuries, when we have been working longer and harder than ever. In an illuminating experiment about how we spend our time, Csikszentmihalyi and LeFevre (1989) found that the lack of flow in leisure is unlikely to be caused by physical exhaustion; more likely, it is due to inability to organize one's psychic energy in unstructured free time; it may also be due to cultural factors, such as lack of socialization in flow activities or perhaps an over reliance on television and other media. Csikszentmihalyi and LeFevre found people had more optimal experiences at work, as opposed to leisure activities. As adults age and may leave the workforce, it is important to create opportunities for them to experience purpose in life. Ideally, there will be a paradigm shift, and the idea of "retiring" will be viewed as a time for new contributions, goals, and gains. Csikszentmihalyi and LeFevre also discussed that although adolescents enjoyed active leisure time, they spent almost ten times that many hours watching television (and cellular phones and tablets). Like adults, inactive children have a high risk of diabetes, obesity, and depression. Csikszentmihalyi (1990) proposed that the goal is experiencing flow that will sustain the good life for you. Somaesthetics, yoga, dance/fitness, strength training, qigong, tai chi, outdoor recreation, hiking, walking, running, sporting activities, and creative movement (especially in group settings) are likely flow-enhancing activities. The idea is to think of voluntary focused activities that are enjoyable at "nonobligatory" times. These "joy of movement" activities provide excellent health benefits for every participant.

Experience: List activities you enjoy doing. What activities have you enjoyed that promoted the feeling of "time standing still," where you became one with the moment? Can you think about activities you enjoyed doing as a child or at other times in your life? Write those in your journal, along with any remembrances about the experiences.

MOVING TOWARD WELLNESS AT WORK

Incorporating wellness programs at work reduces health-care costs and absenteeism, lowers employee turnover, increases productivity, and improves morale (Powell, 1999). Physicians and their patients spend most of their time at work. It is cost-effective for employers, hospitals, communities, and organizations to foster wellness activities and well-being programs on-site. These workplace programs promote goodwill and enhance communication, sustainability, enjoyment, and flourishing on the job.

MOVEMENT SUPPORTS LEARNING AND WELL-BEING IN CHILDREN AND ADULTS

The *Physical Activity and Fitness Digest* reports that nearly 200 studies on the effect of exercise on cognitive functioning suggest that physical activity supports learning (President's Council on Fitness, Sports and Nutrition, 2011). When children exercise and fitness needs are met, students have cognitive energy to learn and achieve. Physical activity programs have been linked to stronger academic achievement, increased concentration, and improved reading and writing test scores. Dr. R. Tait McKenzie's vision about movement and learning has been substantiated. Children who develop basic movement skills are more likely to choose to be physically active later in life. Studies have shown that physical activity levels decrease as children grow, develop, and mature to adulthood, particularly for those who don't have the competence and confidence to engage in a variety of movement activities (Haubenstricker & Seefeldt, 1986). Movement and play are essential to physical, intellectual, and social-emotional development at all ages (Elkind, 2007).

ATCHLEY'S ACTIVITY THEORY

In discussing theories of psychosocial aging, Atchley mentions disengagement theory in older adults, which is in stark contrast to activity theory. Activity theory states that in the absence of poor health or disability, older adults have the same psychological and social needs as younger adults. The more activities older people engage in, the more satisfying their lives will be. The key is to encourage healthy adaptation and a healthy lifestyle.

Experience: Atchley (2004) discusses five components of life satisfaction to adopt in sustaining a positive attitude to growing older. Engaging in enjoyable activity, either in a group or individually, may help you and your patients apply this positive philosophy.

- Harness zest, enthusiasm, and vitality in several areas of life.
- Take responsibility in both good and bad situations in life.
- Don't give up.
- Honor your achievements.
- Think of yourself as a valuable person.

GRATITUDE, APPRECIATION, AND PERSPECTIVE

"Let us rise up and be thankful, for if we didn't learn a lot today, at least we learned a little, and if we didn't learn a little, at least we didn't get sick, and if we got sick, at least we didn't die; so, let us all be thankful." —The Buddha

Creating new positive habits of exercising and movement is a process that can be successfully managed. Applying the transtheoretical model of change, Prochaska, Norcross, and DiClemente (1994) describe six stages of change: precontemplation, contemplation, preparation, action, maintenance, and relapse. During these stages, described in *Changing for Good*, the authors discuss how it is possible to create a climate where positive change can occur, motivation can be maintained, and setbacks can be turned into progress. *Changing for Good* offers strategies for making new beneficial habits, like exercise and a good eating plan, positive and permanent parts of your life.

NURTURING NATURE: GREEN EXERCISE

The term *green exercise* is related to the growing body of evidence that interacting with nature can positively affect our health and well-being, relieving stress and promoting lucidity and concentration. It provides:

> Natural and social connections, including being with family and friends, with pets, and with wildlife, can evoke memories of happier times and may stimulate sacred feelings.

- Breathing fresh air, being exposed to the land and sky and nature's panoply of color, offers us a spirit of sensory stimulation.
- In movement and activities, we learn skill sets, feel the energy of physicality, and enjoy possibilities for goal setting, efficacy, and excellence within our environment.
- We get opportunities for relaxation and escape from modern life. We can reenergize by getting away from stress, giving us time to reflect and gain clarity in thinking.

For information about green exercise, see publications listed by the University of Essex Green Exercise team (2005-2014).

NEUROSCIENCE AND TRANSFORMATIVE EFFECTS OF EXERCISE ON THE BRAIN

In the late 1990s, at the Salk Institute for Biological Studies, Fred H. Gage and his colleagues presented research showing that exercise can improve the performance of the brain by boosting memory and cognitive processing speed. The Salk researchers found that exercise creates a stronger, faster brain (Reynolds, 2007). Regular aerobic exercise increases the conditions that optimal brain functioning requires: plenty of blood flow offering oxygen and the right nutrients, a balance of body chemicals designed to help the brain operate, and an ability to grow new cells and connections in the brain. These results are often measurable within a few weeks after beginning an aerobics exercise program.

In *Spark: The Revolutionary New Science of Exercise and the Brain*, Dr. John Ratey (2008) discusses how exercise strengthens the brain in two major ways. It helps to generate new brain cells, and it strengthens the connections between those cells, providing more mental agility and allowing the brain to stay young even as the body ages. Exercise increases the brain's synaptic plasticity, improving neurogenesis (brain-cell production). According to the author, during exercise, a protein called IGF-1 is conveyed through the bloodstream to the brain, where it helps organize the production of other beneficial chemicals called neurotrophic factors. One neurotrophic factor, brain-derived neurotrophic factor, has been called Miracle-Gro for the brain because of its ability to better equip the brain to process new information. Ratey's compelling evidence demonstrated that aerobic exercise physically remodels our brains for peak performance.

EXERCISE AND PUBLIC HEALTH

Exercise is Medicine

Exercise is MedicineÔ (EIM) is a multi-organizational global initiative that was launched jointly by the American Medical Association and the ACSM late in 2007. The EIM goal is to encourage physicians to include exercise when designing treatment plans for their patients. Exercise is Medicine aims to make physical activity a standard part of the primary care office visit. This new paradigm encourages physicians to discuss the importance of exercising with patients at every visit.

The goal is for exercise to be discussed, assessed, and charted as part of the minimum standard of care. The discussion has begun for the inclusion of (self-reported) exercise as the fifth vital sign (in addition to pulse rate, blood pressure, body temperature, and respiration). Sallis, the founder of the EIM initiative and a Kaiser Permanente primary care physician, has passionately and tirelessly pursued his quest to improve public health and save lives (Young, 2013).

ExerciseIsMedicine.org

With an attractive, layered, and user-friendly Web site, ExerciseisMedicine.org serves medical and health providers, fitness professionals, and the public. There is a handy media section, an international section showing the global reach of this program, and a vast array of resources that are free, accessible, and relatively easy to understand for people of all literacy levels. In addition, there are charts, forms, guides, and initiatives, including a new focus on bringing the EIM message to college campuses.

With a multimedia and social-media presence, including videos, YouTube clips, posters, letters, signs, and e-mails, the EIM message is spreading quickly. Exercise is Medicine has regional centers on six continents. China launched its program last summer. There is also a new Exercise is Medicine Health and Fitness Professionals Action Guide on the Web site. All tools are user-friendly and can easily by customized to your practice.

Exercise as a vital sign

In measuring EIM outcomes, Young (2013) examined the electronic health records of 1,793,385 Kaiser Permanente patients eighteen years and older from April 2010 through March 2011. He found that 86 percent of these patients (1,537,798) had an exercise vital sign in their electronic record. This study had both face and discriminate validity and is encouraging in demonstrating that exercise as a vital sign can be integrated into a primary care office visit as hoped.

Call to action

Exercise is Medicine calls on each person to truly become dedicated to the idea that exercise is medicine, to continue to build, support, and advocate for physical activity as essential for global health and well-being, and to commit to action.

Exercise is Medicine, with its multimedia global outreach, initiatives, and partnerships (including with the Centers for Disease Control and the President's Council on Physical Fitness and Sports), validates the importance of physical activity in whole health care. Exercise is Medicine supports the Healthy People 2020 campaign and has a strong and growing global network. Exercise is Medicine offers education, research, health communications, encouragement, and ultimately the possibility of helping people become healthy, happy, and well.

Experience: Tips to promote exercise to boost exercise retention, adherence, and success

- Set specific long-term and short-term goals applying the SMART goal mode.
- Commit for the long haul. Harness and practice the strength of perseverance (Duckworth, Peterson, Matthew, & Kelly, 2007).
- Exercise to *feel* better. Savor satisfying moments of moving your body well.
- Focus on the intrinsic rewards of exercise.
- Schedule exercise so it becomes a priority. Make a date with yourself. Set a standing playdate with Aristotelian friends (other people who truly care for you and your

well-being, reciprocally). Research shows that starting the day with physical activity is a habit that sticks.

- Try something new. Seek what activities you might enjoy doing. Think outside the box across genres (dance, water fitness, sports, outdoor pursuits, adventure, thrills, relaxation, yoga, martial arts, and play).
- Experience pleasure in moving your body often and well. Strengthen your resolve. Be flexible in your options. Build progression in learning new skills. Promote progression, variety, and balance in movement.
- Make it difficult not to exercise. Move to music. Tap your toes. Lift, twist, and bend. Walk with intention. Check your posture, both seated and standing, and move frequently.
- Exercise with a friend. Make "moving dates."

Finish exercise sessions feeling good, exhilarated, and wanting more.

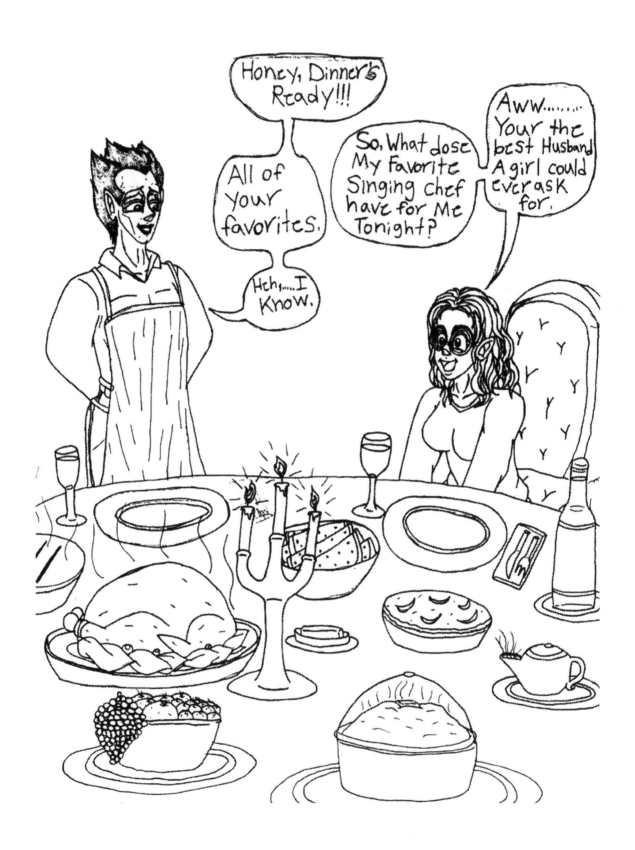

Chapter 5

Positive Nutrition

Guest Author: Lori Lorditch, RD

Believe it or not, you have probably eaten more than 20,000 meals in your life. Without realizing it, your body uses nutrients from those foods to make all its components and fuel all of its activities. How successfully your body handles these tasks depends greatly on your food and lifestyle choices. Nutrition has played a significant role in your life and will continue to play a key role in your longevity.

Nutrition is becoming a primary topic of conversation among many adults, teens, and children. The latest news article and magazine story is likely referring to some new diet or offering some nutrition advice. We know that the word *nutrition* refers to the foods we eat, the nutrients we absorb, and how they function in our body. But why should we eat healthy? What if we are just perfectly content eating processed foods? This may seem fine for the moment, but one day we may visit the doctor for a checkup and be shocked by abnormal laboratory analyses and disease development. We watch what we eat to help prevent this unwanted news and to live our lives to their fullest and greatest potential. Paying close attention to good eating habits now can bring health benefits today and in the future.

Although most people realize that their food habits affect their health, they often choose foods for other reasons. Foods bring to the table a variety of pleasures, traditions, and associations, as well as nourishment. Throughout this chapter, you will learn how to combine favorite foods and enjoyable experiences with a nutritionally balanced diet. You will learn ways to use food as sustenance for yourself, as well as how to give nutritional advice to others. You will learn how to feel positive both physically and mentally through what you eat.

"YOU ARE WHAT YOU EAT"

Even though the body's cells grow and divide more rapidly during infancy and childhood, they are still constantly reproducing in growing adults. An excess or deficiency of specific nutrients may affect how well these cells reproduce, how healthy they are, and how efficiently they work. How well the body functions and how well the organs work depend on how well the cells work, which ultimately depends on if they are adequately nourished (Sears, Sears, Sears, & Sears, 2006).

The body's cells can create a blueprint that determines how cells do their jobs. What we eat affects the cells' metabolic programming. Metabolic programming seems to be especially important for liver cells and brain-cell development. When too much of some nutrients are consumed and not enough of others, the liver cells can become defective. This is of concern due to the important role the liver plays in the body's metabolism (Sears, Sears, Sears, & Sears, 2006). According to one experiment, young, malnourished animals showed less growth of the insulin-secreting cells of the pancreas, a defect that could predispose them to diabetes as adults (Marroqui, et al., 2012).

Our cells reproduce and keep the same genetic makeup by following the code on the DNA. A healthy diet can keep the DNA code stabilized, which in turn allows cells to reproduce the way they are supposed to. An unbalanced diet can predispose to faulty cell reproduction, which can sometimes lead to disease development, such as cancer (Sears, Sears, Sears, & Sears, 2006). Common illnesses can occur to the central nervous system. They can also contribute to metabolic problems, cardiovascular disease, and inflammatory disease. Keep in mind that allowing yourself a soda on occasion will not have an effect on your cell reproduction. But multiple sodas per day, every day, along with other unhealthy lifestyle choices, may contribute to health problems later in life (Whitney & Rolfes, 2005).

One of the newer fields of research is called nutrigenomics, which supports the common saying, "We are what we eat." Nutrigenomics is the study of how nutrition affects our genes. In individuals who are genetically predisposed to a disease, an unbalanced diet may increase their chances for developing the disease to which they are predisposed. For example, someone who is genetically predisposed to type 2 diabetes may be more likely to become diabetic if that person eats a greater amount of sugars (carbohydrates) than the adequate amount that meets his or her needs (King, 2003). This individual would be well-advised to limit sugar intake, especially added sugars, and perhaps even to try some sugar-free food items. Also, this person should follow an exercise plan and the recommendations of a diabetes educator to monitor sugar intake and blood-sugar levels (Escott-Stump, 2008).

Cells communicate with each other using hormones. These hormones carry messages from hormone-producing cells to other cells and organs and tell them what to do. Hormones can be greatly influenced by nutrition. One prime example is insulin sensitivity.

Insulin is the hormone that tells cells to let in glucose for energy. If the body's cells become overwhelmed with sugar, lack of communication can occur within the cells, which makes them resistant to insulin and can lead to development of diabetes. Cells also communicate with each other using neurotransmitters. These are especially important in the brain and gastrointestinal tract. The better nutrition an individual has, the better the brain is able to communicate with the GI tract (Sears, Sears, Sears, & Sears, 2006). This can be seen in individuals who recognize their hunger and fullness cues when eating.

We learned in biology class that the cell is protected by a skin-like structure called the *cell membrane*. The cell membrane has receptors that either help hormones enter the cell or transmit second messages across the membrane so that a hormone or neurotransmitter can have its effect without entering the target cell. Poor nutrition can cause the receptor sites to become defective. The cell is then unable to receive and act on certain messages. When the cell membrane is strong and well-nourished, it has the power to allow the correct and beneficial nutrients into the cell, to exchange nutrients and metabolites with the bloodstream, and to communicate with other cells. Another fact to consider is that the cell membrane is composed mostly of fat. Individuals need a good balance of unsaturated fat and saturated fat. When too much saturated fat is consumed, it can clog the receptor sites on the cells, preventing successful cell communication (Sears, Sears, Sears, & Sears, 2006). Therefore, an individual should have a predominance of unsaturated fats in his or her diet, like those found in olive oil, nuts, seeds, and avocados, and should limit intake of saturated fat, which includes butter, mayonnaise, salad dressings, and baked goods.

Continuing to think about cell structure, we also remember that cells contain mitochondria, which generate most of the cells' supply of chemical energy needed for the cells to work and reproduce. When one's dietary intake is low in nutrients, one's cells cannot make energy efficiently (Escott-Stump, 2008). This is the main reason for the fatigue experienced with poor nutrition. A diet that contains a balanced intake of carbohydrates, proteins, and fats can help cells make and store plenty of energy. Throughout this chapter, balanced eating will be discussed in more detail, along with ways to apply this knowledge to your lifestyle.

Discussion questions

- How does adequate nutrition help prevent disease development?
- If a patient is genetically predisposed to type 2 diabetes, what advice would you give him or her to decrease the chance of developing the disease?
- We know that all the parts of the cell structure function to keep the cell healthy. What are the main parts of the cell that can affect health if nutrition intake is inadequate?

FEED YOURSELF A GOOD-CARB DIET, NOT A LOW-CARB DIET

Over the past several years there has been much misinformation about carbohydrates. Let's clear up this confusion. Carbs are not a bad food. In fact, most adults need at least 50 percent of their dietary intake to come from carbohydrates. Carbs are your main source of energy. They provide fuel for the body and brain. For people who exercise, carbohydrates are vital. Most carbohydrates are abundant in B vitamins. Without B vitamins the body would lack energy, as they help the body use fuel by forming part of the coenzyme that assists certain enzymes in the release of energy from energy-yielding nutrients, such as carbohydrates (Whitney & Rolfes, 2005). They are also stored in the muscles and liver as glycogen for later use once the carbohydrate is broken down into simple sugars: glucose, fructose, and galactose. This also prevents muscles from becoming fatigued during long workouts. Carbohydrates are necessary for protein to fulfill its structural and enzymatic roles. If a person doesn't take in enough carbohydrates, protein will be burned for energy. This may not allow for proper muscle repair, successful production of enzymes and hormones, or the proper formation of new blood cells (McArdle, Katch, & Katch, 1999; Rosenbloom, 2000). Carbohydrates are made up of natural sugars. The single-sugar molecules are glucose, fructose, and galactose. When they are linked, they become disaccharides (two sugars) or polysaccharides, which are built up one sugar at a time (many sugars). Table 5-1 below gives examples of food sources linked to the disaccharide type.

Table 5-1

Disaccharide	Comprised of	Food Sources
Sucrose	glucose + fructose	Fruits, vegetables, and table sugar
Lactose	glucose + galactose	Milk and milk products
Maltose	glucose + glucose	Cereal, pasta, potatoes, etc.

Molecules of many sugars linked together (polysaccharides) are also sometimes known as complex carbohydrates. Starches and fiber are examples of polysaccharides or complex carbohydrates. Starches are found in vegetables such as corn and peas, as well as in rice, potatoes, beans, and grains (Whitney & Rolfes, 2005).

Whole grains are grains with the outer layers, or husks, still on. The outer layers of grains contain most of the fiber, and so cooked whole grains should contain at least three to five grams of fiber per serving to be considered an adequate source of this nutrient. When carbohydrates are eaten, the digestive tract breaks the long chains of starches and disaccharides into single sugars: glucose, galactose, and fructose. All digestible carbohydrates are metabolized to glucose (Whitney & Rolfes, 2005). When glucose enters the body, its level in the blood (blood sugar) rises quickly. To prevent a sugar spike and a quick crash shortly after, eat foods containing both carbohydrates and fiber. Fiber cannot be broken down by humans and is not absorbed in the bloodstream, so it adds bulk to the entire length of the intestinal tract. The bulk contributed by fiber helps the muscles of the intestinal tract move the food and waste through the system. Bulk from fiber contributes to a full feeling and retains water within the intestinal tract (Escott-Stump, 2008; Mahan & Escott-Stump, 2000). This slows the digestion of the carbohydrate and prevents a quick sugar spike. It is important to increase fluid intake along with fiber intake. Foods containing fiber help keep the body fuller longer and prevent hunger shortly after a snack or meal.

Protein takes a little longer to break down and digest than does a carbohydrate. When protein is paired with a carbohydrate, it helps to slow the entry of sugar into the bloodstream and also helps to keep the body feeling fuller longer (Whitney & Rolfes, 2005). The following are some tasty snack combinations with a good balance of carbohydrate, protein, and fiber:

- rice cake with peanut butter and banana
- Parmesan cheese melted on a slice of whole-grain bread
- blueberries in yogurt
- celery sticks with peanut butter
- fruit and yogurt smoothie
- bean dip and veggie sticks
- whole-grain muffins
- cut-up vegetables with salsa and corn chips
- carrot sticks dipped in hummus
- whole-grain cereal with yogurt
- string cheese and a piece of fruit
- handful of raw nuts or trail mix
- popcorn
- cherry tomatoes with cheese cubes
- hard-boiled egg
- homemade oatmeal raisin cookies
- apple slices dipped in peanut butter
- edamame (fresh, cooked soybeans)
- cottage cheese and fruit
- pita bread spread with hummus

The low-carb method of dieting has swarmed the media, food, and weight loss industry for years now. Many have tried the diet and have been successful, while others have tried and failed. It is important to know that there are some dangers to significantly decreasing carbohydrate intake. The body stores carbohydrates in muscles and the liver as glycogen. With each gram of glycogen that is stored, three grams of water are stored. Without sufficient carbohydrate intake, muscles will not have adequate energy or fluid levels. This compromises the ability to exercise and increases the likelihood of injury (McArdle, Katch, & Katch, 1999; Rosenbloom, 2000). Other hazards of low-carbohydrate diets are listed below:

- They are nutritionally inadequate by being low in many vitamins and minerals.
- They are low in fiber, which can lead to constipation.
- Low-carbohydrate diets are typically higher in protein. This can lead to dehydration. A high protein intake forces the body to lose excessive amounts of body water. Symptoms of dehydration that may occur can include headache, fatigue, constipation, blood-pressure changes, and rapid heartbeat.
- Calcium is excreted in the urine with a high animal protein intake, which can lead to calcium deficiency.
- By-products of carbohydrate metabolism are needed to burn fat completely. When carbohydrate is not present, the fat-burning produces ketones, which when present to excess can cause excessive acidity in body fluids. This can also produce an odor called *ketone breath* (Escott-Stump, 2008; Mahan & Escott-Stump, 2000).

Did you ever hear someone say, "I sometimes just crave sugar," or "When I'm stressed, all I want to do is eat sweets"? Some may call themselves food or sugar addicts, but there is some biological evidence that supports our brain developing these cravings. When glucose hits the brain, it triggers the release of serotonin. Serotonin in just the right amount provides a sense of contentment and relaxation (Sears, Sears, Sears, & Sears, 2006). A number of antidepressant drugs such as fluoxetine and citaliopram elevate mood by increasing the amount of serotonin available to stimulate brain cells. With this in mind, can sugar cravings stem from emotions? If carbs contribute to that good feeling, then it can be completely normal to give the brain and body that satisfaction from a small amount of sugar.

The problem that comes when this occurs more frequently and in larger volume is known as emotional eating. Emotional eating can stem from feelings of stress, unhappiness, procrastination, boredom, loneliness, anger, or anxiety. Emotional eating can also be used as a distraction to avoid dealing with other problems. Most of the time these can be seen as "down" feelings, for which the food acts as an "upper." When an individual is experiencing emotional eating due to stress or depression, it can grow to become a primary coping mechanism and can lead to social isolation, obesity, and other health conditions, as well as to a decrease in concentration and brainpower. At this point, an individual may need to seek therapeutic care to help him or her learn other coping skills and help develop a more healthy relationship with food. When individuals find themselves coping in this way, they can stop and ask themselves these questions:

- Why am I eating?
- Am I hungry?
- Is food a reward?
- Am I eating because I am stressed?
- Am I eating because I am bored?

When an individual reaches a point of needing emotional support from a professional, there are plenty of resources available. Therapists, social workers, and psychologists are trained to help individuals sort out their feelings and separate them from the food. Coping skills that can be used include reading a book for pleasure, watching a movie, light to moderate exercise, yoga, meditation, painting, playing a musical instrument, cooking, chatting with a family member or friend, or journaling. Besides these methods of distraction from eating, the individual can learn to practice mindful eating. This will be discussed later in the chapter.

Discussion questions

- Explain the difference between simple and complex carbohydrates. Name some food sources of the different types of natural sugars.
- You have a very hectic and overscheduled lifestyle with work, family, and school. You are trying to make some changes to help develop a healthier lifestyle. Instead of having chips and cookies every day out of the vending machine, name at least three high-fiber-carbohydrate foods and one protein source that you can combine to form a healthy snack. Name three snack combinations other than the ones listed in this section.
- You have a patient in her last year of graduate school. Her planner seems to be filling up with assignments, tests, and papers. Stress levels and anxiety have increased significantly over the past few months. She opens up to you about engaging in a nighttime snacking habit. You notice she appears fatigued and has gained some weight. What type of questions could you ask her to find out if she is engaging in emotional eating? What other mechanisms for coping with stress might she try? What other resources may be options for her to help break her habit?

PROTEIN CONSUMPTION

From the Greek word meaning *primary*, protein is critical for aiding in body growth, repair, and replacing tissues.

The body needs protein to:

- **grow:** Sufficient protein is needed to grow during childhood, during teen years, and during pregnancy to support the growth needs of the fetus. *Proteins are vital as an energy source.* When proteins break down into their constituent amino acids, these amino acids can yield compounds, such as pyruvate, that are key in energy metabolism.
- **repair all tissues in the body:** Protein repairs muscle tissue, forms scars, and contributes to replacing worn-out cells throughout the body.
- **produce new blood cells:** Blood cells last between three and four months. New blood cells are continually being formed in the bone marrow, and protein is continually required for this process. Red blood cells are packed with hemoglobin, a protein that is essential for carrying oxygen around to the cells of the body.
- **keep your immune system strong:** Proteins play a major role in the immune system that serves to combat bacterial infection and even cancer. The immunoglobulins are all proteins.
- **maintain acid-base balance:** Proteins in the blood act as a buffer, preventing dangerous conditions of acidosis (too much acid) or alkalosis (too much alkali, or base).
- **steady blood sugar:** Protein is digested slowly, so the energy from a meal high in protein enters the bloodstream at a slow, steady rate.

Proteins can be classified as either structural or enzymatic. Structural proteins form the scaffolding of skin and cells. Enzymes cause the chemical reactions of the body to proceed at the proper rate for normal body function. Proteins are chains of amino acids, built one amino acid at a time in response to instructions coded in genes. The body can make some of the amino acids, but others must be obtained from food. The ones we must obtain from food are called essential amino acids. These must be present to make the enzymes essential for the body to carry out daily functions. A food containing all the essential amino acids is considered a complete protein. Foods from animal sources and soy provide complete proteins. The amino acids missing in legumes, nuts, and seeds can be found in grains and vegetables to form complete proteins. They don't necessarily need to be eaten together. As long as these foods are eaten within the course of a day, they can form protein in the body (Whitney & Rolfes, 2005; Clark, 1996).

When the body is low on energy intake from carbohydrate sources, it can switch to burning protein as an energy source. When protein is used for energy, it isn't available to fulfill important structural or enzymatic functions. Insufficient energy and protein intake can result in decreased immunity, fatigue, decreased gastrointestinal absorption, and nutrient deficiencies. When the body is extremely deficient in energy, it may start to break down muscles and organs to supply energy to the brain and rest of the body (Evans, 1993).

As mentioned before, low-carbohydrate diets tend to be higher in protein. Excess protein can lead to dietary imbalances, vitamin and mineral deficiencies, and inadequate fiber from lack of other essential food groups. This can lead to constipation and other gastrointestinal distress. Because protein forces release of fluid, it can result in dehydration and increased calcium excretion (Evans, 1993). If protein intake is high, calorie intake can be higher than needed. If the energy from protein is not used, it may be converted to excess body fat.

Protein needs vary depending on age and activity level. A more sedentary adult needs a minimum of 0.8 grams per kilogram of body weight. Teens and exercising adults may need 1.8 to 2.0 grams per kilogram of body weight (Lemon, 1995). Once protein needs are determined, the chart below can be used as a reference on how to consume the right amount of protein. In table 5-2 food types are listed with the concurrent amount of protein per serving.

Table 5-2

Food	Grams of Protein per Serving
Meat, poultry, fish (3 oz.)	21
Egg	6
Egg white	3
Cottage cheese (1/2 cup)	14
Milk (1 cup)	8
Yogurt (1 cup)	8
Cheese (1 oz.)	7
Legumes (1/2 cup) (black beans, kidney beans, chickpeas, etc.)	7–8
Tofu, raw, firm (3 oz.)	13
Peanut butter (2 Tbsp.)	8
Nuts or sunflower seeds (1 oz.)	7
Cereal (1 oz.)	3
Pasta or rice (1/2 cup)	3
Whole-wheat bread (1 slice)	3

How can these food sources be used to help increase protein intake with meals and snacks? Below are some easy ways to add high-protein foods to daily intake to ensure protein needs are met.

Breakfast:

- Make a quick omelet. Mix whole eggs and egg whites.
- Spread peanut butter on an apple.
- Spread almond butter on toast.
- Make a fruit, yogurt, and granola parfait.
- Add walnuts or almonds to a bowl of cereal.

Lunch:

- Make a veggie soup that contains white or black beans.
- Throw chickpeas in a salad.
- Put a piece of grilled chicken on a salad.
- Make a tuna salad sandwich.
- Have breakfast for lunch with eggs, a couple slices of bacon, and whole-wheat toast.

Dinner:

- Add tofu to a stir-fry.
- Add shrimp to a pasta dish.
- Grill chicken or salmon.
- Throw a burger or veggie burger on a roll.
- Mix almonds with green beans.
- Put sunflower seeds in a side salad.

Snack:

- Black bean dip with whole-grain chips
- Cottage cheese with fruit
- Fruit and yogurt smoothie
- Protein shake
- Sunflower-seed butter on a slice of toast

Discussion questions

- Elaborate three reasons why the body needs adequate protein.
- Is it possible for vegetarians to meet their protein needs through nonmeat sources? If so, what kinds of foods should these individuals incorporate into their daily meals to ensure they are meeting their protein needs?
- An individual reports to you that he is feeling increased fatigue and muscle tiredness. He has been developing more colds and viruses than normal. How would you advise this individual to increase his protein intake? Give this individual some ideas for meals and snacks that contain at least one protein source.

IS FAT-FREE THE RIGHT WAY TO GO?

Why is dietary fat necessary? The word *fat* tends to have a negative connotation that can scare people into thinking that if they eat fat, they will get fat. This is highly untrue. Consumers need to watch the portion sizes of their fat sources. Energy from fat can add up quickly to exceed what that person needs. However, every individual needs dietary fat for the following reasons:

- Fats build the brain. The structural components of cell membranes throughout the body are made of fat, and having the right kinds of fats available to form these membranes is especially important in the brain. Fats build myelin, the fatty sheath that insulates nerves. This insulation makes it possible for messages to travel quickly and efficiently throughout the brain and the body (Sears, Sears, Sears, & Sears, 2006).
- Dietary fat provides essential fatty acids, which must be supplied through food. These are necessary to produce hormonelike substances that regulate many body processes, such as blood pressure, immune response, and kidney and gastrointestinal functioning (Sears, Sears, Sears, & Sears, 2006).

Once digested, fat provides an energy reserve, and is a fuel for the body and brain to burn. It can also provide structure for the human body by holding body organs in positions and protecting them from trauma or injury. Fat can also preserve body heat and helps maintain body temperature (McArdle, Katch, & Katch, 1999). Did you ever notice that people with very low body fat frequently suffer from the cold?

Vitamins A, D, E, and K are known as the fat-soluble vitamins. Vitamin A is essential for vision function. Vitamin D is required for calcium absorption and is important for immune function. Vitamin E acts as an antioxidant and helps keep our skin healthy. Vitamin K is necessary for blood clotting and also aids in bone health (Whitney & Rolfes, 2005).

Essential fatty acid deficiency can result in serious illness. Examples are growth retardation, skin lesions, excessive thirst, impaired vision, reproductive failure, fatty liver, and reduced learning. Low fat intake can also have gender-related side effects. In females, insufficient fat intake disrupts hormone balance and menses. This negatively affects bone health, increasing risk of osteoporosis and bone fractures. In men, a very low-fat diet may inhibit testosterone production, which negatively affects muscle building (McArdle, Katch, & Katch, 1999).

A fat molecule is made of three fatty acids attached to a molecule of glycerol. In humans, fatty acids are unbranched chains of carbon atoms with hydrogen attached to each one except the first carbon, where two oxygen atoms are attached to the carbon (the acid group). These fatty acids are either saturated, monounsaturated, or polyunsaturated. Most foods contain a mixture of fatty acids (Whitney & Rolfes, 2005). Table 5-3 depicts the type and definition of fat along with fat food sources.

Table 5-3

Type of fat	Definition	Food Sources
Saturated	The carbon chain has all the hydrogen atoms it can.	Tropical oils: coconut, palm, and palm kernel; high-fat cuts of meat, poultry with the skin, whole milk, cheese, coconuts.
Monounsaturated	The carbon chain is missing one pair of hydrogen atoms, and so has one double bond.	Oils: canola and olive; avocado, most nuts, eggs
Polyunsaturated	The carbon chain is missing two or more pairs of hydrogen atoms, and so has at least two double bonds.	Oils: corn, safflower, sunflower, soybean; soybeans, tofu, fatty fish such as salmon
Trans-fat	Trans-fats are an undesired result of chemically adding hydrogen to polyunsaturated fats (hydrogenation). Trans-fatty acids are more rigid than saturated fatty acids. Essentially these are human-made fats.	Vegetable shortening, stick margarine; partially hydrogenated vegetable oils are in many processed foods.

It is fine to eat foods containing any of the naturally occurring fats (trans-fats do not occur in nature). More of your choices should be from the unsaturated sources, but having some saturated fat is okay also.

Fat serves to add flavor and texture to food. Fat helps satisfy hunger by slowing digestion and helping the body to feel full and satisfied from our food, similar to protein and fiber. Whether your food is creamy, flaky, moist, crispy, tender, or smooth, fat helps contribute to these different textures.

Several years ago the fat-free diet was the newest craze, but is this the healthier way to go? Fat-free or very low-fat diets don't provide satiety. People tend to overeat when trying to maintain a fat-free diet, because they take in excess energy through sugars and other carbohydrates while trying to satisfy their hunger. When fat is removed from a food product, so is the flavor. Food companies then add sugars or artificial sweeteners to make up for the lack of flavor (Escott-Stump, 2008; Mahan & Escott-Stump, 2000).

Fat should never have the title of being a "bad" food ingredient; however, fatty foods should be eaten in moderation. Also, consumers should be aware of hidden fats that may already be in some food combinations or in foods that were prepared by someone else. Table 5-4 shows food sources of all types of fats and their corresponding portion sizes. Each serving size equates about five grams of fat and forty-five calories (Pennington, 1998).

Table 5-4

Food	Serving Size
Oil (canola, olive, peanut, soybean, safflower, flaxseed)	1 tsp.
Soft margarine or butter	1 tsp.
Mayonnaise	1 tsp.
Cream cheese	1 Tbsp.
Salad dressing (regular)	1 Tbsp.
Sour cream	2 Tbsp.
Olives	8–10 olives
Nuts/Seeds (cashews, almonds, peanuts, walnuts, sunflower)	1 Tbsp.
Avocado	2 Tbsp.
Nut butter (peanut, almond, cashew, macadamia)	1 Tbsp.
Nutella	1 Tbsp.
Bacon	2 slices

Discussion questions

- Identify and discuss three reasons why dietary fat is necessary.
- Explain why the fat-free craze is over.
- When asking a client what her twenty-four-hour dietary recall is, you find that it is very high in saturated fat. This may put the client at risk for heart disease and other cardiovascular illnesses. How can you educate this person on the amount and kinds of dietary fat she needs, while giving her some ideas on how to incorporate more unsaturated fats into her daily diet?

BREAKFAST IS THE MOST IMPORTANT MEAL OF THE DAY

Breakfast is probably the most commonly skipped meal. We tend to be rolling out of bed, rushing in the morning, and just running out the door to class or work. The body needs fuel in the morning to run on. Skipping breakfast can lead to overeating at lunchtime or later in the day. It also can lead to fatigue. Think about how the body did not consume any fuel for the eight hours it was at rest during the night. Even if the stomach isn't growling, the body is still starving. It went about eight hours without eating anything! The following are the top three reasons why eating a breakfast is so important.

- **Breakfast perks up metabolism.** Eating a healthy breakfast perks up the body's metabolism. With food intake, the body's metabolic rate increases to facilitate the digestive process. Food in the morning gets the brain working for learning and working. Those who skip breakfast can run out of fuel by midmorning, which can affect concentration (Sears, Sears, Sears, & Sears, 2006).
- **Breakfast regulates blood sugar.** Eating a well-balanced breakfast can help maintain blood-sugar levels throughout the morning. It prevents them from reaching a low point, when the individual may be tempted to make bad eating choices due to low blood sugar. Try to put an emphasis on a balanced breakfast that has a balanced carb-protein-fat ratio (Sears, Sears, Sears, & Sears, 2006).
- **Breakfast helps keep the body lean.** Research has shown that individuals who skip breakfast are more likely to be overweight. The main reason for this is the overeating that occurs later in the day from the body being ravenous. Breakfast can also set the nutritional tone of the day. This research also shows that people who eat a healthy breakfast consume less energy over the course of a day. Energy consumed in the day is used more efficiently, so the body does not need to eat as much later (Leidy, Hoertel, Douglas, & Shafer, 2013).

There are a few main ingredients to keep in mind when planning a balanced breakfast:

- protein
- fiber-filled carbs, which provide a steady supply of fuel
- small amounts of fat, to help maintain nervous-system function
- minerals such as calcium and iron

Protein's breakdown of energy-yielding amino acids can perk up the brain by stimulating the release of neurotransmitters, specifically dopamine and norepinephrine, which give a feeling of alertness. This is especially true of protein that contains the amino acids tyrosine (which acts as a stimulant) and tryptophan (which releases serotonin for a calming effect) (Sears, Sears, Sears, & Sears, 2006). Protein is important at breakfast because of the "fill-up factor." A high-protein breakfast keeps the body from getting hungry as quickly as it does after a high-carb breakfast.

Fiber-filled carbs are like timed-release packets of energy. They give the body and brain a steady supply of fuel that keeps them going all morning long. Carbs low in fiber can spike blood sugar quickly. This can cause attention level to wander and the body to feel jittery. In a balanced breakfast, carbs are always paired with protein and fiber, so the energy from the carbs is released into the bloodstream at a slower and steadier rate.

Time is probably the number one reason why individuals decide to skip breakfast. As mentioned before, most of these folks tend not to be morning people. They wake up at the last minute and hurry off to school or work. But lack of time should never be an excuse. There are plenty of options for good, balanced, "grab-n-go" breakfasts. Below are examples of breakfasts that require a little more prep time, as well as ideas for when you are on the go.

"I am off today, and have plenty of time to have a homemade breakfast."

- whole-grain waffles or pancakes topped with blueberries and peanut butter
- oatmeal with raspberries and yogurt
- whole-grain banana nut bread and a glass of milk
- 1/2 cup of cottage cheese, with sliced cantaloupe and 1/4 cup of granola
- whole-wheat tortilla wrapped around scrambled eggs and diced veggies
- veggie omelet, whole-wheat toast, glass of orange juice
- Strawberry-banana yogurt smoothie with toast

"I really have to get out the door; I have a meeting at 8:00 a.m. sharp."

- granola bar and banana
- drinkable yogurt smoothie and a pear

- bag of dry cereal and box of raisins
- trail mix with dry cereal or granola, dried fruit, and nuts
- whole-grain muffin and small milk carton
- apple with a to-go peanut butter packet
- hard-boiled egg and a peach

Group Discussion questions

- Name and discuss three reasons why breakfast is the most important meal of the day.
- What is the reason for making sure to partner protein with whole-grain carbs at breakfast?
- List three balanced breakfast combinations that you can have when you have time in the morning, and list three breakfast combinations that you can have when you are on the go.

TAKING CARE OF YOURSELF AND BEING A ROLE MODEL FOR OTHERS

Being a healthy role model helps develop rapport with patients and helps develop a long, continued relationship. The message that was engrained in our brains since we can remember is that there should be three meals per day: breakfast, lunch, and dinner. But with our society and how busy we are these days, sometimes our schedule does not work with three structured meals per day. We also don't have a lot of time for food preparation. Some studies have shown that eating smaller, more frequent meals can be a healthy alternative for us. Eating five to six times per day in smaller amounts can keep the body's metabolism constantly working (Palmer, Capra, & Baines, 2006). Making sure not to go more than four hours without eating can help prevent drops in blood sugar and overeating later in the day. The following shows an example of a meal plan that includes three smaller meals with three snacks daily.

8:00 a.m. Breakfast:

- 1/2 English muffin
- 1 Tbsp. peanut butter
- 4–8 oz. 100% orange juice

10:30 a.m. Snack:

- Banana and low-fat yogurt

1:00 p.m. Lunch:

- 2 slices whole-wheat bread
- 3 oz. sliced turkey
- 1–2 cups salad mix for a side salad
- 1 Tbsp. salad dressing

4:00 p.m. Snack:

- 1 oz. cheese and crackers

7:00 p.m. Dinner:

- 3 oz. grilled tilapia
- 1/2–1 cup cooked rice
- 1 cup cooked broccoli
- 1–2 tsp. olive oil

9:00 p.m. Snack:

- blueberries and a/1 cup cottage cheese

The flexibility of meal planning is endless. Later in this chapter we will talk about using our senses to choose what food we really want as opposed to what society is telling us to have. Feel free to switch around meals. Who says we can't have breakfast foods for dinner? Make any adjustments to meal planning that best fit your body's needs.

For many people, especially college students or young professionals paying back college loans, finances can be an issue. Eating healthy on a budget can work; it just takes a little bit of planning and a little bit of time. The following are tips on how to save money on groceries.

- **Plan meals for the week**. Making a list of what food items you need for the week can prevent you from buying items that you really don't need. To save time, write the list to fit the store layout, sorted by aisle (dairy, produce, dry goods).

- **Check your inventory**. Look in your cabinets and refrigerator for special ingredients in the meals you plan to prepare to avoid buying duplicates.
- **Check newspaper ads**. Plan meals around specials (weekly store ads are posted online). Buy extra staple goods when the price is low. Freeze meats purchased during a sale for later use.
- **Plan for some vegetarian meals**. Meats are more expensive than beans, lentils, and tofu.
- **Water**: Consider buying a BPA-free (bisphenol A-free), such as stainless steel, refillable bottle to be green and save money.
- **Clip coupons**. Take coupons to the store only for the items you buy regularly.
- **Eat before you shop**. Fewer impulse buys will save you money.
- **Sign up for a preferred shopping club card**. This will help to save on sale items.
- **Know the store layout** to save time searching for items.
- **Shop the perimeter** for the majority of food items first.
- **Try the store generic brands** that have lower prices, with no national advertising.
- **Use unit pricing to compare** the cost per pound on the shelf label of different brands when comparing products.
- **Buy fresh fruits and vegetables when in season.**
- **Buy frozen vegetables.** They are chopped and ready-to-eat, with a longer shelf life than fresh vegetables.
- **Check dates for freshness.** Avoid food spoilage and waste.
- **Be aware of marketing techniques** to avoid impulse buys in the checkout lane.
- **Cook meals in bulk,** then freeze or refrigerate them and have them as leftovers later in the week.

Discussion questions

- Develop a meal plan according to your schedule that includes five to six meals/snacks, with something eaten every two to four hours.
- What are three ways you can start saving money on groceries?

INTUITIVE EATING

When working with someone on diet, the ultimate goal is intuitive eating. This can generally be described as eating when you're hungry, stopping when you're full, and not letting any social or media messages influence your food choices. All of us have different eating personalities that can be seen through different eating styles. One may be a "careful eater," where one is very health-conscious, or one may be a "chaotic eater," where eating is haphazard. The chaotic eater may also have little to no structure in his or her day. Someone may be an emotional eater, stemming from feelings such as loneliness, sadness, anger, or anxiety. Honoring hunger and respecting fullness are two keys to successful intuitive eating (Tribole & Resch, 1995). Below are two examples for practicing these principles.

Throughout medical school, Jane was dieting on and off. She was always trying to manage her weight. Consistently she would skip meals during the day to keep up with a frantic schedule. By the time her school day was over, Jane was ravenous and found herself eating uncontrollably in her apartment. With this type of eating style, Jane never really felt comfortable with her relationship with food. With practice of being aware of her hunger cues, Jane was able to feed her body adequate energy during the day, which decreased her drive to overeat later in the evening. Jane made it a habit to make time for a lunch break and packed balanced snacks to help satisfy when hunger hit. Jane is now aware of stomach pangs and will honor that by taking time to feed herself.

John enjoyed being social and eating out with friends. He threw parties and attended social events. When he knew he was going to be at a restaurant or a social event where there was to be food, John would restrict his intake during the day to prepare for a large meal later. John loved to eat, but in these situations he sometimes did not know how to stop eating when he felt full. After the meal or even into the next day, John felt overfull and sick to his stomach. Recognizing the body's signals that one is no longer hungry is the key to honoring fullness.

After starving himself, John ate both fast and mindlessly. The body takes about twenty minutes to recognize that it is satisfied from a well-portioned meal. When John would scarf down a meal in ten minutes, he did not allow his body time to register satiety. Because of this, John still felt he could eat more, and so he did. Now John can engage in social eating events while honoring his hunger and fullness. When he knows there is an event coming up, he eats normal meals and snacks throughout the day. He tends either to split entrees with others when eating out, or to order a couple appetizers as his meal. If he orders an individual entrée, he eats until his stomach is satisfied and will take the rest home to have as leftovers. John enjoys conversing while eating. He says it helps him decrease his eating speed and allows him to eat more mindfully, tasting and appreciating the food.

MINDFUL EATING

Mindful eating helps develop a healthy relation with food. Mindful eating can prevent one from undereating or overeating, can reduce stress, and can promote relaxation. Mindful eating involves paying attention to your sensations while you eat. Your sensations can guide you to a greater enjoyment of food and satisfaction with meals.

- **Taste.** When putting a particular piece of food in your mouth, be aware of its taste. Is the food sweet, salty, sour, or bitter? Is it a pleasant taste, or is it a bad taste? Or perhaps it is just a neutral taste. Try to carry out this exercise at each meal and see what type of taste sensations you crave at each meal and time of day (Tribole & Resch, 1995).

- **Texture.** Once that first bite of food has occurred, notice the food's texture. How crunchy is it? If it's too crunchy, does it become frustrating to continue chewing? Do you have any reaction if the food is smooth or creamy? Do you prefer something that involves less chewing, like a liquid-type food? Certain textures may be appealing at different times of the day and at different meals (Tribole & Resch, 1995).

- **Aroma.** Sometimes the smell of a food may have more effect on your desire for it than the taste or texture. Walking by a bakery and smelling the bread being baked, or by a coffee shop and sniffing the brewed coffee beans, can be appealing. Aroma may arouse a craving for that particular item and can influence a food or beverage choice (Tribole & Resch, 1995).

- **Appearance.** Many restaurants and food service companies have a whole department devoted to food appearance. They make sure the menus and sample pictures of the meals look tempting. Look at the food on the plate that's about to be eaten. Does it look fresh and colorful? Think about it, a plate that contains a rainbow of colors such as salmon, red potatoes, and broccoli is more appealing to the eye than a plate that contains plain chicken, white rice, and cauliflower. The presentation of the food on the plate may even contribute to more taste satisfaction just because of the colors alone (Tribole & Resch, 1995).

- **Temperature.** Depending on the season, temperature of food may have an effect on your meal choice. In the summer, a nice cool smoothie or salad may satisfy the palate. But in the winter, a hot and steamy bowl of soup and cup of hot cider may be most desirable when you're shivering from the cold. When choosing a food, decide what temperature best suits the moment. Do you want something hot, cold, or room temperature? (Tribole & Resch, 1995)

- **Volume.** This is where deciphering hunger cues comes into play. Is your stomach growling every few minutes? Has it been more than four hours since the last time you ate? This may mean you will feel satisfied from a large pasta meal, despite taste, texture, aroma, or temperature. If you just feel a little hungry, you may be satisfied with something a little lighter, like a soup or salad that contains a small amount of protein (Tribole & Resch, 1995).

Keep in mind that people have different senses and like different types of foods. One way to work on finding your own likes, dislikes, and food satisfactions is by asking yourself the following questions the next time you feel like eating.

- What do I feel like eating?
- What smells appeal to me right now?
- Does this food look favorable?
- Do I want something sweet, salty, sour, or even bitter?
- Do I want something crunchy, smooth, creamy, soft, or a fluid?
- Do I want something hot, cold, or in between?
- Do I want something light, airy, heavy, filling, or in between?
- How will my stomach feel when I'm finished eating?

With all this information about healthy eating, the basic principle for increasing longevity is to honor your health. There are many lifestyle changes that other health professionals discuss about keeping healthy. These may include getting adequate sleep and exercise, practicing meditation, educating clients on the dangers of smoking, and emphasizing moderate use of alcohol. But it is almost impossible to talk about health and taking care of oneself without discussing nutrition. This topic can, however, be quite frustrating to the consumer.

The role of nutrition in preventing chronic disease has been clearly established by the scientific community. But this country has engraved in our minds that eating a traditional Thanksgiving meal or a dessert should inflict guilt upon the consumer. One does not need to be a chronic dieter to be worried about nutrition and food. Every day there is a new headline on the news or a commercial that a little bit of butter is horrible for you, and if you don't eat organic tomatoes, you can develop an illness. None of these claims has been proven scientifically, so let's develop our own food-attitude adjustment. Eating healthy should feel good both physically and psychologically. This can be defined as eating balanced meals with a variety of foods, making sure all the food groups are balanced in a day, allowing oneself all foods (including desserts) in moderation, and having a healthy relationship with food. With all the information discussed in this chapter, take some time to develop a healthy meal plan to help live your own healthier life, and pass along these practices to others.

Breakfast Recipes

Egg Burrito

2 large eggs
1 whole-wheat tortilla
1 tablespoon salsa
1 tablespoon shredded cheese

1. Beat the eggs in a small microwave-safe bowl.
2. In the microwave, cook the eggs on high for 1 minute, and then stir. If the eggs are not yet set, microwave for another 30 seconds. When finished, the eggs should not be runny.
3. Place the tortilla on a plate and heat for 30 seconds in the microwave.
4. Wrap the eggs and other ingredients in the tortilla and enjoy!
5. Add a glass of milk and piece of fruit to make this meal complete.

Nutty Breakfast Sandwich

2 frozen waffles
1 tablespoon peanut butter
1/2 banana, sliced
2 teaspoons strawberry jam

1. Toast both waffles.
2. Spread one waffle with peanut butter and top with banana slices.
3. Spread the other waffle with strawberry jam and place on top to make a delicious and nutritious breakfast sandwich.

Lunch Recipes

Tuna Sandwich

1 (3-ounce) can light tuna in water, drained and flaked
1/4 cup carrots, chopped or shredded
1 small apple, peeled, cored, and coarsely chopped
1–2 tablespoons mayonnaise
2 slices whole-wheat bread, toasted if desired
1–2 slices tomato

1. Combine the tuna, carrot, apple, and mayonnaise in a medium bowl and mix well.
2. Spread the tuna mixture evenly over one bread slice.
3. Top with tomato slice and other slice of bread.

Salmon Melt

1 (3-ounce) can pink salmon in water, drained

1/2 large carrot, peeled and shredded

1–2 tablespoons mayonnaise

1 whole-wheat English muffin, sliced in half

1 tablespoon shredded cheddar cheese

1. In a small bowl mix together salmon, carrot, and mayonnaise.
2. Toast the English muffin halves in the toaster.
3. Place toasted muffin halves on a microwave-safe plate.
4. Spread the salmon mixture on each muffin half; sprinkle with cheese.
5. Heat on high in the microwave for 1 minute or until cheese is melted.

Dinner Recipes

Chicken Tortilla Soup – 6 servings

4 corn tortillas (6-inch) cut in strips

2 1/2 tablespoons canola oil

1 1/2 cup red or green salsa of choice

2 1/2 (10.75-ounce) cans low-sodium chicken broth

2 cups cooked boneless skinless chicken breast, cubed

2 cups yellow corn, canned or frozen, drained

1 cup black beans, canned, drained

1 medium red pepper, diced, sautéed

1 large zucchini, halved lengthwise and cut into fours, sautéed

1. Cook tortilla strips in hot canola oil until crisp. Set aside and drain on paper towel.
2. Combine salsa and chicken broth in a large saucepan and bring to a boil over medium-high heat.
3. Reduce heat to medium; add chicken breast, yellow corn, black beans, red pepper, and zucchini; heat all the way through.
4. Serve in bowls; top with tortilla strips and a dollop of sour cream (optional).

Pineapple Chicken – 4 servings

2 teaspoons canola or sesame oil

1 (10-ounce) package frozen broccoli (or stir-fry vegetable mix), thawed

1/2 cup stir-fry sauce

1/4 cup pineapple juice; use reserved juice from canned pineapple

1/4 teaspoon garlic powder

1/4 teaspoon crushed red pepper (optional)

1 (15-ounce) can pineapple chunks or tidbits, drained (reserve the juice)

2 cups diced cooked chicken or 2 (10-ounce) cans chicken breast, drained and flaked

1. Heat the oil in a large skillet over medium-high heat. Add all the ingredients except the pineapple and chicken. Cook and stir until heated through, 5–6 minutes.
2. Add pineapple and chicken; cook another 2 minutes.
3. Serve over instant brown rice or whole-wheat pasta.

Snack Recipes

Tasty Trail Mix – 4 (1-cup) servings

2 cups low-fat popcorn

1 1/2 cups honey nut cheerios

1/2 cup raisins

1/4 cup almonds

1/4 cup dark chocolate chips

Combine all ingredients together. Mix well. Serve in 1-cup portions.

Salsa Bean and Corn Dip – 4 servings

1 cup frozen corn, thawed

1 (15-ounce) can black beans, rinsed and drained

1 small jalapeno pepper, chopped

1 medium tomato, diced

1 small onion, diced

1/4 cup red-wine vinegar

2 tablespoons canola or olive oil

1. Throw everything in a medium bowl and mix.
2. Refrigerate for one hour to let the flavors mix.
3. Serve with baked tortilla chips.

Dessert Recipes

Almond Apricot Bars – 18 servings
2 cups white baking chips, divided
1/2 cup butter, softened
1/2 cup sugar
2 eggs
1 teaspoon vanilla extract
1 cup all-purpose flour
3/4 cup apricot jam
1/2 cup sliced almonds

1. In a microwave, melt 1 cup chips; stir until smooth. Set aside.
2. In a large bowl, cream butter and sugar until light and fluffy. Add eggs, one at a time, beating well after each addition. Beat in melted chips and vanilla. Gradually beat in flour.
3. Spread half of the batter into a greased 8-inch square baking dish. Bake at 325° for 15–20 minutes or until golden brown. Spread with jam.
4. Stir remaining chips into remaining batter. Drop by tablespoonfuls over jam; carefully spread over top. Sprinkle with almonds. Bake for 30–35 minutes or until golden brown. Cool completely on a wire rack. Cut into squares, and then cut squares in half.

Chocolate Peanut Butter Mousse – 6 servings
1 milk-chocolate candy bar (5 ounce), chopped
1 cup heavy whipping cream
1 cup creamy peanut butter
1/3 cup chocolate-covered peanuts, chopped

1. In a microwave-safe bowl, combine the candy bar, cream, and peanut butter. Microwave at 50 percent power for 2–3 minutes or until smooth, stirring twice. Transfer to a small bowl. Cover and refrigerate for 1 hour or until chilled.
2. Beat until soft peaks form. Spoon into dessert dishes; sprinkle with chocolate-covered peanuts.

Author's Note: I strongly suggest that, with the knowledge you have learned so far, you begin to keep a daily Health Habits Journal. This is not a time-consuming activity and may only take several minutes of your time each evening prior to retiring. The journal can contain many things that will help you maintain awareness of your positive health habits and help you to stay engaged in positive health practices. Such things include a journal of the healthy foods you eat each day and/or meal planning for the week, and exercise/movement accomplishments and plans. With each chapter that follows, you might find additional ideas or suggestions to add to your health habits journal, such as reflections on meaning, purpose, gratitude or three good things. Rather than an exercise in frustration, I have made my health habits journal a welcome place to plan, organize, and think deeply.

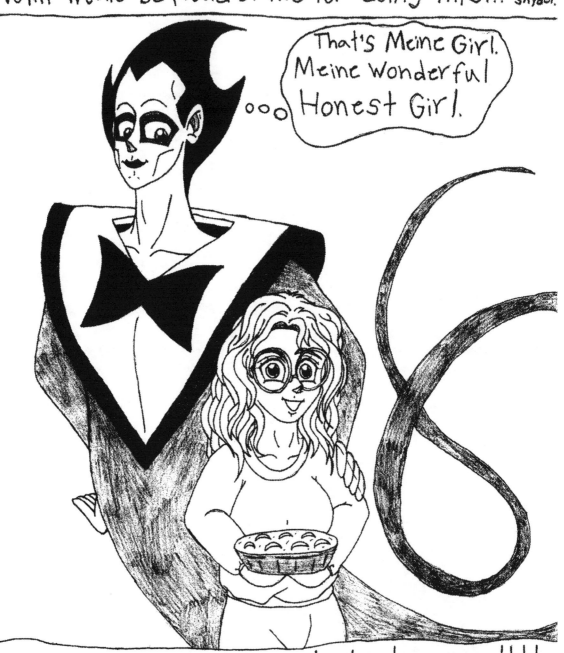

102

Chapter 6

Identifying and Building Strengths

An unfortunate culture of medical student and physician mistreatment was discussed in chapter 1 of this book. Abuse, harassment, and belittlement establish a culture in which teaching is most commonly accomplished through tactics of public humiliation, shame, and fear. The damaging effects of these tactics are seen worldwide in significant problems of physician ill-being.

The science of positive psychology focuses on the development of human potential and allows us to take a different approach to teaching and to growth than has been the norm in the medical-education setting. Positive psychology is an umbrella term for the study of positive emotions, positive character traits, and their enabling institutions (Seligman, Steen, Park, & Peterson, 2005).

To promote a science of human strengths, Peterson and Seligman catalogued the human character strengths that make the good life possible, with the domain of concern being psychological health. They developed a classification system in a volume entitled *Character Strengths and Virtues: A Handbook and Classification*, which was designed to be comparable to the Diagnostic and Statistical Manual (DSM) or the ICD classification for illnesses, but instead, aimed at wellness or the good life (Peterson & Seligman, 2004). The six virtues are the core characteristics valued by moral philosophers, religious thinkers, and wise men globally throughout time. The twenty-four character strengths are the psychological ingredients, processes, or mechanisms that make up the virtues.

Knowledge and use of one's character strengths, particularly one's "signature" strengths, creates a sense of well-being and benefits both oneself and others. This chapter will introduce the character strengths and virtues, their classification, and their beneficial applications to a physician's professional and personal life.

Each reader should begin by taking the survey known as the VIA (Values in Action). To access this survey, go to the Web site www.creatingpositivehealth.org. Look for the link labeled VIA character strengths. Please access the survey and complete it before proceeding further with this chapter. Once you have completed the survey, print out your results and set them aside. Later on in the chapter, you will be given further instructions and guidance regarding the survey. Please return to this point once you have completed the above instructions.

THE VIRTUES

Peterson and Seligman began with a classification of virtues as the foundation of good character. A large-scale literature search explored not only psychology, but also related areas of philosophy, politics, education, and religion. The search was given further focus by centering on the three most influential thought traditions in human history—that is, China, South Asia (primarily India), and the West (Peterson & Seligman, 2004). Within these cultures and thought traditions, primary attention was paid to the dominant spiritual and philosophical traditions originating in each: Confucianism and Taoism in China, Buddhism and Hinduism in South Asia, and Judeo-Christianity and Islam in the West. Once virtues from all sources were collected, those that were thematically similar were grouped together. This search and grouping process revealed a set of six core moral virtues that were consistent across both time and culture: courage, justice, humanity, temperance, transcendence, and wisdom. We will now take a closer look at each of these six core virtue categories.

Courage, or the capacity to overcome fear and fearsome situations, is universally valued across cultures and history. Courage can be further broken down into three types: physical, moral, and psychological.

Physical courage is directed at overcoming the fear of physical injury, pain, disease, or death in order to do good or save others or oneself. The father who runs back into his burning home to rescue his young baby still lying in her crib displays physical courage, as does the patient diagnosed with cancer who chooses to undergo disfiguring surgery and distressing chemotherapy in order to save her life.

Moral courage, on the other hand, has more to do with maintaining ethical integrity and personal authenticity in the face of pressure to do otherwise. The risks involve deep personal losses, such as friends, employment, privacy, or prestige. The display of moral courage can be not readily apparent to others, but can take a deep toll on the self and on others when it is not displayed. For example, because health-care workers are human and humans are not perfect beings, errors occur in hospitals. The moral courage to admit an error, at the risk of losing one's job, one's livelihood, and the respect of one's colleagues, allows for corrective measures to be instituted for those who may have been affected and allows the institution of safety measures to protect against further recurrence of the same error. On the other hand, covering up the error can result in harm to those patients and personnel affected, a likelihood of repetition of the error, and many sleepless nights for the health-care worker who lacks the courage to be truthful.

Psychological courage involves facing our deepest inner fears, such as death, a destructive habit or situation, loss, or a debilitating illness that robs us of our freedom of function. We as physicians, taking care of the sick or bearing a life-threatening diagnosis to a patient, have seen the remarkable difference that a patient's psychological courage can make on prognosis and recovery. Because we are exposed to illness and death as physicians, we also grapple with our own inner demons and fears. Suppressing or not acknowledging them leads to stress, pathology, and ill-being. It is important for us as physicians to understand our fears and to build the psychological courage to face them before we ever get to a patient's bedside.

Justice refers generally to that which makes life fair; however, we know that life is not always fair. The concept of justice in Western industrialized nations instead refers to the concept of equity: the belief that rewards should be given according to contributions or merit and that people should ultimately get what they deserve. This does not apply to all cultures, however, as there are cultures that favor the notion of equality or need when making fairness-based decisions (Peterson & Seligman, 2004, pp. 393-397).

The identification of justice as a core virtue reflects the shared belief that a standard practice should exist to protect that which is fair for all. Justice is a virtue concerned with relating to others equitably. Perhaps the greatest and most important example of this in the medical setting is that of the multidisciplinary health-care team (see chapter 15 for further information). Hospitals traditionally have a vertical hierarchical structure, in which each discipline reports through its own hierarchical chain of command. In this structure there is little, if any, communication among disciplines; little, if any, equality; and little opportunity for disciplines to cooperate with one another. With a more horizontal organizational structure, power to take action is given to the frontline multidisciplinary teams, and each team member, regardless of discipline, is empowered to act positively on behalf of the team and the patients he or she serves. As a result of this climate of equity and a focus on service, care becomes more easy, efficient, and pleasant. The seemingly impossible becomes possible!

Like justice, *humanity* is a virtue that is focused on relating to others and improving the welfare of others. Humanity, however, focuses on the interpersonal strengths that go beyond fairness and impartiality, to those that lie within the realm of altruism and pro-social behavior. Humanity involves showing compassion, sympathy, or consideration to another human being. The highest examples of humanity go beyond what might be expected, asked for, or imagined. Such examples might include showing generosity when an equitable exchange would suffice, demonstrating kindness even when it cannot or will not be returned, and showing understanding even when punishment is due. The ability to have and display empathy is essential and underlies the virtue of humanity.

While humanity is one virtue that is uniquely important to patient care, it unfortunately is often missing in an overworked, burned-out doctor. When a doctor is stressed, pressured, ill, angry, rushed, distracted, hungry, or tired, humanity is a casualty. Stress leads to withdrawal into the self and feelings of detachment that prevent people from accessing their humanity. As far back as early medical training, we doctors are taught to be tough, detached, and impartial. The critical skills of empathy and communication are, sadly, absent from early physician education.

Temperance refers to the virtue of moderation in action, thought, or feeling. In psychological terms, temperance refers to the ability to monitor and manage one's emotions, motivations, and behavior in the absence of outside regulators (Peterson & Seligman, 2004, p. 431). Those who are consistently able to exercise appropriate self-control tend to avoid hurting themselves or others. This results in significantly greater success, happiness, harmony, and inner peace for those who possess temperance.

Because temperance is a form of inhibition or self-denial, it is virtuous only to the extent that it results in benefit to the self or to others. Obsessively controlling behavior, by its nature, is intemperate and not virtuous, resulting in harm to self or others. For example, a doctor's drive to achieve, along with fear of malpractice litigation or of making errors, can lead to obsessive overwork and a loss of life balance. This does not qualify as virtuous behavior, nor is it beneficial for the doctor or any of his or her patients.

The virtue of *transcendence* refers to the quality of being beyond the limits of human experience or knowledge. Transcendence can apply to acting on a belief that there is a meaning or purpose to life beyond survival or mortal existence.

There is more to transcendence than religious thought or belief or spirituality. Transcendence can also refer to something or someone in our daily reality that deeply inspires awe, hope, or gratitude. Such a person or act will make our everyday, trivial concerns seem inconsequential. At the same time, transcendence will elevate us out of feelings of insignificance, particularly when we are committed to a noble purpose that has deep meaning for us and allows us to make a significant contribution to our fellow human beings. (See chapter 8 on meaning and purpose.)

Transcendence is the virtue that allows us to keep sight of our life's meaning and purpose despite our daily frustrations and problems. The loss of this transcendent virtue is a major contributor to burnout and ill-being in a physician or medical student. It is similar to going to a museum to view a beautiful painting, only to be distracted by a detail in the foreground that either you do not understand or you dislike. In your dismay you become so focused on this annoying detail that you leave, never having looked at the rest of the painting or enjoyed its overall beauty. You leave the museum feeling disheartened and frustrated. However, had you taken time to step back and view the painting as a whole, you might have better appreciated how that detail actually complemented the painting or added to its deeper meaning. In medicine, we often have to step back from the distractions of bureaucratic annoyances and remind ourselves of the beauty and hope implicit in serving others and helping them thrive.

Wisdom is a type of intelligence that goes far beyond general knowledge, IQ, academic achievement, and general intelligence. The virtue of wisdom is a broad and deep understanding of the human condition applied to situations requiring reflective judgment. Most wisdom is acquired through living one's life, encountering hardship, making mistakes, winning small victories, and appreciating accomplishments (see chapter 12 on posttraumatic and post-ecstatic growth). Wisdom is a form of noble intelligence, inevitably used for good, which creates feelings of appreciation from those with whom it is shared (Peterson & Seligman, 2004, p. 95). Young doctors have a wonderful opportunity to appreciate the wisdom of the older adults whom they treat. In the therapeutic exchange, the young doctor can listen to the life wisdom of the older patient, and in exchange teach important principles of positive health.

The character strengths

The character strengths are the psychological ingredients, processes, or mechanisms that define each of the six virtues. Each strength within a given virtue category represents a way of displaying that virtue.

The processes by which candidate character strengths were identified were similar to those used to identify the virtues: brainstorming by groups of scholars; literature searches into fields such as psychiatry, philosophy, and youth development; and surveys of history, education, sociology, and cultural contributions throughout time. Once redundancies had been eliminated from the list of candidate strengths, a final list of ten criteria was generated. These criteria would need to be satisfied by the final list of character strengths. These criteria were articulated after many dozens of candidate strengths had been identified, and criteria were needed to consolidate the list and look for common features. Of the twenty-four character strengths, half meet ten criteria, with each of the remainder missing only one or, at the most, two (Peterson & Seligman, 2004, p. 17).

The criteria for character strengths are:

1) A strength is a positive aspect of character that facilitates achievement of the good life and positivity for oneself and for others. Although character strengths can help an individual more effectively cope with adversity, the primary function of a strength is to facilitate achievement of flourishing. Therefore, well-being grows from exercising one's character strengths.

2) Although strengths can produce desirable outcomes, each strength is morally valued in its own right, even in the absence of obvious beneficial outcomes. It is in this way that they differ from talents and abilities. For example, a talent such as athletic prowess or an ability such as good memory has no moral value and no value beyond the direct benefits it produces. If I am a great runner, I benefit only by my ability to win my race. If I have a good memory, I benefit by being able to remember a friend's address and phone number when I get lost going to my friend's house. However, a strength such as kindness is valued not only for its direct benefits, but for the moral and human value it represents. Strengths encourage a variety of positive tangible outcomes, including self-acceptance, mental and physical health, respect by and for others, positive and supportive social networks, satisfying work, and subjective well-being.

3) The display of a character strength does not in any way diminish others who are close by or are party to the action. In most cases, onlookers are elevated by the moral and virtuous action of their fellow human beings. They witness behavior to which they, too, can aspire, as opposed to behavior that creates either jealousy or resentment.

4) For something to be regarded as a character strength, its opposite could not be manifested as a positive action or behavior.

5) A character strength needs to manifest across a range of behavior, including thoughts, feelings, and actions, and in such a way that it can be assessed reliably. It should have a degree of generality across situations and stability across time in a given individual.

6) Each individual strength is distinct from every other one in the classification and cannot be broken down into a combination of any other of the twenty-four strengths.

7) The existent culture highlights strengths of character through stories, parables, songs, and poetry that feature role models for a given positive strength, be they real or mythic.

8) Prodigies exist within the culture with respect to these strengths. Although this criterion cannot readily apply to all strengths, it does apply to most.

9) Conversely, another criterion for a character strength is the existence of individuals who demonstrate the selective absence of that given trait.

10) The final criterion is that the larger society creates and provides institutions and associated rituals for cultivating a given strength, and then for sustaining and maintaining its practice. These rituals are like trial runs or simulations, where strengths can be developed safely and with guidance, particularly in youth with the help of adults. For example, the high school sports team practices teamwork, overseen by an adult coach who carefully monitors the team's activities. The high school student council exercises leadership skills, overseen by an adult faculty member who monitors the students' development. This shows us that virtues and strengths, such as leadership and teamwork, can be taught, nurtured, and cultivated in others (Peterson & Seligman, 2004, p. 27).

Classification of character strengths

In table 6-1 you will find the full classification of all six virtues and their twenty-four character strengths as they are distributed under each of their representative virtues. A brief definition of each character strength is given (Peterson & Seligman, 2004).

Measuring character strengths

To develop a science of human strengths, including tools that can accurately evaluate the impact of interventions, validated instruments for measuring character strengths must be readily available.

The VIA is a self-report questionnaire designed to measure the twenty-four character strengths. The questionnaire asks individuals to report the degree to which statements reflecting each of the character strengths apply to themselves, using a five-point Likert scale to measure the degree of agreement. The VIA contains five items for each of the twenty-four character strengths, with a total of 120 (120) items. Responses are averaged within scales, all of which have satisfactory internal consistency (Cronbach's alpha > .70) and substantial test-retest correlations over a four-month period (r ~ .70) (Peterson, Park, & Seligman, 2006).

The aims of measuring one's character strengths are to facilitate an awareness of what is best and most naturally strong in oneself, to embrace these qualities, and to increase their use. With increased use of character strengths, positive goals such as building positive relationships, increasing achievement of life goals, and greater overall life satisfaction become more easily accessible.

As you have already seen, a website for the VIA Institute exists on which any individual can freely access the VIA inventory. After completing the survey, a consumer-friendly

Table 6-1. The VIA Character Strengths and Virtues

The VIA Classification of Character Strengths

(© Copyright 2012,VIA Institute on Character; www.viacharacter.org)

1. Wisdom and Knowledge – cognitive strengths that entail the acquisition and use of knowledge
    o **Creativity** [originality, ingenuity]: Thinking of novel and productive ways to conceptualize and do things; includes artistic achievement but is not limited to it
    o **Curiosity** [interest, novelty-seeking, openness to experience]: Taking an interest in ongoing experience for its own sake; finding subjects and topics fascinating; exploring and discovering
    o **Judgment** [open-mindedness; critical thinking]: Thinking things through and examining them from all sides; not jumping to conclusions; being able to change one's mind in light of evidence; weighing all evidence fairly
    o **Love of Learning**: Mastering new skills, topics, and bodies of knowledge, whether on one's own or formally; related to the strength of curiosity but goes beyond it to describe the tendency to add systematically to what one knows
    o **Perspective** [wisdom]: Being able to provide wise counsel to others; having ways of looking at the world that make sense to oneself/others

2. Courage – emotional strengths that involve the exercise of will to accomplish goals in the face of opposition, external or internal
    o **Bravery** [valor]: Not shrinking from threat, challenge, difficulty, or pain; speaking up for what's right even if there's opposition; acting on convictions even if unpopular; includes physical bravery but is not limited to it
    o **Perseverance** [persistence, industriousness]: Finishing what one starts; persevering in a course of action in spite of obstacles; "getting it out the door"; taking pleasure in completing tasks
    o **Honesty** [authenticity, integrity]: Speaking the truth but more broadly presenting oneself in a genuine way and acting in a sincere way; being without pretense; taking responsibility for one's feelings and actions
    o **Zest** [vitality, enthusiasm, vigor, energy]: Approaching life with excitement and energy; not doing things halfway or halfheartedly; living life as an adventure; feeling alive and activated

3. Humanity - interpersonal strengths that involve tending and befriending others
    o **Love** (capacity to love and be loved): Valuing close relations with others, in particular those in which sharing & caring are reciprocated; being close to people

- o **Kindness** [generosity, nurturance, care, compassion, altruistic love, "niceness"]: Doing favors and good deeds for others; helping them; taking care of them
- o **Social Intelligence** [emotional intelligence, personal intelligence]: Being aware of the motives/feelings of others and oneself; knowing what to do to fit into different social situations; knowing what makes other people tick

4. Justice - civic strengths that underlie healthy community life
   - o **Teamwork** [citizenship, social responsibility, loyalty]: Working well as a member of a group or team; being loyal to the group; doing one's share
   - o **Fairness**: Treating all people the same according to notions of fairness & justice; not letting feelings bias decisions about others; giving everyone a fair chance
   - o **Leadership**: Encouraging a group of which one is a member to get things done and at the same time maintain good relations within the group; organizing group activities and seeing that they happen.

5. Temperance – strengths that protect against excess
   - o **Forgiveness** [mercy]: Forgiving those who have done wrong; accepting others' shortcomings; giving people a second chance; not being vengeful
   - o **Humility** [modesty]: Letting one's accomplishments speak for themselves; not regarding oneself as more special than one is
   - o **Prudence**: Being careful about one's choices; not taking undue risks; not saying or doing things that might later be regretted
   - o **Self-Regulation** [self-control]: Regulating what one feels and does; being disciplined; controlling one's appetites and emotions

6. Transcendence - strengths that forge connections to the universe & provide meaning
   - o **Appreciation of Beauty and Excellence** [awe, wonder, elevation]: Noticing and appreciating beauty, excellence, and/or skilled performance in various domains of life, from nature to art to mathematics to science to everyday experience
   - o **Gratitude**: Being aware of and thankful for the good things that happen; taking time to express thanks
   - o **Hope** [optimism, future-mindedness, future orientation]: Expecting the best in the future and working to achieve it; believing that a good future is something that can be brought about
   - o **Humor** [playfulness]: Liking to laugh and tease; bringing smiles to other people; seeing the light side; making (not necessarily telling) jokes
   - o **Spirituality** [religiousness, faith, purpose]: Having coherent beliefs about the higher purpose & meaning of the universe; knowing where one fits within the larger scheme; having beliefs about the meaning of life that shape conduct and provide comfort

report is issued, including lists, graphs, practical exercises related to one's top character strengths, and suggestions how to enlarge on their use. All this is available from the Web site for a minimal fee. Your top strengths or signature strengths are available free of charge.

On the report generated by the VIA, the individual receives a top-down ranking of his or her character strengths, based upon the responses given when completing the survey. The absolute score of a given character trait indicates the degree to which that strength is expressed in one's life.

An individual's five highest-ranking strengths are generally referred to as his or her "signature strengths." These are an individual's dominant strengths, those that form that individual's essential core. Expressing one's signature strengths tends to be effortless, natural, and comfortable, and builds feelings of positivity.

Character and character strengths occupy a central role in positive psychology because good character enables pleasure, flow, and other positive experiences. Furthermore, there is a strong connection between the use of signature strengths and well-being because strengths help us meet our basic needs for independence, relationship, and competence. Individuals who use their character strengths experience greater well-being related to both physical and emotional health. Therefore, it can be said that character strengths also play a central role in positive health and in resilience. Use of one's character strengths, particularly signature strengths, is associated with less stress and burnout, increased positive affect, and increased self-esteem.

It is important to note that there is no single preferred top strength, nor a top category of strengths that is indicative of superior functioning. It is extremely unusual to find one individual who is strong in all twenty-four character strengths. Those strengths that rank toward the bottom of an individual's list do not indicate an absence of those character strengths. Instead, the lower-ranking strengths tend to be used only in specific situations, or otherwise tend to be used infrequently. It is important to note that character strengths can be cultivated through enhanced awareness, use, and effort.

Why the identification and use of character strengths is crucial for doctors

It is likely readily apparent from the preceding chapters of this book that the philosophy of and approach to medical education must be radically improved in order to promote well-being and overcome the epidemic of burnout and discontent in the physician population. Specifically, an emphasis on and ample reinforcement of each doctor's character strengths will promote self-esteem, increase competence and confidence, increase overall well-being, and help avoid burnout.

An understanding and appreciation of character strengths is also important in a crisis situation, such as facing a life-threatening illness or encountering death, which doctors and their patients do on a daily basis. For example, immediately after the events of September 11, the character strengths of faith, hope, and love showed a significant increase in the United States population (Peterson & Seligman, 2002).

A crisis, particularly when it is overcome, can lead to remarkable growth, including the building of character and the emergence of a new understanding of one's life priorities. The commitment to act in accordance with these priorities creates the emergence of new character strengths.

A study done in 2002 of 2,087 adult volunteers from the VIA Web site taking the VIA was supportive of these findings (Peterson, Park, & Seligman, 2006). In those volunteers who had experienced recovery from a serious physical illness and a return to high life satisfaction, the character strengths of bravery, kindness, and humor seemed to be important contributors to their recovery state. A physical illness compromises function and increases awareness of personal mortality. Bravery helps the individual face death and loss directly. Kindness and humor augment life satisfaction and help the ill persevere despite challenges. Those who are ill may become more aware of the needs of others (empathy) and become more willing to help them. This results in more acts of kindness, which lead to a more meaningful and satisfying life. In those who had recovered from a psychiatric disorder, strengths including appreciation of beauty, creativity, curiosity, gratitude, and love of learning showed predominance and growth. Reviewing this list, it is notable that the strengths for responding to psychological disorders are primarily cognitive and intellectual. Of these, the two that are also related to life satisfaction are appreciation of beauty and love of learning. They involve a turning inward, as one does when dealing with a psychiatric disorder (Peterson, Park, & Seligman, 2006).

Just as these character strengths help the sick recover from an illness and regain life satisfaction, these and other character strengths have a similar impact in health-care workers who are stressed and who confront illness and death daily in their work. By using one's signature strengths and developing the strengths that lead to posttraumatic growth and well-being, physicians can grow and thrive in their work of healing and teaching positive health to patients.

The circumplex of character strengths

Another important way in which character strengths can be viewed is along two orthogonal dimensions. These are the heart/mind dimension and the self/others dimension (Peterson C., 2006, p. 158; Niemiec, 2014, p. 32). When we map these two dimensions on one character map (called the *circumplex*), we see a characteristic pattern of character strength (see table 6-2 below).

Two Factor Balance Graph

This report offers another view of the character strengths. Scientific studies have found the 24 VIA character strengths cluster in particular ways. One way to conceptualize them is across two primary dimensions. One dimension is Heart-Mind, which describes the degree to which a given character strength is based in mental activities (e.g., thinking, logic, analysis) or in matters of the heart (e.g., feelings, intuitions). Strengths that are closer to the left are the highest mind strengths (e.g., judgment, prudence) while those closest to the right are the highest heart strengths (e.g., gratitude, love). The other dimension is the continuum of Intrapersonal-Interpersonal, which describes the degree to which a character trait focuses attention on oneself or on others; "Intrapersonal" strengths generally only require oneself in order to express the strength (e.g., creativity), while "Interpersonal" strengths generally require other people in order to use the strength (e.g., team-work).

Important points to remember about this graph:

- The dots are in the exact same position for everyone as this is the result of scientific findings.

- The individual's highest strengths are shown in red.

- The circles are a way to orient visually to the graph.

- There is no "ideal" profile in that one should have signature strengths in each quadrant or all in one quadrant.

- Two strengths close together on the graph are more likely to comfortably co-occur, while strengths that are far apart are more likely to be traded off in that it is less likely this person habitually shows both at the same time.

Questions for exploring this graph:

- How might this graph inform this individual as they think about the balance of strength expression in their life?
- Does this individual approach life more from a "heart" or from a "mind" perspective, as noted in this graph?
- How might strengths be turned inward towards oneself, e.g., practice more self-kindness or self-forgiveness?

21

The heart/mind dimension describes the degree to which a given character strength is based in cognitive activities (such as thinking, logic, and analysis) or in emotion-based activities (such as feelings and intuitions). This dimension is displayed vertically on the circumplex, with mind strengths being closer to the top and heart strengths being closer to the bottom.

Very clearly, medical education as it is now structured tends to favor use of the mind-based strengths, while patient care and self-care tend to require development and use of those strengths that are heart-based.

With regard to the self/others dimension, those character traits that focus attention on oneself and only require oneself to exercise them lie toward the "self" end of the scale and are called *intrapersonal strengths*. Those strengths lying toward the "others" end of the scale generally require the presence of other individuals for their successful use. They tend to be group-focused strengths and are called *interpersonal strengths*. This self/others dimension is mapped horizontally on the circumplex, with "self" or intrapersonal strengths to the right side of the diagram and "others" or interpersonal strengths to the left.

The current structure of medical education emphasizes self-strengths, while de-emphasizing, if not outright discouraging, interpersonal strengths (see chapter 1). However, doctoring in today's multidisciplinary team setting, as well as with patients and families, requires the mastering of interpersonal skills. More importantly, positive and meaningful relationships with others are keys to the good life and to flourishing.

It is important to note that the location of each character strength on the circumplex was determined scientifically and remains static for all situations and across all individuals. Character strengths do not change location or placement with an individual's score or signature strengths. However, if we locate our signature strengths on the diagram, we are provided with additional information regarding the areas in which we work best. There is no "ideal" profile nor should one expect to be strong in all four quadrants. In fact, it is more common to see a clustering of strengths in one or two quadrants of the diagram. It is important to note that the "self" strengths are in no way related to being selfish or negative. All strengths are equally positive.

Discussion questions based on the circumplex

- Dr. Smith has signature strengths that tend to be high in a "mind" perspective. How might she use these strengths in dealing with patients? In what areas might she tend to have difficulties?
- Dr. Jones has signature strengths that tend to be high in a "heart" perspective. How might Dr. Jones use his signature strengths with patients? Are there areas in which Dr. Jones might tend to have difficulties?

- Drs. Smith and Jones decide to join forces and go into practice together. Brainstorm creative ways in which they might use their combined strengths to help one another, their patients, their employees, and their practice.
- Very often, we readily direct heart-based strengths, such as kindness and forgiveness, toward others, like our patients. How might we learn to direct those toward ourselves (e.g., self-kindness, self-forgiveness) on a regular basis?
- What might the circumplex tell you about the balance of your own signature strengths and their expression in your life?

In-depth look at specific character strengths

You have taken the VIA character strengths survey, and you have learned valuable background information about the origin and value of character strengths. The next step in the process will be to view and understand the results of your own individual survey and to learn how to use and apply those results toward future success, growth, and well-being.

Statistically, the five character strengths most highly related to life satisfaction in the general population are hope, zest, gratitude, curiosity, and love (Park, Peterson, & Seligman, 2004). Of these five, we will now take a closer look at two, curiosity and zest. The purpose of this examination is to provide a template for the in-depth exploration of your own signature strengths. Once we review curiosity and zest, you will be given guidelines and exercises regarding your own signature strengths. The general information that follows, as well as additional general information on character strengths, is available on the VIA Institute Web site (www.viacharacter.org).

Curiosity

Curiosity contributes to the virtue category of wisdom and knowledge (Kashdan, 2009). Curiosity can be described as an avid interest in ongoing experience or in new subjects or topics. It is an intrinsic desire for experience and knowledge, which results in fulfillment when an answer is found, a new fact is learned, or new understanding develops. When an individual uses curiosity advantageously, his or her mind is alive with wonder and interest, actively seeking information and asking appropriate questions. This can be a tremendous asset for a physician attempting to diagnose a patient in an initial visit or planning a therapeutic intervention. An alert mind, avid interest, and a desire for knowledge will help the doctor seek relevant information that will guide him or her to the problem's identification and solution.

Curiosity, similar to other character strengths, can be used excessively by an individual who tends to favor its use, but is unaware of the impact it is having on others. For example, a curious doctor may either ask questions persistently to the point of annoying patients, or might pursue information that is not appropriate for him or her to know (personal boundary violations). Unchecked curiosity might also lead to a lack of focus, distracting from the primary therapeutic task or goal. The skills of social intelligence, empathy, and active listening may help a doctor counterbalance overwhelming curiosity. By allowing a patient the time to fully respond to your question, and then empathizing with the emotional tenor of his or her response, you will have a wealth of information regarding how to most effectively proceed in your effort to help your patient.

Group discussion questions about curiosity

- How might your circumstances or the people you are with affect your ability to express the strength of curiosity in a professional setting? In a personal setting? How can you facilitate its expression in some of the more difficult situations?
- When you begin to wonder about something, what, if anything, gets in the way of pursuing or expressing your curiosity? How can you overcome these obstructions?
- How can curiosity be used to your advantage in areas of your life other than medicine?
- How would you use the character strength of curiosity to help motivate a noncompliant patient who is feeling powerless over his or her own care?

Individual exercises: New ways to use curiosity

- Make a list of new places or activities that you have never experienced, and then pick one each week and commit to the firsthand experience. What did you learn? How did you grow? What did you enjoy?
- Travel on a vacation to a new city or country to have fun, to learn, and to explore new customs, languages, food, and ways of living. Do this several times each year. Reflect on your learning and what was most fun for you. In learning about new places and people, did you learn something new about yourself?
- Think of a favorite topic (other than medicine) and then make a list of things you do not, as yet, know about the topic, but would be interested in learning. Use your curiosity to learn about two new things from your list each week.

Zest

Zest is a character strength that supports the virtue of courage. Zest refers to an approach to life filled with excitement and energy. Individuals with zest tend to live life as an adventure. As much a property of the body as it is of the mind, zest refers to a feeling of aliveness, high energy, and enthusiasm for life and all its activities and involvements.

Although individuals who are high in zest feel physically at ease and psychologically content, it is important to note that this measure is independent of health status. Thus, an individual who has had a prior serious illness or has a chronic illness but has made a successful recovery or adaptation to that state may well be high in the character strength of zest.

Individuals with zest tend to experience deep meaning and purpose in life and are likely to view their work as a calling and extremely fulfilling. They live life as an adventure with great enthusiasm, which tends to draw other people to them. Looking forward to each new day, they inspire others, providing opportunities for fun and meaningful relationships, and encourage others to undertake and complete positive projects.

Clearly, zest can be an asset to physicians: high energy coupled with a deep sense of meaning and purpose, seeing medicine as a calling to help others. The strong association of zest with happiness and life satisfaction makes it protective against the burnout and ill-being that is all too common among medical professionals.

As with curiosity and other character strengths, zest can be overused. When displayed in a constant and strong fashion regardless of person or situation, zest can be overbearing to others, particularly those who tend to be more quiet and introverted. Particularly in a hospital setting when around those who are sick and suffering, a doctor who strongly displays zest in an unchecked fashion can create feelings of jealousy, resentment, and lack of trust in patients. Social intelligence, empathy, and self-regulation skills are particularly helpful in such a situation (see chapter 11 on professionalism).

Group discussion questions about zest

- How do good health habits influence zest, and vice versa?
- How is zest affected by disease or illness? How is illness affected by the strength of zest? Is it possible to teach and build zest in those who must live with chronic illness? How might that affect prognosis or the course of illness?
- What situations or people tend to suppress the expression of zest when its use might otherwise be beneficial? Why? How might you remedy these situations?
- How does zest lead to positive things in one's life?

Individual exercises: New ways to use zest

- Select one routine activity you do daily. Deliberately try to do it with more energy, vigor, and sense of purpose. Practice that daily for one week. Then select another activity, and continue the process for the next week. Continue to find a new activity each week to handle with zest.

- Monitor the timeliness and regularity of your sleep routine. Work on getting eight hours of restful sleep per night. How does this impact your energy level and zest? If one is so focused on and so dedicated to work that one does not have time for meals during the day, what will happen to zest? Using self-awareness, self-regulation, and self-directed kindness, how can busy doctors best organize their days to preserve and maintain zest?

- Identify one routine assignment or task in your work life and one in your personal life. Write each down. Brainstorm ways to make these tasks more exciting or engaging. Practice these new ways daily for a week. Then identify two additional new tasks and begin the exercise again. Imagine the following scenario. You notice that you are finding the routine task of taking patient histories becoming tedious. You decide to approach it in a new way by, instead of asking your usual line of routine questions, just asking one open-ended question and then allowing the patient to speak while you listen. You may find that you learn many interesting things about your patients that you had never learned before, without even speaking a word! In this event, your interest and enthusiasm for taking patient histories would increase, and you would be able to relate better to your patients while gathering better information.

Looking at your individualized results

Look carefully at your individual results from the VIA survey at this time. If you took the survey for free, you will only have your character strengths in rank order. However, if you paid for the VIA-ME or the more in-depth VIA profile, you will see the definition of your signature strengths.

As discussed above, it is important to understand the definition and meaning of each of your signature strengths. In addition to understanding the meaning and value of each of your signature strengths, several additional thought/discussion questions and exercises may be particularly useful in maximizing your ability to create well-being in your life and work using your signature strengths. Some questions and exercises follow.

Discussion questions for each character strength

- What situations contribute to the ability to use and express this character strength? Which situations detract? Brainstorm ways to appropriately maximize your use of this character strength.
- How does this character strength help you pursue the various aspects of flourishing, that is, PERMA (positive emotions, engagement, positive relationships, meaning and purpose, and accomplishment)?
- How will use of this character strength help you improve your skills and well-being as a physician? How will it help you care for others? How will it help you promote well-being in others?
- How can use of this character strength help you take better care of yourself and implement the principles of positive health in your daily life? How can it help you avoid burnout?
- What are the ways this strength might be overused? What do you need to be aware of to avoid overuse of this strength? What sort of feedback might be helpful?

General exercises

- Think of the usual ways in which you use this character strength. Then brainstorm a list of five new ways to use the same character strength, in a new setting, with new people, in a new form or way. Implement one new way to use the character strength each week and practice that for the week. If you run out of new ways to implement a single strength, brainstorm new ways to use two of your signature strengths together as a pair.
- Although you cannot routinely administer the VIA survey to your patients and others for whom you are a role model of positive health, think of ways you might get some clues as to their signature strengths. How can you, then, reinforce these strengths in others? Observe carefully what happens when you sincerely reinforce the character strengths of another. How does that person feel? How well does he or she learn? How do you feel?

Your character strengths and the lessons learned in this chapter about them lay a very important foundation of health, strength, and wellness upon which the remaining chapters will build. You will find that use of your signature strengths will be relevant to and a natural asset in positive health, resilience, and professionalism, as well as being a thriving, happy physician and human being.

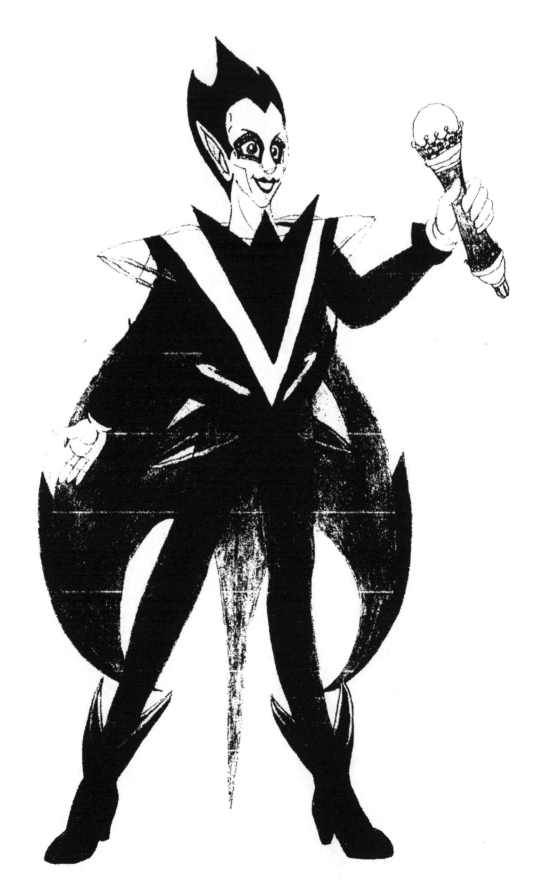

122

Chapter 7

Identifying, Defining, and Building Resilience

Resilience is a central focus in this curriculum for success and well-being of physicians, as well as of the general population. Chapter 1 of this book identifies resilience as an important skill that is needed by physicians, frequently recommended to physicians, yet never clearly defined nor formally taught in medical school or any continuing medical education offering. To redress this deficiency, this chapter will clearly identify resilience, review its definition (as well as those of related terms), and discuss various tools and models for building resilience through case examples and related activities. Seeking to build resilience in the physician population makes great humanistic and financial sense. Resilient physicians are able to be more compassionate and more empathetic and more involved with patients, and enjoy greater job satisfaction. They experience far less depression, stress, and burnout. Furthermore, physicians practicing resilient thinking will tend to teach that mind-set to their patients (to the benefit of the entire population).

Resilience is a term that has several definitions depending on the perspective of the researcher. From a developmental perspective, resilience arises from basic adaptation systems that protect human growth through the diverse conditions and challenges of childhood (Masten, Cutuli, Herbers, & Reed, 2009). Among children, resilience refers to patterns of positive adaptation during or following significant adversity or risk, which might otherwise be associated with negative outcomes. Instead of succumbing to the negative outcome, resilient children employ internal resources to make a positive adaptation (Masten, Cutuli, Herbers, & Reed, 2009).

Resilience among adults is a natural recovery process after loss or trauma, which is relatively common in the population. (Bonanno, 2004). Resilience reflects the ability to maintain one's equilibrium after a threat, and it involves protective factors that foster the development of positive outcomes.

As part of a healthy reaction to trauma or loss, resilient individuals can exhibit overt symptoms of sadness or upset, or subthreshold symptoms such as restless sleep or sporadic preoccupation. Nonetheless, they are able to maintain psychological and physical functioning (Mancini & Bonanno, 2006). They generally exhibit a stable trajectory of healthy functioning across time, as well as the capacity for generative experiences and positive emotions.

There are several pathways to resilience. Hardiness, a healthy personality trait, is characterized by a commitment to finding meaningful purpose in life. Self-enhancement, a cognitive process with less healthy effects, involves an unrealistic or overly positive bias in favor of the self, which can lead to high self-esteem. However, because unrealistically high self-esteem leads to narcissism and a tendency to evoke negative impressions in others (leading to longer-term deleterious effects), one may question the overall health of this cognitive process (Bonanno, 2004).

According to Lindstrøm (2001), salutogenesis is a sociologically based concept that explains how people can successfully respond to difficult life conditions. It differs from resilience, which is psychologically based. The salutogenic model, originally developed by Aaron Antonovsky in the 1970s, is based on two underlying assets: general-resistance resources and sense of coherence. The *general-resistance resources* represent both internal and external manifestations of character that aid the individual in life management. They are psychological mechanisms that are ineffective in isolation (sociologically based). The ability to use these general-resistance resources is based solely on one's sense of coherence. *Sense of coherence* is a global and pervasive feeling that whatever happens in life can be made understandable and can be managed, that there is a purpose and meaning attached to everything. The perception of coherence is based on cognitive, behavioral, and motivational factors (Lindstrøm, 2001).

The difference between resilience and salutogenesis is subtle, but it is particularly relevant with regard to issues of health. Unlike the absoluteness of the classic definition of health, Antonovsky viewed health as a relative concept. Therefore, instead of emphasizing the presence or the number of general-resistance resources, the important issue is one's ability to use the general-resistance resources that one does possess, powered by a sense of coherence. Here is an example of salutogenesis in an actual patient. A forty-four-year-old single woman, employed, and the single parent of two older dependent, disabled children, has a chronic, disabling autoimmune disorder, and all medications for her condition, including experimental drugs, have become ineffective. There is not even a prospect of a possible new treatment for a minimum of a year. Looking at this patient from the classic definition of health, she would appear quite unhealthy. However, from the standpoint of salutogenesis, we instead focus on her available resources and her cognitive, behavioral, and motivational strengths to put them to work. This patient's resources include high intellectual abilities, creativity, relative financial stability, a career, and prior excellent good health and physical conditioning. More importantly, she has the desire to be well, the knowledge of how to use what is available in her environment to best maintain her health, the determination to maintain her health so that she can continue to serve others, and the desire to enjoy life as an adventure. Although she is lacking in absolute health, she is relatively rich in resources and has a strong sense of determination of how to best use those resources to benefit herself, her family, and those she serves.

There is no disagreement that physicians, residents, and medical students pursue a career that involves high levels of stress. However, high stress does not automatically result in emotional distress and burnout. Hans Selye (1950), when describing his theory of general adaptation syndrome, indicated that the same stressor that produces a maladaptive response in one individual can be tolerated with impunity by another. Exposure to a stressor can produce disease if the defense reaction is inadequate or when the general adaptation syndrome is prevented from evolving in a normal manner (Selye, 1950).

Resilience is more common in the population than was previously thought, allowing individuals to bounce back from stress (Bonanno, 2004). Recent research has begun to identify the environmental, genetic, epigenetic, and neural mechanisms that underlie resilience and has shown that resilience is mediated by adaptive changes in several neural circuits, involving numerous neurotransmitters. These adaptive changes alter functioning of pathways related to reward, fear, emotional reactivity, and social behavior, and mediate successful coping with stress (Feder, Nestler, & Charney, 2009).

For example, early life stress has been linked to chronically high levels of corticotropin-releasing hormone from the hypothalamus, leading to excessive activation of the hypothalamic-pituitary-adrenal axis and the release of chronically high levels of cortisol from the adrenal. Sustained exposure to abnormally high levels of cortisol can lead to harmful states, such as hypertension, immunosuppression, and cardiovascular disease. Thus, reduced corticotropin-releasing hormone release and adaptive changes in corticotropin-releasing hormone receptor activity might promote resilience (Feder, Nestler, & Charney, 2009).

Over time, an individual's genes and their interaction with the environment shape that individual's neural circuitry, which gives expression to the behaviors identified as resilience. Various impinging systems, such as limbic reactivity and prefrontal-limbic connectivity, influence the initial response to negative or traumatic events, as well as one's capacity for cognitive reappraisal of these events. Further, the integrated circuits that mediate mood and emotion play a role in stress resilience. More adaptive functioning of fear, reward, emotional regulation, or social-behavioral circuits is thought to underlie a resilient individual's capacity to face fears, experience positive emotions, positively reframe stressful events, and derive benefit from supportive social relations. Thus, resilience is an active process that can be enhanced by promoting protective factors and using interventions aimed at maximizing stress resistance (Feder, Nestler, & Charney, 2009).

Marsha W. Snyder, MD., MAPP.

RESILIENCE AND POSTTRAUMATIC GROWTH

Posttraumatic growth describes the positive personal changes that may result from the struggle to deal with severe trauma and its psychological consequences (Tedeschi & McNally, 2011). The idea that tragedy and suffering can trigger personal transformation is not new. This has been a recurring theme in both secular and religious literature. Posttraumatic growth and resilience are distinct concepts, although posttraumatic growth can lead to increased resilience in the face of subsequent adversity. Five elements are known to contribute to posttraumatic growth. The first element is to understand the response to the trauma itself, including the shattered beliefs about the self, others, and the future. The second element is anxiety reduction, which includes techniques for controlling intrusive thoughts and images. The third element is constructive self-disclosure, including telling the story of the trauma. The fourth element is creating a trauma narrative in which loss and gain, grief and gratitude, happen together. The narrative also details the strengths demonstrated, improved spirituality, relationships solidified, and how life has been better. Finally, the fifth element is the declaration of strengthened positive life principles (Tedeschi & McNally, 2011).

Posttraumatic growth has been noted in response to life-threatening physical illness. In a review of fifty-seven published journal articles, Hefferon, Grealy, and Mutrie (2009) found elements common to instances of illness-related posttraumatic growth. The fifty-seven studies included a range of illnesses, including cancer (35), HIV (8), myocardial infarction (4), rheumatoid arthritis (3), multiple sclerosis (3), and other illnesses (each represented by one study). Key themes arising from the studies included the following: (a) restructuring of prior priorities, including a reduced obsession with appearance and money; (b) reappraisal of relationships with family members and close friends; (c) thankfulness for the simple things in life and for life itself; (d) reevaluation and change in life goals (e.g., going back to school, achieving new goals); (e) spiritual, emotional, and psychological transformation to a new authentic self; (f) increased emotional connection to humanity and a need to give back; (g) meaning and purpose in life; and (h) a new heightened awareness of the physical self, and a need to reduce stress through healthy behaviors (Hefferon, Grealy, & Mutrie, 2009).

Evidence-based methods for teaching resilience

Resilience skills are crucial in leading a successful life. Reivich and Shatté (2002) note that humans have four fundamental uses for resilience: (1) to overcome the obstacles of childhood; (2) to steer through everyday adversities; (3) to deal with major setbacks or life-altering events, enabling the individual to regroup and move forward; and (4) to reach out to others, enabling the individual to find renewed meaning and purpose in life and to facilitate achievement.

Resilience is a skill set that can be taught. Several studies demonstrate that individuals taught specific psychological resilience skills subsequently engage in behavioral changes that enable them to become more resistant to psychopathologies such as anxiety and depression (Reivich & Shatté, 2002; Brunwasser, Gillham, & Kim, 2009). To accomplish this goal requires focusing on a strengths-based, rather than a deficit-based, approach, proactively leveraging psychological strengths rather than reactively mitigating weaknesses (Reivich & Shatté, 2002).

There are several factors that contribute to a resilient mind-set. Optimism wed to reality is a major driver of resilience, as it stimulates a set of behavioral responses characterized by seeking and testing alternative approaches until one that works is found, rather than giving up at the first sign of failure. Flexible and accurate thinking is also essential. This is because thoughts that influence our emotions and subsequent behaviors can be distorted by incomplete data or shortcuts in thinking. Empathy and connection, impulse control and self-regulation, and emotional intelligence and awareness are all important components of resilience (Reivich & Shatté, 2002).

The Penn Resiliency Program is an example of a program that has effectively taught resilience to older children and adolescents. It is a "train the trainer" program in which clinicians from the Penn Resiliency Program come in to working classrooms to teach teachers the skills and techniques of the program. Its major goal is to increase students' ability to handle the day-to-day problems that are common during adolescence, promoting optimism by teaching students to think more realistically and flexibly about the problems they encounter (Reivich, Gillham, Chaplin, & Seligman, 2005). The Penn Resiliency Program also teaches assertiveness, creative brainstorming, decision making, relaxation, and other vital coping skills. It is one of the most widely researched depression-prevention programs in the world. Outcome studies have shown that the Penn Resiliency Program reduces and prevents symptoms of depression, reduces hopelessness, prevents clinical levels of anxiety and depression, reduces conduct problems, and improves health-related behaviors among at-risk young adults and adults (Gillham, Brunwasser, & Freres, 2008; Roberts, Kane, Thomson, Bishop, & Hart, 2003). Individuals who complete the program have fewer symptoms of physical illness. Furthermore, the decrease in depressive symptoms remained for twelve months post-intervention (Brunwasser, Gillham, & Kim, 2009).

Building resilience

We learn through resilience research that the principal roadblocks to tapping into our inner strength lie not in our emotions, but in our **cognitive style and in the ways we process information**, processes that are amenable to change through learning. When adversity strikes or when we are too busy and suffering from cognitive overload, we tend to use mental shortcuts to process the abundance of information that barrages us. Unfortunately, these shortcuts can lead to processing errors and misperceptions that can lead us astray, causing self-defeating emotions and behavior. However, simply by learning to understand our thinking style, including the mind traps that lead to misperceptions, we can correct errors in thinking. This, in turn, leads to a broadening of perspective and the elimination of self-defeating consequences. In other words, resilience refers to a positive thinking style that is realistic and supports well-being. This includes seven specific thinking skills that can be easily learned and readily used, and that support a resilient mind-set (Reivich & Shatté, 2002).

Of the seven, two of these thinking skills seem particularly relevant and are frequently misused by doctors who are in cognitive overload, frequently stressed, and trained in a culture of harshness and negativity. Each of these will be introduced, explained, and reviewed using a single case example. One case involves a forty-year-old female physician who electively presented for coaching over a six-month period to improve her communication skills. She will be referred to as "Dr. or Doc Rock." The coaching-session examples are being used to highlight how coaching, as opposed to psychotherapy, can often be a more effective and acceptable tool for physicians whose interpersonal problems result from lack of knowledge, awareness, and prior education.

Doc Rock and learning your ABCs

Doc Rock (a pseudonym) is a forty-year-old female medical doctor from the Western United States who had a successful career as a physician and chair of radiology at a large health network. After receiving her master's in business administration, she began a second successful career as a health-care executive. Doc Rock's signature strengths include curiosity, creativity, spirituality, love of learning, and appreciation of beauty. Temperance and humanity are two areas of relative weakness. She entered into coaching to improve her communication skills.

The following coaching session took place via Skype.

Following opening greetings …

Coach: Doc, as you well know from all of the ups and downs and challenges you have faced in your career, resilience skills are crucial in leading a successful life. Humans have four fundamental uses for resilience:

- to overcome the obstacles of childhood
- to steer through everyday adversities
- to help deal with a major setback or life-altering event (job loss, divorce, illness) so that one can regroup and continue to move forward

- to reach out so that one can find renewed meaning and purpose in life and achieve all of which one is capable (Reivich & Shatte, 2002).

The ability to develop and build resilience skills is based on four important pillars:

- Life change *is* possible—people can change positively and permanently.
- Thinking is the key to boosting resilience. Thoughts that influence emotions are the core of who we are; they represent our essential humanity.
- Accurate thinking is the key, as opposed to incomplete data or shortcuts to process them, which can lead to biased appraisals.
- It is important to refocus on one's human strengths, the basic strengths underlying all the positive characteristics of a person's emotional and psychological makeup (Reivich & Shatté, 2002).

Can you recall a significant event in which you used resilience skills to deal with adversity?

Doc: Yes. After the problems and disagreements I experienced with my superiors when I was chair of radiology, I could have felt that I was not good enough and that everything was my fault. However, I had a lot of confidence in my skills and abilities and I knew that the recommendations I was making were correct and beneficial. Instead of staying frustrated and angry, I went out and reinvented my career, getting a job as a health-care executive in another company.

Coach: That was a great example. So, resilience, then, is the basic strength underpinning all the positive characteristics in a person's emotional and psychological makeup. Resilience requires certain characteristics in a person. Can you think of some?

Doc: Sure (she laughs). Be certain that it's other people's fault so you can stick it to them and know that it has nothing to do with you.

Coach: Really?

Doc: Only kidding. Humor. Also, feeling good about myself.

Coach: Good. The six major underpinnings include:

- optimism—this should be optimism wed to reality,
- flexible and accurate thinking,
- empathy and connection,
- self-efficacy (I can)—which you mentioned,
- impulse control and self-regulation, and
- emotional awareness and emotional intelligence (Reivich & Shatte, 2002).

Are there any of these six areas that you feel might be particularly challenging for you?

Doc: As you know, I have some difficulty with impulse control. I get angry easily if I have a lot of tasks to do and I feel that other people are bugging me or preventing me from getting those tasks done.

Coach: So, it sounds like one of the important lessons you have learned about yourself is to regulate your schedule so that tasks do not pile up and cause you to feel pressured or uncomfortable.

Doc: Absolutely.

Coach: There are seven skills of resilience that fall into two basic categories. The two categories are know-thyself skills and change skills (Reivich & Shatté, 2002).

Know-thyself skills are those that guide you toward a better understanding of how your mind works. In other words, they help build self-awareness.

One of these skills is what we will focus on today—the ABC model. This model helps to give you an awareness of your thoughts, feelings, and behaviors and how they are interconnected. The name of the model, *ABC*, is an acronym for **a**ctivating events, **b**eliefs, **c**onsequences.

The ABC Model starts with an activating event (A) that elicits push-button thoughts and behaviors. There are both positive and negative events on this list. As you can see, even positive events can present challenges at times, thereby making objective responses difficult. Below is a list of some examples of activating events in Fig. 7-1.

Figure 7-1: List of some activating events (Reivich & Shatte, 2002)

Conflicts at work with colleagues or authority

Conflicts with family members or friends

Receiving positive or negative feedback

Success or lack of success

Loneliness or not having enough time alone

Taking on new responsibilities

Managing a hectic schedule or juggling too many tasks at once

Adapting to change

Attending social functions

Responding to negative emotions or positive emotions in others

Dealing with your own range of emotions (anger, sadness, anxiety, etc)

Savoring happiness or contentment

Criticism

Coach: What are some of the positive and negative events that push your buttons? Explain what happens during these events.

Doc: Attending social functions is an example of a positive event that pushes my buttons. When I am around a lot of people I don't know and no one bothers to make introductions, I feel as if people look at me as though I'm unimportant and don't matter. If I try to say "hi" and they have nothing to say, it makes me feel angry, and I wonder why I made the effort in the first place. As I told you before, a negative event that always pushes my buttons is when I don't have enough time for myself or when I have a lot of tasks to complete and people keep interrupting me so that I can't get my tasks done.

Coach: Yes, you explained that.

Doc: Yes. It also pushes my buttons when people treat me with disrespect.

Coach: Do you feel that people intentionally treat you disrespectfully?

Doc: Not always. But I do dislike being treated disrespectfully, and it is something that pushes my buttons.

Coach: "B" in this model stands for beliefs. These are heat-of-the-moment thoughts. We all have a running ticker tape of thoughts, even though we are not always aware of their presence. When an activating event occurs that pushes our buttons, we tend to have two categories of thoughts or beliefs:

- Why: beliefs about what caused it
- What next: beliefs about the implications.

These beliefs lead to C, or consequences. Consequences are emotions and behaviors that result from beliefs about the activating event. With A's that push our buttons, the B's tend to be negative, leading to the C's, consequences, which also tend to be negative, unproductive emotions and behaviors (Reivich & Shatte, 2002).

The value of this model is that we often find ourselves repeating negative or unproductive behavior patterns or repeatedly experiencing unproductive emotions without understanding why. If we can understand both the unproductive beliefs we associate with activating events and the consequences that result, we might be able to correct distortions in our thinking. It is often difficult, however, to remember the exact thoughts that are going on in your mind at the time of an event. What we tend to remember are the consequences—the emotions and behavior.

There are characteristic beliefs and emotional consequence pairs that follow one another. These belief-consequence pairs commonly occur together (see figure 7-2).

For example, if you can pinpoint that anger is a frequent emotion you feel in push-button situations, you may infer that this is brought on by the belief that someone has intentionally violated your rights or has set out to harm you.

Figure 7-2: Typical Belief/Consequence Pairs (Reivich & Shatte, 2002):

YOU FEEL (C):	YOU BELIEVE (B):
Anger	Your rights have been violated
Sadness, Depression	True loss or loss of self-esteem
Anxiety, Fear	Future threat
Guilt	You hurt or violated another's rights
Embarrassment	You are being compared neg. to others
Hope	Bright future with pos. change

*Coach:*Is there one particular "C" that you tend to experience more frequently than any other? Can you directly recall the beliefs associated with it?

Doc: Definitely. The C that I experience more than any other is anger. According to what you just explained, I must think that someone is either intentionally violating my rights or deliberately harming me. When I think of a time in which I felt disrespected, for instance, when I left my job as chairman of radiology.

Coach: Good work, Doc. Although that must be a painful memory, perhaps we can now learn to take this process a step further.

Let's now take a look at a step-by-step plan of how to use the ABC exercise. Step 1 is to describe the activating event (A) as objectively as possible (who, what, where, when). The goal is to separate the facts from any beliefs or judgments.

Step 2 is to identify the consequences (C) of the event. What did you feel and how did you react as the event unfolded? Include both emotions and behaviors. Note the intensity of the emotions.

Step 3 is to figure out the beliefs (B) that connect the A to the C. If you can directly recall your thoughts, this is best. What was I thinking that caused me to feel C? Use your knowledge of the B-C connections to make a mental check of your logic.

Pattern detection, when accurate, enables you to anticipate and prevent non-resilient beliefs and reactions.

Let's try some examples from your list of push-button activating events.

Doc: Okay. Here's the A: I went to the post office today to mail an envelope to Switzerland. I had written both the postal code and Switzerland on the envelope. The clerk told me I had to rewrite "Switzerland" on the envelope because the country had to be the last thing on the envelope. The C is that I was angry at the stupidity of having to write Switzerland again and that she did not offer to do it herself. So, there's that old anger again. My thought at the time was how lousy she was at her job.

Coach: Can you say more about your thoughts? What have you learned about anger?

Doc: I had already given her the money to mail the letter and was about to walk out. Rather than pointing out the error and making a big deal about it, she could have corrected the error herself and written Switzerland at the bottom of the envelope herself. It seemed like she was a disagreeable person who wanted to make my day as disagreeable as hers was.

Coach: Can you say more about your exact thoughts?

Doc: She went out of her way to make me feel bad and treat me poorly because she was a disagreeable person. That made me angry.

Coach: That is an unfortunate way to feel. I'm sure it must have taken awhile before you felt better.

Doc: Yes, about half the day.

Coach: Do you think it is possible that your thoughts and conclusions might have not been correct? What could be some other causes of her behavior?

Doc: Well, I'm sure she was just following protocol and procedure.

Coach: Anything else?

Doc: (after much thought) I guess she could have been sick or not feeling well. (Another long pause) Or perhaps she was having a bad day because she lost someone or something in her life went wrong or her boss just yelled at her …

Coach: So, in reality, there is no way for you to know for certain the cause of her suboptimal customer service. However, by falling into the thinking trap of personalizing, you gave yourself an unnecessary six hours of misery.

Doc: Yes, I can see that I tend to personalize a lot. Maybe that is why some of these events set me off.

Coach: Wonderful, Doc. Good work. So, what can you do that would be more resilient?

Doc: Try not to assume that the negative behavior has anything to do with me, so I don't let it ruin my day.

Coach: Excellent, Doc. It gets easier with practice.

Doc: Yes.

Coach: Doc, how do you suppose you can use some of your signature strengths to make it easier to get control of or modify your thoughts to make them more resilient?

Doc: One of my strengths is creativity. If I am more creative in my thinking, I can challenge myself to come up with three alternative explanations for a person's negative behavior every time I find myself starting to personalize things. Another strength of mine is curiosity. If I have doubts about someone's motives, I can always ask appropriate questions to get clarification.

Coach: Bravo, Doc. You rock! Do you have any questions or comments about resilience or the ABC model and how it works?

Doc: No. I think I've got it. I'll report back next month on progress.

Doc Rock and subsequent coaching session on the traps to avoid

Coach: Since you have obviously understood the ABC model and are working well with it, we will move ahead to a discussion of *thinking traps*: what they are, and how you can avoid them. Finally, we'll work together with the ABC model and thinking-trap avoidance. Does that sound good to you?

Doc: Absolutely.

Coach: Our senses are constantly taking in large quantities of information, far more than our brains can possibly process. We need to somehow simplify this information in order to use it, so we often cut corners and take shortcuts in our thinking to better handle the load. This makes our thoughts and beliefs about the world vulnerable to error. We are particularly prone to errors during periods of adversity.

Eight of these errors, called thinking traps, directly interfere with our resilience and how effectively we handle stress in our daily lives. Therefore, thinking traps are common patterns of thinking that cause us to miss critical information (Reivich & Shatte, 2002).

Any questions so far?

Doc: None.

Coach: I will now briefly review all eight thinking traps. When we get to the three traps that are most relevant to you, we will broaden the discussion.

Thinking trap 1 is jumping to conclusions. This is the thinking trap of making assumptions without complete data. It involves believing that one is certain of the meaning of a situation despite insufficient evidence. It is the umbrella error, since all of the thinking traps involve making assumptions of one kind or another. When one jumps to conclusions about the meaning of a message and then acts as if one's own interpretation is certainly correct, one cannot respond in a resilient fashion.

Can you think of situations in which you tend to jump to conclusions?

Doc: Yes. I tend to do it when I am in a hurry or under time pressure. I do it when I think the other person doesn't know what he or she is talking about. I do it if I think I am being treated disrespectfully.

Coach: People who habitually jump to conclusions respond impulsively to situations because they act before they have full and accurate information.

Doc: Yes. At the post office (again referring to the event we discussed in detail at our last meeting), I decided that the clerk was deliberately trying to ruin my day. That was a perfect example in which I jumped to a conclusion with inadequate information and responded inappropriately. It made me angry for no reason, and I ruined my day feeling bad about it.

Coach: Good thinking, Doc. In a few minutes, we will discuss strategies to avoid these thinking traps. For now, we'll continue.

Thinking trap 2 is tunnel vision. This involves focusing on the less significant details in a situation while screening out the more important aspects. Tunnel vision is most often directed toward negative outcomes and is the result of sampling from the environment in a biased way, resulting in incorrect conclusions. With tunnel vision, you are only registering small bits of what is going on around you, and you can only remember those things that you register. Do you have any questions about it?

Doc: None.

Coach: Can you think of an example of tunnel vision?

Doc: Yes. When I was a resident, I covered the service of a private attending who was a fanatic for perfection. No matter how great a job I did with his patients, all he focused on was the minor negative events. I made rounds with him one morning after a night of being on call. Every patient was in excellent condition, despite the fact that we had several ICU patients. When we got to the last patient's bedside, the nurse came in stating that the patient's glasses appeared to be missing. The attending blew up at me as if a terrible crisis had happened and I was to blame. Would that be an example of the attending's tunnel vision?

Coach: Good example, Doc. Next, we'll go on to magnifying and minimizing.

Thinking trap 3 involves errors in evaluating events in which, most often, the negative aspects of a situation are magnified and the positive aspects are minimized. This differs from tunnel vision in that you register and can remember most of the events that have occurred, but overvalue some and undervalue others. Rarely, people magnify the good and minimize the bad, causing them to underestimate problems and the need for change. Magnifying the negative can lead to low mood and can undermine success in work, relationships, creativity, problem solving, and thinking skills. Resilience rests on accurate appraisal of one's life.

Personalizing is thinking trap 4. This is the tendency to attribute problems to one's own doing. Explanatory style is our habitual way of explaining the events in our lives.

A "personal" or "me" explanatory style is a known risk factor for depression (Reivich & Shatte, 2002). This individual's reflex is to automatically blame himself when something goes wrong. People who do this not only blame themselves but also often allude to some character flaw within themselves as the cause. The B-C connection often involves thoughts about the loss of self-worth or thoughts of violating the rights of others, which then leads to feelings of sadness and guilt. Resilience comes from believing realistically that one has the power to control one's behavior and to change what needs to be changed. Only in that context can personalizing be helpful in making positive change. An individual who tends to fall into the thinking trap of personalizing might have responded to the harsh attending in your story by feeling responsible for the patient's glasses being lost and believing the attending's accusations of incompetency.

Thinking trap 5 is externalizing. This is the flip side of personalizing. It is the tendency to automatically attribute the cause of an adverse event to other people or circumstances (Reivich & Shatte, 2002). Externalizing tends to be more common in physicians and most people with responsibility in the hospital. People who externalize fail to locate those elements of an adversity that are of their doing and within their control. Therefore, they miss an opportunity to improve their situation or make things better. Although they avoid sadness and guilt, externalizers tend to find themselves prone to anger. Any questions, Doc?

Doc: No.

Coach: Thinking trap 6 is overgeneralizing. This involves "always" and "everything" explanations. It involves developing global beliefs about a topic based on a single situation. Personalizers who overgeneralize tend to assassinate their own characters. Externalizers who overgeneralize tend to assassinate the characters of others.

Thinking trap 7 is emotional reasoning. This occurs when one draws conclusions about the world based on one's emotional state as opposed to more objective, realistic thinking. For example, the proximity in time of an anticipated threat affects our perception of how dangerous it is. The day before it occurs, it seems more dangerous than a month before it occurs.

Thinking trap 8 is mind reading. With this thinking trap, we believe we know what others around us are thinking and then act in accordance with our possibly false beliefs. The corollary to the belief in one's own ability to read the minds of others is the belief or expectation that others can read one's mind and truly know one's thoughts. This is a common thinking trap of relationship partners. When we "read" minds, we often read them wrong and jump to erroneous conclusions.

When we are using the skill of avoiding thinking traps, we are trying to find ways to get more balanced, correct, and complete information. Let's review the three thinking traps that you felt were most relevant to you. The process starts with an analysis of the

ABCs of an activating event as we reviewed last meeting. Once you have figured out your ticker-tape beliefs (B), compare them to the list of thinking traps, which are listed on Table 7-3. Try to identify the thinking trap that is embedded in your ticker-tape beliefs.

Table 7-3:

THINKING TRAPS (Reivich & Shatte, 2002):

Jumping to Conclusions: Believing one is certain of the meaning of a situation despite little or no evidence to support it

Tunnel Vision: Focusing on less significant details in a situation, while screening out the more important aspects

Overgeneralization: Developing global beliefs about one's general lack of worth or ability on the basis of a single situation (either self or others)

Magnifying and Minimizing: Errors in evaluating events in which the negative aspects of a situation are magnified and the positive aspects of a situation are minimized (or the opposite)

Personalizing: The tendency to automatically attribute the cause of an adversity to one's personal characteristics or actions

Externalizing: The tendency to automatically attribute the cause of an adversity to other people or to circumstances

Mind Reading: Assuming that you know what another person is thinking, or expecting another person to know what you are thinking

Emotional Reasoning: Drawing conclusions about the world based on one's emotional state as opposed basing one's conclusions on rational thinking and objective facts.

Coach: If you jump to conclusions, speed is your enemy. Your goal should be to slow down. (See the list of Thinking Traps and the skills needed to avoid them in Table 7-4 below). Then you can check for evidence upon which to base your conclusions. How might that have worked with the clerk in the post office?

Doc: Instead of assuming that she wanted to ruin my day, if I had slowed down and looked around, I would have noticed that she was the only employee there to help customers, that the line of customers was getting long, and that she had to deal with it all by herself. Therefore, she was probably a bit on edge and tired. Perhaps I could have even reached out and been helpful to her.

Coach: That might have made both of you feel better. With the thinking trap of externalization, ridding yourself of this unproductive thought pattern starts with holding yourself accountable. Ask yourself what you might have done to contribute to the situation. Try asking, "How much of the problem is due to others and how much to me?"

To avoid the thinking trap of mind reading, we must learn to speak up and ask questions of others instead of assuming we know what they are thinking. We also must make our own beliefs known directly and clearly and convey all pertinent information instead of assuming that others can read our thoughts. Ask yourself if you are expecting others to figure out your needs or goals.

By practicing catching your thinking errors in real time and asking yourself the appropriate questions, you will become much more resilient and avoid costly errors. Do you have any questions about ABCs or thinking traps, Doc?

Doc: No. It all seems pretty clear to me, and I have been finding the ABC model increasingly easy to use. I like it. I think it has helped make my thinking more resilient.

Coach: How wonderful to hear this. Do you have any questions regarding our work today or anything we have covered?

Doc: No, none. I will keep practicing my resilience skills.

Table 7-4: Thinking Traps and the Skills Needed to Avoid Them (Reivich & Shatte, 2002):

Jumping to Conclusions: Speed is your enemy. Avoid this by trying to slow down. Then check for evidence upon which to base your conclusions. What is the evidence?

Tunnel Vision: Try to refocus on the big picture. How important is this one aspect to the big picture? What salient information might I have missed? How important is this one aspect compared to the overall view?

Overgeneralization: Look more closely at the behaviors involved. Is there a specific behavior that explains the situation? Is there a more specific explanation?

Magnifying and Minimizing: Strive for better balance. Try to be more evenhanded. Find the good (bad) things that happened as well as the bad (good).

Personalizing: Learn to look outward. Did anyone or anything else contribute to the situation? How much of the problem is due to me and how much to others or extenuating circumstances?

Externalizing: Learn to look inward. Start holding yourself accountable. What might I have done to contribute to this situation? How much of the problem is due to others and their actions and how much to me and my actions?

Mind Reading: Learn to ask questions of others. Did I express myself? Did I make my beliefs known? Am I expecting others to figure out my needs? Did I ask the questions needed to understand the needs of those around me?

Emotional Reasoning: Practice separating feelings from facts. Do I draw conclusions based upon the facts? Do my feelings accurately reflect the facts of the situation? What questions must I ask to know the facts?

Group discussion questions

- What is resilience? Why is it important to doctors to have resilience?
- Discuss the factors in your current work life that tend to discourage resilient behavior. What could you do to change them?
- Describe a recent professional incident in which you exhibited reflexive reactive or non-resilient behavior. Describe the adverse event, the consequent behavior, the beliefs behind the behavior, and the thinking trap(s) involved in distorting your thinking. What was the cost of the behavior to you? To others? What might you do differently next time to have a more positive outcome?
- If, as in table 7-4 there are relatively simple ways to avoid these thinking traps and consequent non-resilient behavior, why do we keep repeating the same unproductive behavior? What can we do to change this?

Individual observation

In your health habits journal, begin to keep a record of episodes of non-resilient behavior in the work setting. Go through the steps of noting the A and C, figuring out the B, and identifying the thinking trap involved. Then make a note of what you could have done differently that might have produced a more resilient outcome. Try doing at least three of these per week. The more you do, the more easily resilient behavior will come to you. Soon you will learn to exhibit resilient patterns of thinking and behaving even in adverse situations.

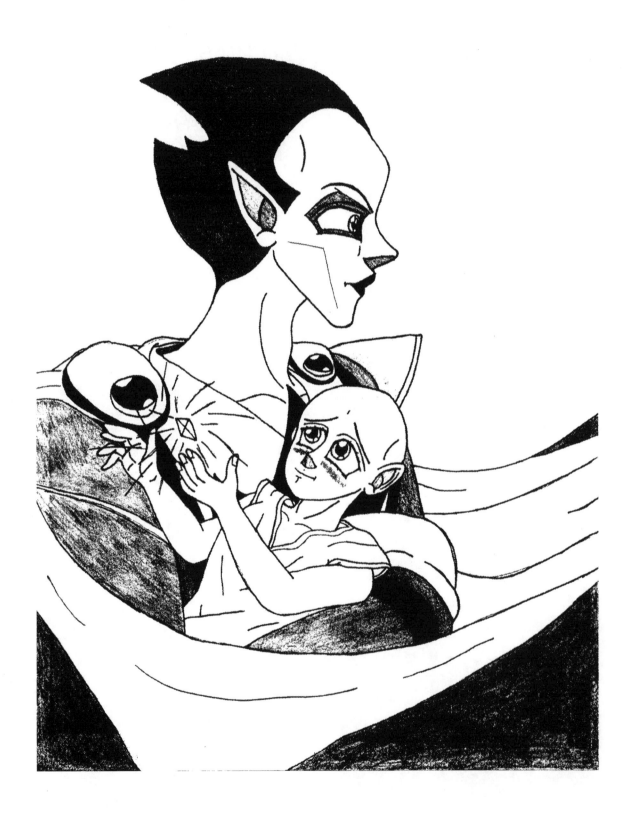

Chapter 8

Meaning and Purpose

Coauthored by: Dr. Barry Heermann and Dr. Marsha W. Snyder

In his book entitled *Flourish*, Dr. Martin Seligman introduced a major change to his underlying theory of positive psychology, from the authentic happiness theory to the well-being theory (2011). The authentic happiness theory was predominantly mood-based, with the goal being increased life satisfaction, which he later came to regard as somewhat unidimensional. In its place, Seligman offered the construct of well-being, realizing that life satisfaction does not take into account the important role of engagement with work and loved ones, and deep meaning and purpose in life, both of which are also essential to flourishing.

Seligman defines meaning as belonging to and serving something that you believe is bigger than the self (2011, p. 17). To attain and maintain a state of well-being, therefore, one must clearly understand the important role of meaning in one's life and know how to connect to it and stay connected to it. When most high school and college students envision a career in medicine, they are deeply connected to the purpose of healing and helping others. That is how the overwhelming majority of doctors-to-be enter medical school. And yet, starting by the middle of the first year of medical school and continuing throughout training and a professional career, a high rate of burnout, discouragement, and loss of meaning and purpose afflict a frighteningly high percentage of doctors-in-training and doctors. (These statistics are reviewed in chapter 1.)

Why is it that so many doctors become burned out? Why is it that work is so burdensome and unfulfilling for so many of the individuals who are employed in the health-care setting? The growing body of positive organizational research documents the possibility of joy and fulfillment at work (Heermann, 1997). In chapter 15 on the empowered frontline multidisciplinary health-care team, we explore some of the external realities of hospital and health-care organizational structure that can detract from an empowered frontline multidisciplinary team, whose common mission is to provide outstanding, error-free, compassionate care to patients and one another. However, when that team is ignited with meaning, spirit, and a passion to serve, extraordinary outcomes result in spite of external barriers.

The study of spirit can be applied at the individual level as well as at the team level. This chapter will focus on the spirit that lies at the heart of extraordinary individuals, which include each of us. This chapter will introduce you to a more schematic way of looking at the different parts of yourself, a way that may lead you to rediscover your sense of purpose.

Meaning and purpose lie within you. You may feel burned out, unhappy, or disheartened right now. But your meaning and purpose remain inside you. The critical journey for you is to uncover your purpose, so that your goodness may be released to the world. You will then be in a place of *noble purpose*—a term used frequently in this chapter. Noble purpose, from Dr. Barry Heermann's book of the same name (2004) refers to purpose that offers the potential of great benefit to someone other than one's self. This chapter will introduce a path to such purpose.

THE PATH TO NOBLE PURPOSE

All human beings yearn to contribute. Regardless of who we are, at a deep level we are each called to serve. As human beings, serving others brings us joy and meaning. So, while noble purpose is socially responsible behavior of the highest order, it brings great gifts to both the giver and the recipients. In the words of Dr. Heermann, "When you are connected to your Noble Purpose you gain a deeper knowledge of yourself and access a wider dimension of your gifts. Alignment of who you are in the world with your unique gifts allows you to make important contributions to others regardless of the scale. You are simultaneously freed and able to experience unbounded joy, vitality and a sense of accomplishment." (2004, p. 11).

Noble purpose is fundamentally a matter of the heart. Although it may seem remote to a doctor who is burned out, fatigued, and questioning his or her decision to remain in clinical medicine, perhaps doctors can, yet, begin to find ways to uncover and unlock it.

For the purposes of this discussion, consider the following tripartite model of the self (figure 8-1). This model is not offered as a theory of the mind, and it is not based on any empiric scientific evidence. Instead, it is simply intended to be a schematic way of looking at the self that results from a lifetime of experiences and living.

Figure 8-1. The tripartite model of the self. (from *Noble Purpose*, QSU Publishing, 2004)

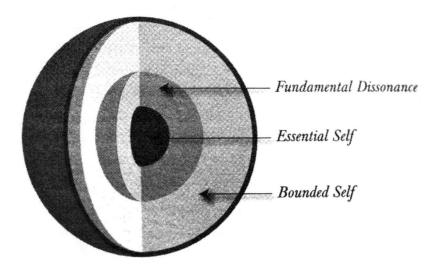

In figure 8-1, you can see concentric circles. The innermost layer or circle represents the *essential self*. The essential self is essence and unlimited potential of a new infant, swaddled with unconditional compassion and love, that each of us brings with us into the world. The essential self is much like the classic archetype of the loved child; he or she thrives in the goodness of everything, including his or her own perfection and infinite potential. The essential self is ensconced in harmony and perfect consonance. From the perspective of the essential self, the universe is a place to be trusted, and it is unfolding perfectly, as it should. The essential self is where one's noble purpose lives, thrives, and is accessible.

As we all know and have experienced, painful and challenging events can happen throughout life. These are often unintentional events, though some are more intentional or evil. To protect the essential self, a strong protective layer builds up. This layer of protection tends to grow with the depth and frequency of wounding and persists throughout life, protecting the essential self, yet keeping it completely out of our reach and awareness. This layer immediately surrounding the essential self is the *fundamental dissonance*. Out of this layer come fear, self-doubt, resignation, cynicism, and self-diminishment. The abuse and bullying (both the giving, but especially the receiving) that are so high in the medical culture (see chapter 1) are examples of a fundamental dissonance and a wounding that add thickness to this layer, keeping our meaning and purpose hidden away behind the scars.

Because we must live in a relatively safe way that protects us from these dissonances, we develop a hard outer veneer that becomes the third layer. This layer, called the *bounded self*, serves as a boundary to protect you from the unpleasant dissonances around you. It encapsulates the pain of your dissonance, giving you a degree of safety and protection from it. However, by walling you off from your goodness, it limits your existence to one of superficiality.

Let's take a closer look at what the bounded self might look like. Your bounded self includes any and all of the superficial aspects of the self that we mistake for part of our identity. Examples include your job title, your profession, your possessions, your social status, your money or financial status, your physical appearance, your ability to dance, ski, run, or play golf, and so much more. If someone had asked me to describe myself ten years ago, my response likely would have been something like, "I am a young, athletic, and vibrant doctor and single parent who is chair of psychiatry for a large northeastern health network. I love to sing, dance, ski, and run. My passion is caring for others, especially my two autistic children and my patients and employees." Little would I know that within a year or so of making that statement, all those things that I thought defined me were lost because of an illness.

Because the bounded self is constantly fighting to keep the pain of fundamental dissonance at bay, it is constantly on edge and in a defensive posture. This leads to the use of unhealthy defenses, such as power, control, and manipulation, to manage your environment and others in it, in a feeble attempt to avoid yourself. The compassion of the essential self is removed and remote, virtually inaccessible, leaving you numb. This is the picture of the classic, burned-out physician.

The good news is that the hard outer veneer of the bounded self can be pierced to once again regain access to the essential self, one's life purpose and joy. One way is more or less involuntary in nature. A second way is a process that we can explore.

This first process involves a radical life transition or trauma. Examples of such events include the loss of a job, the death of a loved one, or a catastrophic illness. As doctors, we frequently see our patients experiencing this sort of crisis. When one undergoes such a crisis oneself, there is a radical cracking open of the bounded self (see figure 8-2). Perhaps this occurs because there is no longer energy available to fortify the defenses of the bounded self. Perhaps, as in my case, it is because that superficial self simply disappears.

Figure 8-2. Cracking open (from *Noble Purpose*, QSU Publishing, 2004)

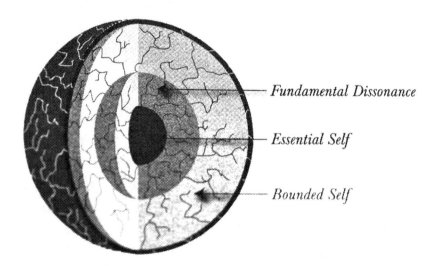

Fundamental Dissonance

Essential Self

Bounded Self

My story

The first event that broke through my denial was when I was walking down the street with some friends and I could not keep up with them. As a runner, that got my attention. I was frightened. And I went to see a rheumatologist because I had been experiencing keratoconjunctivitis sicca and fatigue for the previous eight years. Although I was experiencing no symptoms of a mental health disorder, the rheumatologist suggested I see a psychiatrist, which I did not do. Next, over the subsequent two years, I saw a series of eight different neurologists as I gradually lost my ability to walk, work, care for my children, sing, dance, ski, and run. Because I had considered myself invincible, I had no disability insurance and lost most of my savings supporting my children and myself through this period. Therefore, my financial security was also at risk. Without a diagnosis and having lost everything that I thought was the essence of my identity, I was in a true crisis. My bounded self had literally crumbled away. This rapid destruction of my bounded self and the resulting identity crisis fortunately left me nowhere to go but to my own essential self.

Thankfully, most people do not experience the sudden jolting path described above. Instead, you can choose to follow a process that lets you connect with your fundamental dissonance, opening the door to your essential self. "These pathways lead you to a clearing within you. The clearing is a space wherein you come to terms with who you are—returning to your essential self. In this space, or clearing, you purge yourself of toxicities that interfere with experiencing your Noble Purpose. You release the old, dysfunctional, automatic response patterns and rigidities of the bounded self, gaining access to your essential self and the instinctive knowledge that allows you to move mountains." (Heermann, 2004, p. 22).

We will now begin this journey together, using a brief look at this pathway that you will see again in chapter 15, "The Spirited Multidisciplinary Health-Care Team." This pathway is a spirit-based journey to access your essential self. Ultimately, it will reveal how you can use your strengths to bring thriving to self, others, and the world. For more information on this process and meaning and purpose in healthcare go to www.creatingpositivehealth.com.

Figure 8-3. The noble purpose spiral

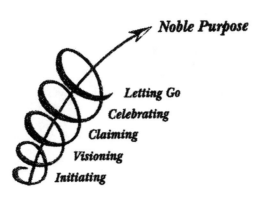

Initiating

Initiating is beginning the passage to a deep inner knowledge of the perfection of the universe. Initiating is choosing the path of trust, knowing that your universe is perfectly unfolding. For a burned-out physician, with years of working within an imperfect health-care system, this might sound totally absurd. However, it is important to distinguish what is within you and what you choose to be part of you, from what is external to you.

It is through initiating a path of trust that we can begin to make sense of the good and bad things that happen to us throughout life. A sense of belonging and trust in the universe encourages deeper relationships, which allow us to seek the support of others even when life events are not positive.

Trusting relationships with colleagues starts with a positive self-image and trusting one's strengths. Accomplishing this requires letting go of constant self-evaluation and the anxiety attached to it. Embracing your dissonances without blame is a big step toward reaching this goal. In addition, it is necessary to suspend judgment of others. Doubting yourself in the world around you leads to needless depletion of your energy. We see this energy depletion all too frequently in the health-care arena.

Summary of initiating actions

- Choose to release all evaluation of yourself, others, and circumstances.
- Become conscious of gifts and blessings in your life.
- Embrace learning from the dissonances in life.
- Affirm perfection in your life, trusting that nothing is missing from your universe.

Discussion questions related to initiating

- How does one realistically choose to trust in a benevolent universe in spite of negative events that might be impinging?
- When you choose to trust in a benevolent universe, in whose universe are you trusting?
- Why is it important to know and trust your strengths and gifts?

Initiating in your routine

Choose one or more of these suggestions to help you incorporate initiating into your life.

- Create an affirmation that strengthens initiating in your life. Write it on a 3 × 5 index card and carry it with you, repeating it upon arrival at work, before lunch, before leaving work, and before bed. An example of such an affirmation might be, "I experience the universe as benevolent, completely supporting my well-being, my life journey, and my career as a physician."
- Where do you feel most at peace and attuned with the world around you? In a special room? A place of worship? In nature? Consciously go to that place and allow yourself to feel a deep connection with the blessings of your life. If you cannot physically get to that place, close your eyes and visualize being there. Feel the fullness of your experience of connection with the perfection around you.
- Identify loved ones or wisdom figures, alive or dead, real or fictional, who have lived life as if the universe is innately good and wonderful. Make a list of these incredible people in your journal, and reflect on how each one demonstrated belief in a benevolent universe.
- Find a favorite piece of music, poem, or painting whose artistic expression exemplifies initiating. Spend the day with that work of art, listening/viewing/reading it many times throughout the day. Try to take in the qualities of initiating through this art form. An example of music that reminds me of initiating is the opening chorus of J. S. Bach's "Christmas Oratorio." John Denver's "Sunshine on my Shoulders" incorporates many aspects of initiating.

Visioning

Visioning is the revealing of imaginative new possibilities, which can manifest in a new reality when put into action. It is the capacity to bring your noble purpose to light. The ability to vision only comes with successful initiating, having the trust in the universe and in oneself and the limitless possibilities of great acts.

Your vision is the energy that animates your noble purpose. Discovering your vision often comes from considering the answers to several key life questions. As these questions are reviewed, suggestions for journaling will be offered. Begin by folding five sheets of paper in half, lengthwise, and pick up a pen. On each of the five pieces of paper you will write a list, going down the left-hand side. For each question, simply make the list without comment or elaboration. Once all lists are complete, return to each list and, on the right-hand side, write one or two feelings associated with each item on the left.

Make the following five lists (one on each of the five pages):

- From childhood: list your earliest hopes and dreams, things you liked to do, possessions you liked having, adventures you enjoyed taking, fantasies you enjoyed, and people with whom you liked to interact.
- From your adult experience: list your dreams, things you like to do, possessions you value, favorite adventures, people with whom you enjoy interaction.
- List your favorite books and movies from childhood through adulthood in the left column, adding a hero, heroine, or storyline that was memorable, and why, in the right column.
- List on the left "mountaintop" experiences you have had throughout life, when you felt life-changing or ecstatic experiences.
- List your greatest accomplishments in the left column. In the right column, write the contribution embedded in each and the strengths used to achieve it.

Once you have created each of these lists, go through each of them again. As you reread them, you will find that certain items stimulate more energy within you. Underline each of the items that stimulates unusual energy.

Now, take time to review those items that you have underlined. Do you see any common themes? How does your energy link them together? Notice the part of your spirit from which this energy is emerging. Take some time to journal about this motivating energy. What is inspiring you? How does your inspiration reflect on your uniqueness? What might it suggest about your noble purpose? Write down whatever thoughts come to mind without judging yourself.

In successful visioning, you allow what animates you to move you and become you. It is the ability to effectively use energy to access your potential for good.

Do not feel discouraged if your vision is not clear after one or two reviews of your list. Have a one-on-one discussion with a coach, an advisor, or a trusted friend who can help clarify points that were initially confusing. Use the exercises at the end of this section to aid you in your visioning practice. Resist judgment to come up with an answer. Instead, relax and enjoy the journey of self-discovery.

Summary of visioning actions

- Become conscious of sources of energy, from experiences, activities, projects, or interests in your life or work.
- Discern images/urgings that are related to your source of energy that inspire you.
- Visualize your purpose and your inner call to serve.

Visioning discussion questions

- What is the relation between these newly discovered sources of energy and your career in medicine?
- When you consider the most energizing ways in which you use your talents to make a positive contribution to the lives of others, consider if you are currently using these energizing talents in your work as a doctor. Creatively imagine how you can add more of those energizing talents to your daily life and work.

Visioning in your routine

Pick one or several of these suggestions to help you understand and incorporate visioning in your life.

- Affirmation: Create an affirmation that emphasizes visioning, and write it on a 3 × 5 index card. Read and repeat the affirmation before leaving for work, before lunchtime, before leaving work, and before bed. An example of such an affirmation might be, "I attract everything I need—information, understanding, and perspective—necessary to envision my extraordinary noble purpose."
- Journaling activity: Close your eyes. Envision five remarkable achievements you would like to have happen in your life over the coming six months. Think big, and allow yourself to dream, knowing that these things can and will occur. Notice how your spirit feels regarding these achievements. Journal about these feelings. On your calendar, mark six months from today's date and make a notation to return to the entry you have just made in your journal. Six months from now, add to your journal entry the feelings attached to your wish list and your accomplishments.
- Ritual: Visioning is about bringing your noble purpose into the light. This evening, find a quiet place away from others. In a darkened space, light one or more candles, viewing the light of the candles as the glowing expression of your noble purpose. Sit quietly with the light of the candles, letting in the light of your strengths and the noble purpose for which they will be used.
- Rekindling visioning awareness through aesthetic appreciation: Find a favorite piece of music, a poem, or a painting that emphasizes elements of visioning. Place it where you can listen to it/view it several times a day. For example, "Easter Morning in Wales," a poem by David Whyte, embodies the ideas of visioning. Here is an excerpt:

"I have waken from the sleep of ages and I am not sure
        if I am really seeing, or dreaming,
        or simply astonished
        walking toward sunrise
        to have stumbled into the garden
        where the stone was rolled from the tomb of longing."

Claiming

Claiming can be defined as *the manifestation of the contribution you envision in its tangible form and structure.* It includes embodying your unique purpose while staying soundly grounded in your essential self.

Whereas in visioning you dream big and create your magnificent purpose, claiming is the phase in which you responsibly manifest your vision, making it come alive. Claiming focuses on action. Claiming is the marriage of inner peace with intention. It is keeping your word and getting the job done. Inspired claiming makes your vision come alive by implementing and acting on all the steps necessary to make the vision a reality.

With the energy of your vision driving you forward as you take action and implement the steps needed to reach your goals, you can accomplish more than you ever imagined.

A young physician, Dr. M., came from a wealthy family. He graduated medical school and completed his residency in surgery at a prestigious surgical training program. When he began his practice, a private practice in a wealthy suburb of a major city, he cared for many upper middle class patients who were financially secure. One day, he was called to the hospital and asked to consult on the case of a young impoverished child from a poor African nation with a marked facial deformity. The child had been brought to the United States by a charity specifically for the purpose of having the deformity corrected. Dr. M. immediately agreed to perform the surgery. In getting to know this frightened young girl and her family, he was deeply moved by their strength, their hope, and their love. Realizing the degree of poverty that she lived in and the fact that his young patient could never have gotten this kind of care in her own country, the doctor was sad, but motivated to take action. It started with a vision that he could help by making this surgery available in the girl's country and in other such poor countries. With the power of this vision and his openhearted desire to serve, inspired claiming began. Dr. M. contacted the charity that had brought the young girl to the United States and presented his vision to them. They were thrilled, and in turn, knew other key stakeholders to bring into the project to make it successful. Before long, the doctor had raised sufficient funds to begin a surgical clinic fixing facial deformities in the young girl's country. He flies there once a month to operate on children in need of his skills.

There are three motivations that can quickly undermine great claiming. They are desire for power and control, fixation on results, and the need to look good to others. Unfortunately, the culture of medicine values all of these motivations by encouraging competitive excellence. However, exploring these behaviors more closely reveals that each is rooted in your fundamental dissonance, making you feel as though you are not enough, they are not enough, and it is not enough. Fear undermines one's noble purpose. It is the antithesis of trust in the goodness of people. Claiming is devoid of fear. It is a place of quiet effectiveness and fierce resolve. At its best, claiming combines inner peace and confidence with inspired action and high performance.

In summary, the essentials of claiming include the following actions:

- Be present to your purpose.
- Establish action plans to realize your purpose.
- Identify human resources to accomplish your goals.
- Be responsible for the resources you need to accomplish your purpose.
- Follow up on service provided to others.

Claiming discussion questions

- Dr. X took the VIA Character Strengths Survey and scored high in creativity, zest, and love. He easily was able to vision his meaning and purpose as a physician. What character strengths might facilitate excellent claiming?
- What do patience, persistence, and consistency have to do with inspired claiming?
- How does the need to win or come out on top interfere with accomplishing your purpose?

Claiming in your daily routine

- Affirmation: Create an affirmation that strengthens any aspect of claiming in your life. For example, "I live my purpose, realizing my vision through generating and sustaining service in the world." Write your affirmation on a 3 × 5 index card and carry it with you throughout the day. Repeat it before going to work, before lunch, prior to leaving work, and before retiring for the evening.
- Body exercise: Take ten to fifteen minutes to sit quietly, releasing your thoughts, closing your eyes, and focusing on relaxing your body and being aware of its sensations. Embodying your purpose requires a generative strength that is grounded

in a place of effortless peace. Great claiming occurs with ease and grace. Scan your body and notice how so many functions occur automatically. Notice how you are the rhythm of your breath, the beat of your heart, and the digestion of your food. Your body provides these functions without toil. Feel this capacity that serves you without a thought. Model your claiming as a similarly transparent process that is quietly, yet brilliantly, amazing.

- Journaling: Close your eyes and think of all the individuals you have known in your life. Choose one or two of these individuals who took ideas and brought them to life with the utmost peace and equanimity. Journal about these two people. What were their inner strengths and resources? What was unique about each individual? Journal about how you might access such inner strength in your own life.

- Claiming through aesthetic expression: Find a favorite piece of music, a poem, or a work of art that evokes the qualities of claiming. Listen to this music, view this work of art, or read this poetry frequently, reflecting on the thoughts and emotions that it evokes in you. "The Journey," a poem by Mary Oliver, includes the following excerpt, which embodies claiming:

"One day you finally knew
what you had to do, and began,
though the voices around you
kept shouting
their bad advice …

But you didn't stop.
You knew what you had to do."

Celebrating

Celebrating is a key step for achieving great purpose in life. However, nothing could be further from the medical culture, a culture where flaws are quickly pointed out, but victories are rarely celebrated.

I have fond memories from my medical training of congregating with colleagues at the end of the workday each Friday for what we called *liver rounds*. Liver rounds involved beer, camaraderie, and sharing war stories of the prior week. Though fun, it is not what is meant by celebrating, in the context of meaning and purpose.

Celebrating is the experience of profound gratitude for the gifts of the universe that allow the achieving of noble purpose. Living from this place of deep appreciation is key to deep meaning and purpose. It is the awakening to the reality of the goodness in your life and work, which is a new and healthier attitude for most doctors.

Celebrating actually encompasses both an inner and an outer component. The outer component of celebrating is the tangible expression of regard, respect, recognition, and acknowledgment of others with whom we live and work. We celebrate others by giving full expression to our appreciation of them, their contribution, their talents, their strengths, and their purpose. This comes from an open heart with unconditional regard for colleagues. This ability to celebrate others is closely linked to one's ability to celebrate oneself, which is the inner component of celebrating. This inner component is the deep gratitude for the goodness in the universe, your personal gifts, and the goodness in your life and work. Experiencing the awe and wonder of life positions you for a deeper fulfillment of your life's purpose.

Celebrating requires consciousness. Telling your story of growth is an important expression of celebrating. Cynical stories, on the other hand, deplete you and are disempowering. This reinforces negative realities in your world, distancing you from your noble purpose. You can't ignore your negative stories, but you can rewrite them. Even the most traumatic experiences of loss contain the seeds of new learning and growth. I realize how easy this is to say and yet how difficult it is to do when the life-changing loss belongs to you. However, it can improve the lives of all concerned.

Dr. S. was a resident in psychiatry and had married prior to beginning her residency. She was full of hope about her new career. She became pregnant during both her second and fourth years of residency, giving birth to first a girl, then a boy. Becoming a mother added new meaning and tremendous joy to her life. Like all parents, she had high hopes for a life filled with joy for her beloved children. Unfortunately, when her daughter became age three and then four, it became increasingly obvious that she was not achieving key developmental milestones. Dr. S. took her daughter for evaluation by a team of experts at her local school district's evaluation unit. Once the evaluation was complete, Dr. S. learned that her daughter had a severe form of autism. The team recommended immediate intervention for Dr. S.'s daughter, but they also suggested evaluation of her son because of the increased risk of autism in siblings of those affected. After her son's evaluation, Dr. S. was devastated to learn that both of her children had autism and would never lead a normal life. She grieved for the devastating losses this news carried for her precious children, for herself, and for her family.

Now, when Dr. S. looks back on this experience in her life and the lives of her children, she tells quite a different story. "My children have been a unique and special gift in my life and to the world. Each one has special gifts that are unique to them and not commonly seen in most other people. In spite of the fact that each one has had to deal with a great deal of hardship, including teasing, exclusion, and the breakup of the family, they are remarkably gifted, warm, and loving individuals. We have always been, and continue to be, very close. I celebrate, and am grateful for, these two adored human beings, who have been a true blessing and have brought so much love and meaning to my life."

As you can see, powerful celebrating has you looking with an appreciative eye for the good in others and in the situation.

In summary, the essentials of celebrating include the following:

- Be conscious of what you have been doing and who you have been that helps to advance your purpose.
- Allow yourself to take in and experience gratitude for your strengths, gifts, and accomplishments.
- Actively celebrate those gifts and accomplishments.
- Acknowledge the gifts and accomplishments of others and honor their personhood.

Celebrating discussion questions

- What is the relation between celebrating and the character strength of gratitude?
- What is the difference between celebrating one's gifts and accomplishments and bragging or being boastful?
- How is celebrating related to the fulfillment of extraordinary noble purpose?
- Does celebrating exclude the possibility of sadness and loss in one's life? Why or why not?
- Dr. Y. is a medical oncologist who treats primarily cancer patients. Dr. Z. is a geriatrician who treats primarily the frail elderly. What role might celebrating play in each of their lives, given their practices?

Celebrating in your daily routine

Choose one of the following suggested processes for integrating celebrating into your daily routine:

- Affirmation: Create an affirmation that emphasizes or strengthens the concept of celebrating. For example, "I experience great gratitude for my gifts of intelligence, insight, and empathy, which allow me to deliver compassionate healing and pain relief to patients." Write the affirmation on a 3 × 5 file card and carry it with you throughout the day. Repeat the affirmation prior to leaving home for work, prior to lunch, prior to leaving work, and prior to retiring at the end of the day.

- Anchoring activity: Explore celebrating by expressing your appreciation to one colleague or coworker weekly in the following manner:

  - Recall the details of what they did or said that made a difference to you.
  - Contact the colleague and arrange a time to meet.
  - Tell your colleague what he or she did that you valued so highly and why you are so appreciative.

- Journaling activity: In a relaxed and quiet space, consider your greatest gifts. What are they? What is it that you just can't help but provide to those with whom you work and those you care for? What would your closest friends and colleagues identify as your greatest gifts? Write in your journal the thoughts that come to mind regarding your gifts and strengths. Make sure you have come up with a minimum of three or four gifts or strengths. Allow yourself to bask in the wonder of these strengths. Consider what life would look like if you consistently lived out of these gifts. Record the responses in your journal.
- Celebrating through aesthetic experience: Different forms of aesthetic expression can be used to heighten your awareness and understanding of celebrating. Find a favorite piece of music that exemplifies the different aspects of celebrating in your heart and mind and listen to it often. A favorite poem that you can read often or a favorite piece of art that you can view that evokes the qualities of celebrating works equally well. For me, the "Gloria" movement from the "Mass in B-Minor" by J. S. Bach evokes deep feelings of celebration. I often listen to it when I want to remind myself of the importance of celebrating in my life.

Letting go

Letting go is about becoming aware of, and releasing, emotions that are blocking access to your essential self. Because life is not a linear process, the noble purpose process exists as a spiral through which we are continuously evolving. It is when we find ourselves getting stuck in our boundedness or avoiding a difficult or painful situation, that work on letting go is needed. The bounded self is focused on superficiality, control, and approval. Letting go involves the release of such desperate clutching, fear, and the need for power, control, and approval.

Similar to celebrating, letting go has both an inner and an outer level of understanding. At the outer level, letting go is entering into and resolving difficult or painful situations with others with whom you interact in life and work. This includes relinquishing the need to safeguard and protect oneself, and allowing complete freedom and openness with others. The benefits of this outer level of letting go are multiple, as you will learn in other chapters, as the resultant positive emotions and positive relationships have been linked with longer life and increased flourishing.

At the inner level, letting go is the understanding and releasing of pain associated with a personal wounding, whether that wounding is from a past childhood experience or a recent experience with a coworker. This is accomplished through a process of becoming conscious of the feelings and surrendering to the painful emotions. Allow your feelings to have space, and notice what is happening in your body at the same time. Record your feelings in a journal or discuss them with a trusted friend. You will find that when you accept the dissonance fully as an event over which you had no control and for which you had no responsibility, it becomes part of the past. You are no longer the victim of it nor are you compelled to act out your resistance to it. Instead, it becomes a learning and growth experience from which you gain wisdom. Thus, through letting go, you release bounded behaviors.

Letting go is a crucial part of the noble purpose spiral. At least two major negative outcomes may result from resisting a major dissonance in one's life. To avoid the dissonant situation, you inadvertently give it a central role in your life as you go out of your way to avoid any situation that remotely resembles the initial wounding or deals with the individuals involved. Both you and your life become immobilized, restricted, and disempowered.

The second possible negative outcome, which is seen far more commonly in physicians, is that you tenaciously work to go beyond or compensate for your dissonance or wounding. You become superman or superwoman in an effort to overcome and get beyond your pain and imagined inadequacies. For example, a child who was always made to feel second-best and not as smart as his older brother grew into an adult who has to be an academic "hero," first in his class, and to always know all the answers at all times and at all costs. While the tenacity is a testament to the human capacity to get beyond any obstacle, the great price of such behavior is depletion and separation from one's essential nature, purpose, goodness, and significant relationships with others.

In conclusion, a summary of letting-go actions includes the following:

- Identify your conflicts from both childhood and the present, allowing yourself to completely feel these feelings.
- Be aware of episodes of withdrawal into your bounded behaviors, the need for approval, the fear of failure, and other dissonant behaviors.
- Notice, as well, when you begin to use power, control, and manipulation and become aware of the fear that is provoking these tendencies; fully feel the fear without resisting it.
- Communicate authentically with others, without melodrama, disclosing your true feelings and providing constructive feedback.

Letting-go discussion questions

- Dr. X. is a resident in internal medicine. He loves his work, and he enjoys interacting with patients and families. However, every night that his team is on call, he avoids taking any admissions with neurologic problems and hands these off to another team member, using various excuses for the handoff. How might letting go be helpful to Dr. X. in this situation?

- When Dr. R. went through medical school and residency training in OB-GYN, she felt she had become hardened by the fact that "everyone was quick to point out what I was doing wrong, and no one seemed to care about all of the things I did that were right." Now, she finds that she constantly looks for approval from others in both her personal and her professional life, feeling insecure when it is not forthcoming. As her trusted friend, she asks you for help and guidance. How might you advise her?

- St. Francis is a large suburban health network that has been slowly acquiring most of the local private physician practices. Dr. W. and his partners sold their practice to St. Francis, fearing they could not compete with the rapidly growing network. Since the acquisition, Dr. W. has felt increasingly burned out, seeing many more patients in a day than he did before and than he feels is safe. He feels disrespected by the practice manager who was placed in position by St. Francis, but Dr. W. has silently tolerated all of these changes for two years, feeling helpless. The situation has begun to take a toll on his health and his homelife, in addition to his sense of joy and purpose at work. Why might Dr. W. feel helpless? Is Dr. W. helpless? What can he do to help himself? How can Dr. W. help himself through good communication and positive relationships, instead of silence and withdrawal?

Letting go in your daily routine

Choose one of the following suggested processes for integrating letting go into your daily routine:

- Affirmation: Create an affirmation that emphasizes or strengthens any aspect of the letting-go process and that will aid you in your journey to meaning and purpose. For example, "I let go of all fear, anxiety, worry, or concern about my noble purpose, knowing that the fruits of my gifts and my open heart can powerfully effect change in the world." Write your affirmation on a 3 × 5 index card and carry it with you. Repeat the affirmation before leaving for work in the morning,

before going to lunch, immediately prior to leaving work for home, and just prior
to retiring for sleep at night.

- Ritual: Take a notebook-size piece of paper and fold it in half lengthwise. In a
  quiet place, contemplate your essential self and the noble purpose that is already
  deep within yourself. As you do this, notice any feelings of tension, lack of ease,
  or any blockages that you are experiencing. List these tensions on the left-hand
  side of your paper. These tensions and dis-ease represent sources of frustration and
  worry. On the right-hand side, next to each tension, write the frustration or worry
  associated with it. With a scissors, cut each tension-and-worry pair into a separate
  strip of paper. In a fireplace, ritually burn each individual strip of paper. As you
  light each paper identifying a frustration or blockage, allow yourself to release all
  tension and worry related to that doubt or roadblock. Do this until all pieces of
  paper are burned and all tension is safely released.

- Journaling activity: What is the greatest obstacle or frustration that is blocking you
  from your deep meaning and purpose? Allow yourself to fully bring this obstacle
  to mind, including the disappointment, worry, concern, or anger you feel about it.
  Journal about these feelings, including how they might relate to key dissonances
  in your life. Now, try to view the obstacle in a different light. How has it been an
  opportunity? How has it promoted growth, creativity, or wisdom within you? Write
  a second paragraph about the opportunities and gifts that have come as a result of the
  frustration. Now, think about actions, both actions that diminish or eliminate the
  frustration and actions that make your noble purpose a reality. Write a list of actions
  you can take to overcome your obstacles and bring your noble purpose to the world.

- Increasing awareness of letting go through aesthetic appreciation: Different forms of
  aesthetic expression can be used to heighten and help you explore emotions related to
  letting go. Find a piece of music, a poem, a movie, a work of art, or any artistic creation
  that exemplifies letting go to you. Exposing yourself to that work of art, and opening
  your mind and heart to its message will help to enhance letting go in your daily life.

Noble purpose

The process that has been described thus far in this chapter is about realizing your potential
and your calling, your meaning and purpose, by working through the different phases of a
spiral we have called the *noble purpose spiral*. The spiral and process is highlighted as noble
because it focuses on the generous giving to and serving of others, bountifully reciprocating
and inspiring high-level purpose and meaning in life and work while taking care of oneself.
One's calling and potential become clear through embracing the qualities of the spiral.

We know from research on optimal work performance that when you are fully engaged in the expression of your unique gifts, time seems to disappear (Csikszentmihalyi, 1990). The ego seems to vanish, and craft and person harmonize in perfect consonance their joyful song of service to others.

Noble purpose involves the perfect marriage of both serving oneself and serving others. When you discover and live your noble purpose, your physical health and well-being flourish. As you learned in chapter 1, an overwhelmingly large percentage of physicians suffer from burnout and exhaustion (40–60%). The remedy for exhaustion is personal renewal, feeling fully alive, and the passion that comes from having meaning and purpose in your life and work.

It is not unusual to, at times, feel removed or distanced from your noble purpose. Not only is this expected, but also it can be beneficial. Once you understand that this arid space can be nurturing and mysterious, allowing the discomfort and dissonance to flow in and through you can be generative of new ideas and new directions.

The culmination of your breakthrough to your essential self is the discovery of your noble purpose. The following three exercises will assist you in formulating your noble purpose statement. For each of these exercises, it is advisable to take adequate time and space to complete it in a relaxed manner. A quiet place is ideal, perhaps accompanied by calming music that creates a contemplative mood.

Before completing the exercises, it might be helpful to review your prior journaling regarding the five phases of the spiral, so as to be fully present and participating from your essential self and with an open heart.

Exercise 1

Draw two vertical lines down your journal page or notepad, creating three separate columns. Title the first column "Noble Purpose Figure," the second "Noble Purpose Contribution," and the third "Learning."

Begin with the first column. Reflect on individuals in life whom you regard highly. This includes those you respect greatly because of positive contributions or what you have learned from them. These can be family members, friends, colleagues, wisdom figures, heroes, famous people, or mythic figures. Make your list as complete as possible, listing one name per line. Feel free to continue to add names as you continue the exercise.

Now close your eyes and fully relax. Take a deep breath in and blow it out, letting go of all tension. When you feel relaxed, turn your attention to the second column. In this column, next to each name, record in two to three words the contribution you associate with each noble purpose figure. For example, for daughter Mary, it might be "fun-loving and generous." Be sure to look beyond the role played by each of these figures to their actual essences as human beings. As you complete this, become aware of any tension that is developing in your body. Take a moment to release it with some deep breathing.

Move on to the third column, and write there the lesson you have learned from each of your noble purpose figures. Keep in mind that what you learned from them might differ from their contribution to society or your life.

When you have completed the three columns, go to a blank page in your journal. What have you learned through completing this exercise? How does what you learned reflect on your own noble purpose? Take as much time as you need to consider and journal about these questions.

Exercise 2

Now choose the single noble purpose figure whose teaching or contribution stands out the most for you. On a new page of your journal, reflect on this individual with regard to the aspects of the noble purpose spiral discussed in this chapter:
- initiating: trust in the goodness of life and sense of belonging;
- visioning: ability to reveal new possibilities;
- claiming: commitment to realizing results;
- celebrating: capacity to fully appreciate and be grateful for life and work; and
- letting go: ability to release power or control, and to discuss negative feelings.

Add anything else that comes to you with regard to this noble purpose role model that relates to your high regard for him or her.

Now, take a deep breath, relax, and contemplate that you share the same remarkable traits and characteristics, zeal, and relationship to the world that your role model possesses. Understand that, to a large extent, you embody the greatness you so admire in your role model. Reread everything you wrote in your journal about your noble purpose role model and about all other noble purpose figures you listed in exercise 1. Accept these positive aspects of your noble purpose figures as your own, taking them deep into your heart and mind. As you do this, record any feelings and realizations that come to mind. What have you learned about yourself? Answer this question in your journal.

Exercise 3

With the learning obtained from exercises 1 and 2, complete the following steps using a new page in your journal:

- Express your noble purpose in a few words as an affirmative statement about your intended contribution, using an action verb.

- Try to expand your statement beyond your immediate job or role in the world.
- Begin with a statement of purpose, for example, "My purpose is to serve the elderly with compassion, presence, and encouragement." In the case of the author (B.H.), the statement is, "My purpose is to foster deep belonging, unbridled freedom, and service in the workplace."

Once you have finalized your statement, write it on a 3 × 5 file card that you can carry with you; refer to it throughout your day.

Work on meaning and purpose is a wonderful journey of deep learning and self-knowledge, discovering and embracing the essential self. This journey often takes time, patience, and helpful guidance. Thus, the work introduced in the chapter material above is only a beginning. Particularly for those who have never been guided through purpose-based work before, additional learning, particularly with a knowledgeable guide, is recommended. We invite you into a special section on the Creating Positive Health Web site, where opportunities for continuing and further work on meaning and purpose can be found. Access to this site is available at www.creatingpositivehealth.com, under meaning and purpose.

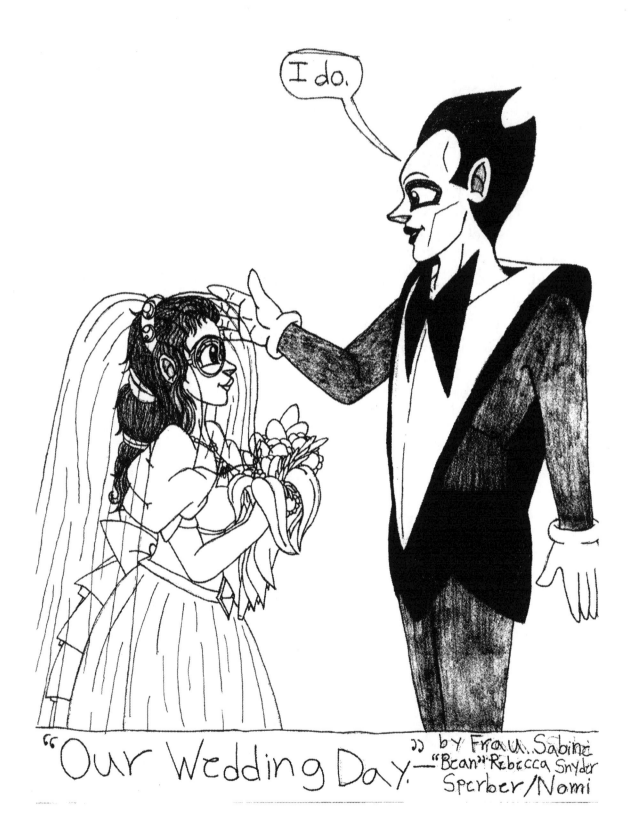

Chapter 9

Positive Relationships

In 2011 Dr. Martin Seligman introduced his well-being theory, a replacement for his former authentic happiness theory. In well-being theory, Seligman posits five primary aspects of human well-being, for which he created the acronym PERMA (see chapter 3 in this book for a more complete review of this topic). In PERMA, each letter signifies one of the five primary aspects of well-being. The "R" of PERMA signifies positive relationships, which is the focus of this chapter. Seligman has stated that very little that is positive is solitary, and that other people are the best antidote to the downs of life and the single most reliable up (2011, p. 20). Seligman further notes that doing a kindness for others produces the single most reliable momentary increase in well-being of any exercise his group has tested (2011, p. 20). If all of that is true, one wonders how doctors and medical students, who continuously work around people in a helping profession, could be so lacking in well-being and so high in burnout, depression. and other associated problems and stresses.

In this chapter we will look at the importance of positive relationships, including various theories of what makes them successful and health-giving. The value of this information is clear and will be reinforced throughout the chapter. Positive relationships are consistently associated with good health and increased happiness, which, in turn, promote success and satisfaction both at work and in one's personal life.

Dr. Christopher Peterson, a prominent thought and research leader in positive psychology, often summed up the field in three words: "Other people matter." (2006, p. 249).The capacity to love and be loved is an inherently human tendency from infancy through old age that results in improved health and well-being. Large-scale epidemiologic studies have demonstrated that social isolation, on the other hand, is associated with a substantial increase in all-cause mortality risk. Further, poor-quality relationships or lack of social ties is associated with poorer functioning in the cardiovascular, immune, and endocrine systems (2006). Thus, both the empirical data as well as common experience support the idea that forming and maintaining stable and positive relationships is a crucial component of health and well-being. Processes that can promote high-quality relationships and support well-being will be discussed later in this chapter.

There is a clear neurochemical basis underlying the capacity for love and positive relationships in humans. For example, the release of the hormone oxytocin from the posterior pituitary occurs in response to social contact and touch, and plays a particularly prominent role during childbirth and early infancy. Oxytocin has been linked to the creation of bonding behavior between two individuals. The neurochemical root of this behavior emphasizes the primary importance of positive relationships in human well-being. In addition, as you may recall from chapter 2, oxytocin is one of the positive biological health assets that contribute to an overall state of positive health. If oxytocin is released and increased with positive social contact, then positive relationships become a direct contributor to positive health!

Among the most valued resources exchanged in a positive relationship is social support, or how others help us cope with stressful or challenging events. Social support actually includes several different types of positive support. Appraisal support is that which includes constructive feedback and affirmation of our ideas and actions. Emotional support is the empathy, trust, and caring we receive from those who are close to us. Informational support includes advice and helpful suggestions, and instrumental support is the contribution of tangible aid and service in times of need. Unwanted and negative advice and suggestions obviously do not qualify as support. It is easy to see how positive social support can buffer against the effects of stress and be linked to good health.

However, research has also shown that perceived social support, that is, the perception that one has supportive others who would be available in times of need, is also consistently associated with good health. In fact, studies have linked perceived social support with positive health and well-being, decreased incidence of anxiety and depression during stressful events, positive adjustment to illness, and decreased heart rate and blood pressure during a stressful speech task (Gable & Gosnell, 2011). Exactly how this effect occurs is uncertain, although theories of its efficacy vary from a direct effect of social integration in a large social network to a buffering model, in which effective support protects an individual from the negative effects of stressful events when they do occur. This is because high levels of perceived social support can decrease the number of perceived stressors and calm reactions to those stressors. The presence or perception of friends can alter the perception of challenges, making those challenges more manageable. The perception that problems are manageable is associated with an improved sense of self-efficacy: "My problems are manageable, and I am strong enough to manage them." (Gable & Gosnell, 2011).

Even with only the perception of social support, problems and challenges become far more manageable, and your trust and confidence in your ability to handle those challenges increases substantially. This clearly points out how important positive relationships can be in a high-stress profession such as medicine, or in a high-stress situation, such as being an ill patient in a hospital. It is unfortunate, therefore, that the medical culture has consistently emphasized competition, which has given rise to a culture of abuse and bullying (see chapter 1). This clearly needs to change in order to eliminate the epidemic of burnout and ill-being among physicians at all career levels. For example, adopting a collaborative and team-based learning approach from the very first year of medical training would set the stage for the development of positive working relationships, social support, and the important skill of learning to work in medical teams (see chapter 15).

Positive relationships with others favorably impact aspects of the good life other than those already described. For example, pleasures are enhanced in the presence of friends and loved ones. Married people tend to score higher on measures of life satisfaction than do their single counterparts.

Positive relationships come in many different forms. Two people can enjoy a monogamous intimate loving relationship, a friendship, a business relationship, an affiliation, membership in a common group, or a family tie, to name a few. Positive relationships can involve two people or groups of people.

A friendship is a relationship of respect, mutual liking, mutual perception of similarity, and expectations of reciprocity and equality. Consistent with other positive relationships, having friends positively correlates with life satisfaction and well-being.

Christopher Peterson describes an unpublished study that he performed with Tracy Steen (Peterson C., 2006, p. 266). They examined the phenomenon of "best friends" in a study in which 289 respondents, mostly middle-aged and college-educated Americans, answered a series of questions about an individual in their lives they would describe as a best friend. Ninety-seven percent of the respondents affirmed that they had had a best friend at some point during their lifetime, and 76 percent remained best friends at the time of the study.

In some cases, these friendships had been lifelong, having been formed in childhood. In this study, best friends tended to be close in age and of the same gender, although some cross-gender best friendships were noted as well. These relationships were described as sustained and reciprocal, and were marked by shared positive emotions. Words that were used to describe best friends included dependable, honest, loyal, committed, kind, loving, playful, and fun. Most respondents felt that their best friend tended to bring out their own best self (Peterson C., 2006, p. 267).

Adults in marriages, similar to adults in friendships, are physically and emotionally healthier than their single counterparts, statistically speaking. These benefits are greater for males overall than they are for females. On the other side of that reality, nearly 50 percent of all marriages end in divorce in the United States. Divorce is a painful and disruptive experience, and we see an increase in depression, alcohol abuse, and physical illness occurring in its aftermath (Peterson C., 2006, p. 270).

The experience of intense love that forms the basis of deep connections between significant others is a phenomenon experienced as highly positive, and yet one that tends to be filled with emotional highs and lows, at least in part due to the deep emotional investment of each partner in the other and the emotional risks and benefits of that investment. This creates a question of interest: What portion of this web of feelings is actually love, versus, for example, self-protection due to vulnerability?

Dr. Barbara Fredrickson, a positive psychologist who has done extensive research in the area of positive emotions and positive relationships, theorizes that the love we crave as humans occurs within momentary and limited experiences of connection with another or others. These moments are mind-expanding, allowing participants to become more aware, more knowledgeable, more resilient, more socially integrated, and healthier. In other words, they broaden and build, setting off upward spirals of growth that allow participants to blossom into better individuals (Fredrickson, 2013).

In Fredrickson's theory, love can blossom anytime two or more individuals, even strangers, connect over a shared positive emotion, whether it is mild or strong (2013). This connection over a shared positive emotion results in the momentary creation of a swell of positive resonance among participants. This "positivity resonance" consists of shared positive emotions, biobehavioral synchrony, and patterns of mutual care. Positivity resonance involves mirroring the joy and good feelings in one another's emotions, gestures, neurochemistry, and caring impulses. Each becomes a reflection and extension of the other. Fredrickson explains that love unfolds and reverberates between and among people—within interpersonal transactions—and, thereby, belongs to all parties involved, though temporarily (2013, p. 17). Positive relationships, as described by Fredrickson, tend to emerge in certain circumstances, particularly those in which there is a perception of safety, as well as a sensory and temporal connection.

One of my most memorable experiences of positivity resonance occurred over thirteen years ago at a continuing medical education seminar for physicians that I attended in Cape Cod, Massachusetts. Unlike most typical continuing medical education offerings, this one was a five half-day workshop with a class size limited to twenty-five participants. The workshop was presented and led by Dr. Barry Heermann, an expert in spirit-based team building and servant leadership, on the subject of team spirit (see chapter 15). The atmosphere created by Dr. Heermann over the five days was one of safety, deep sharing, and a mutually shared spirit of excellent service to patients. With an abundance of open discussion, working together in pairs and groups to vision the ideal multidisciplinary health-care team to deliver that outstanding service, the entire group became very strongly connected. The result was the development of a deep closeness among all participants in that workshop. On the final day, many tears were shed as we said good-bye to one another and prepared to go our separate ways. I believe that although some of those tears were tears of sadness, most were tears of gratitude for the love and growth we experienced together as a group.

In her theory of love and positivity resonance, Fredrickson highlights the neurochemical underpinnings of this phenomenon. Love is associated with increased release of oxytocin (principally from the posterior pituitary) into the bloodstream. Traveling throughout the body, oxytocin leads to an increase in bonding behavior, such as increased eye contact and greater responsiveness to the smiles of others. Increased levels of oxytocin also create an increased sensitivity to environmental cues that are linked to positive social connections (Fredrickson, 2013).

Oxytocin also affects the amygdala, an area of the brain that is linked to the processing of emotions. Oxytocin affects the amygdala by calming fears that might steer one away from social interactions, particularly with strangers.

Incredibly, that is far from the end of the amazing roles played by oxytocin in our well-being! As was noted above, one of the three important aspects of positivity resonance is biobehavioral synchrony. It has been shown that one individual's oxytocin flow and discharge can trigger the discharge and flow of oxytocin in a partner in a biochemical synchrony that supports mutual engagement, care, and responsiveness (Fredrickson, 2013).

The wonder of how the emotions, the body, and well-being fit together goes further. A high level of oxytocin is not the only positive biological health asset that increases love and is increased by love. Those individuals who experience the most positivity resonance have also been found to demonstrate significant increases in heart-rate variability (due to increases in vagal tone), which is yet another positive biological health asset. High vagal tone independently fosters an openness and receptivity to love and positive synchrony. Therefore, love, by Fredrickson's definition, creates better health! (2013, pp. 84-86).

Despite all the scientific knowledge available on the causal connections between positive relationships and good health, experts in doctors' health continue to scratch their heads at the ever-increasing rate of burnout and ill-being among physicians in a competition-based and adversarial culture that, seemingly, no one wants to deal with or change. Even today, as many as 80 percent of medical students report being affected by some form of harassment or bullying, even victimization (see chapter 1 of this book). In addition, the divorce rate among physicians remains high, symptomatic of the high stress within medical marriages. What skills are physicians lacking? What are we not being taught? What distorted sense of priorities is reinforcing this unhealthy and unproductive behavior?

Because the process of getting into medical school is highly competitive, future doctors begin early to prioritize work and success in their lives. Once they are accepted into a medical school, they are suddenly competing with "the best of the best" in a system that teaches, "You need to get that top residency position," and then the top fellowship position. Then the emphasis might switch to getting a top faculty position, publishing more papers, earning more money, gaining more prestige, and so on throughout a doctor's career. The obvious message is that career success must be a top priority at all costs and that your fellow doctors are the competition keeping you from your goal. The resulting isolation and deprivation is a perfect setup for developing burnout, stress, and depression. The likelihood of any positive relationships taking hold is poor. Viewing your colleagues in this negative light results in a self-protective attitude toward others. Further, the macho doctor image of working twenty-four hours around the clock without food, sleep, family, or friends teaches physicians that relationships, in general, are of secondary importance. Therefore, doctors lose connection with their patients, their friends and family, and, ultimately, with themselves. This unrealistic and unproductive system of values instilled in physicians helps no one, and hurts many, including the doctor and the many patients he or she might have helped had he or she remained healthy.

Some forward-thinking and progressive medical schools are beginning to challenge this unhelpful approach to medical education by providing rotations in which students are able to form extended relationships with a family doctor and his or her stable group of patients over time. We can see that building positive relationships, at least in part, requires a series of skills that can be taught. It also requires values and priorities that honor the importance of relationships in one's personal and professional life, so that one's time, attention, and energy can be focused on developing and maintaining them.

The remainder of this chapter will be devoted to viewing two different models of positive relationships, minding theory and active-constructive responding. These are offered for their illustrative and skill-building value. Their principles can be applied to both personal and professional positive relationships.

"MINDING" IN RELATIONSHIPS

The theory known as *minding* in close relationships is aimed at developing and enhancing closeness between two individuals over time. Minding can be defined as a reciprocal knowing process that occurs in an ongoing fashion, involving a complexity of interrelated thoughts, feelings, and behaviors (Harvey & Pauwels, 2009).

There are two major components to a relationship in minding theory. The first is a focus on gaining information about your relationship partner and then taking action that reflects a positive response to the information you have obtained. Thus, knowing and allowing oneself to be known at a deep and intimate level is of key importance in minding. This open exchange of information, ideas, thoughts, and feelings early in a relationship encourages and facilitates the building of trust and confidence in one another and in the relationship itself, which can then continue to grow over time. It also avoids the holding back of important information for fear that it might be unacceptable or judged negatively by the relationship partner. However, it is important to point out that the emphasis in the minding relationship is on actively seeking self-expression from the other, not on expressing oneself. This overt desire to truly know and focus on the other is what encourages and allows for more and better communication.

It is extremely difficult to demonstrate a genuine focus on, and desire to know, another, be it a patient in a hospital or a loved one at home, when one is stressed, rushed, exhausted, or preoccupied. This is why the doctor who takes a rushed ten-minute history, standing at the foot of the bed, making no eye contact, and asking question after question will not make a connection with his or her patient and will likely not get an accurate history. Actively seeking self-expression in another requires one's total presence. This means you are comfortably seated, with your mind and heart fully focused on this wonderful opportunity of interacting with another human being. You create the space for the other's self-expression by opening your mind, focusing your attention on him or her, being silent to give the patient space to express himself or herself, and occasionally asking open-ended questions or offering encouragement to show empathy and care. This concept is also extremely important in marriage and other personal relationships. However, at the end of a long workday when we come home exhausted, how many of us remember to take time to give this personal focus to our family members? If you do not take the time habitually, start today to change your habits. Both you and your loved ones will benefit.

The second important relationship component in the minding model is relationship-enhancing attributions. Relationship-enhancing attributions are those that assume positive motivations to dispositional causes. For example, today is Dr. X.'s birthday, and she has taken the day off to celebrate with some well-deserved rest and relaxation. Her husband, who usually comes home at 6:00 p.m., surprises her and shows up at the house at 4:00 p.m. She immediately assumes, "My husband came home from work early today in order to celebrate my birthday and spend more time with me."

Enhancing this positive thought is the assumption that negative behaviors, when they do occur, can be attributed to external and unavoidable causes, thereby giving the other person the benefit of the doubt. Thus, a week later, when Dr. X. and her husband had arranged a dinner date at a mutually loved restaurant on Friday at 7:00 p.m. and she was late getting home from work, Mr. X. assumed, "My wife was late for our date because she had car trouble." (Harvey & Pauwels, 2009).

It is easy to see how actively seeking the other's self-expression and relationship-enhancing attributions can be helpful in both professional and personal relationships. However, this requires some investment of time and energy, and must, therefore, be given a high priority if it is to occur. The rewards of that investment are great in both personal and professional arenas, possibly lifesaving in the professional arena.

Imagine for a moment that you are a patient in the hospital. You are sick, scared, in pain, your condition is worsening, and yet no one is sure what is wrong with you. Dr. Jones enters your room suddenly and with rapid steps. It is quite obvious that she is in a hurry based upon her rapid-fire questions and the tone of her voice. She stands at the foot of your bed, making little, if any, eye contact. Once her specific questions are answered, she immediately leaves your room. You feel even more isolated and frightened, particularly because very few of her questions were related to your pain, and you feel as if no one cares what is happening to you or has even the smallest desire to accurately diagnose your condition. About an hour later, Dr. Smith comes to visit you. Dr. Smith is another member of the team of doctors assigned to your care. He comes into the room and comfortably sits down in the chair that is closest to the head of your bed, after introducing himself and asking your permission to sit down. Dr. Smith makes immediate and continuous eye contact with you. He touches your arm lightly and invites you to explain, in your own words, the recent changes in your health and how he might be of help. He acknowledges your pain and anxiety, offering his pledge that the team will be devoting their attention and resources to uncovering your diagnosis so treatment can begin. He focuses on your story of your illness as you tell it, giving reassurance and acknowledgement, and asking occasional guiding questions. Ultimately, both doctors spent about fifteen or twenty minutes with you. Who, do you think, has a more accurate and informed view of your illness? How do you, as the patient, feel about each of these physicians?

In addition to the two major components of the minding relationship discussed above, other positive emotions and behaviors are also important relationship tools. Acceptance and respect are important in minding relationships and in all close, positive relationships. As we all know, no human being is ideal or perfect in all ways. Acceptance is coming to know the aspects of another that, to us, are less than ideal, and respecting that individuals have differences and weaknesses, and yet are still worthy of our honor and love. Positive behaviors that support an atmosphere of acceptance and respect include such things as listening respectfully to each others' needs and opinions, working out compromises that are considerate of both individuals' needs, and being respectful of the other's feelings during conflicts while trying to resolve them. Relationships that lack acceptance and respect, in which pervasive criticism, contempt, defensiveness, and poor communication prevail, have little chance of long-term survival.

Forgiveness is another important aspect of the minding relationship. Even the most satisfying relationships and the closest friendships will encounter misunderstandings or stressful events that lead to confusion or mistrust. Forgiveness allows a relationship to survive such a stressor and, once again, thrive.

There is a strong sense of equality and reciprocity in a minded relationship. It involves the sharing of affection, respect, quality time, support, and assistance, when needed and requested. Also key in relationships is appreciation. Appreciation includes providing genuine positive feedback and expressing deep thanks and gratitude for the wonderful gift that you share. Although expressing gratitude is a strength that comes more easily to some than to others (see chapter 6 on character strengths), it is an important strength to nurture in promoting one's well-being and nurturing one's relationships (Seligman, 2011).

The minding relationship model highlights the importance of prioritizing relationships as a focus of time and energy investment, encouraging open communication and positive attribution, encouraging your partner's communication, and honoring the information you learn from your partner.

I am sure it is not surprising to learn that good communication is a key part of many different theories and models of positive relationships. After all, it is through communication that we can explore areas that we have in common, share feelings, share stories, and form many of the bonds that we share with another. Although we know that positive social connections at work, home, and elsewhere figure prominently in our well-being, it is the close relationships characterized by mutual understanding, caring, and validation that generate the most happiness.

Active-constructive responding

Social connections at work, at home, and in other aspects of our lives figure prominently in our well-being. As noted above, close relationships characterized by mutual understanding, caring, and validation tend to generate the most happiness. These relationships offer security in which partners can share intimate details about themselves and can count on one another for support. Secure attachments of this nature have multiple benefits. They include greater physical and emotional health, an increased sense of self-worth, lower blood pressure, a stronger immune system, longer life, and increased well-being, generativity, and creativity. They also guard against indecisiveness, burnout at work, and difficulties dealing with stress.

Interestingly, a partner's positive response to good news (referred to as capitalization) is actually a better predictor of relationship well-being than any support given in response to bad news (Gable, Gonzaga, & Strachman, 2006). This successful technique, described by Dr. Shelly Gable, is called active-constructive responding. It involves responding enthusiastically, asking positive questions, and sharing in another person's joy. By doing so, you help the teller of the good news to bask in his or her good fortune, while your active-constructive response confirms to the teller the importance of the event and its implications to you as well as to him or her. Further, it demonstrates your intimate knowledge of, and caring about, the partner.

Exchanges of this type increase positive emotions in both partners (coworkers, friends) and generate greater satisfaction with the relationship. They also lead to a decrease in daily conflicts and an increase in relationship trust, and result in the ability and desire to engage as a pair in additional enjoyable activities on a daily basis. Relationship research has shown that, in men, only perceived responsiveness to positive event disclosure predicted future relationship health. The partner's response to negative events had no bearing whatsoever. In women, on the other hand, perceived responsiveness to both negative and positive events was important for relationship well-being, but only responsiveness to positive events predicted future relationship health (Gable, Reis, Impett, & Asher, 2004).

There are four possible ways that people respond when others share good news, talk about a positive experience, or describe a success. Of the four, only one, active-constructive response, leads to stronger secure relationships. The positive experience can be either big or small. It is important to remember that the bearer of the good news is the one who determines the meaning of the experience. You, as the listener, are there to positively reflect on, and amplify, your partner's celebration and joy.

Table 9-1: The Four Possible Responses to a Capitalization Experience

	Constructive	Destructive
Active	Authentic interest, elaborates experience; person feels validated and understood	Squashing the event, brings conversation to a halt; person feels ashamed, embarrassed, guilty, or angry
Passive	Quiet, understated support; conversation fizzles out; person feels unimportant, misunderstood, embarrassed, or guilty	Ignoring the event; conversation never starts; person feels confused, guilty, or disappointed

Active-constructive responding is not inauthentic cheerleading. It must be authentic happiness for the teller's good news. Body language, facial expression, and affect must be consistent with your words. Your response should be properly attuned to the needs of the teller. It is important to modulate your response so that it feels comfortable to both you and the teller.

Demonstration of active-constructive responding

This is a conversation between two good friends, Mary and Bob.
Bob: "Hey, Mary, my wife called and told me she got a great job."
Mary's responses using each response style are below.

	Constructive	Destructive
Active	That's great! What is the new job? When does it start? What did she say about it? How are you planning to celebrate?	So, who is going to let your dogs out so they don't pee in the house? With two incomes, I bet you'll be in a higher tax bracket!
Passive	That's nice. (Yawns.) Boy, am I tired.	My sister called yesterday. Just wait until you hear what she's been up to!

Of all the possible responses to a capitalization opportunity, only active-constructive responses validate the discloser and demonstrate caring and affective investment in the relationship. Close relationship partners are often active participants in each other's personal development and goal pursuit through affirmation of the partner's "ideal self." Partner affirmations are, in turn, associated with personal well-being and high relationship quality. Thus, the time and effort you invest in active-constructive responses to capitalization opportunities rebounds to your benefit in well-being and high-quality relationships.

Group discussion questions

- According to Dr. Barbara Frederickson's definition of love, how does love create better health and thriving?
- You have just been appointed Dean of X University School of Medicine. One of your top priorities is to change the culture of the medical school to one that emphasizes positive relationships. What is the first and most important change you would make?
- How do the principles of minding theory impact the medical marriage that is now at risk and in danger of dissolving?
- Why is it important to include group discussion as part of this learning process?

Small group exploration

- Divide into groups of three. This is a role-playing exercise in which the three roles are observer, teller, and responder. The individual in the role of the teller has a discussion with his or her dear friend, the responder. The discussion involves the telling of a piece of good news. The discussion should last for no more than three minutes. The observer's role is, once the discussion is complete, to characterize

175

the response (active/passive, constructive/destructive) and the emotions that were observed in the teller due to the response. Then, roles should be switched and the procedure repeated until each person has had an opportunity to play each role. What did you learn from this experience?

- Divide into small groups of three or four to discuss and propose solutions for the following situation. The Dean of Students at X Medical School has called you in as an expert consultant to help solve a problem. A large number of students have been experiencing feelings of isolation, loneliness, and being overwhelmed with the work they have to do. The dean wonders what is causing the problem and what he can do to improve the situation. In your team, come up with some answers to the dean's question and a plan he might begin to implement to make positive changes. Emphasize interventions that will directly affect the students. Once you have completed your plan, discuss the following question: Which of these positive changes, if implemented today in your current setting, might create a more positive work environment for you and your colleagues? Take those to which you responded affirmatively and create an implementation plan at your worksite.

Individual journaling

- Refer to the scenario earlier in this chapter in which you were asked to imagine yourself as a patient (who is visited by both Dr. Jones and Dr. Smith). Reread that page. Before beginning, close your eyes and relax your body and mind so that all your focus and attention can be directed at imagining what it might feel like to be that patient, suffering from a painful illness with no known diagnosis. Imagine what it might feel like to be lying in a hospital gown in pain, and with multiple faces of strangers coming in and out of your room, touching you, asking questions, rarely explaining why. Now, imagine what you feel you would need and how you would want to be treated in that situation. What would your ideal doctor be like? What would he or she do or say? How would he or she approach you? When you are ready, open your eyes and, in the greatest detail possible, journal about your vision of your ideal physician and what that interaction would look like. How can you apply these ideals in your clinical work? Discuss this topic with a clinical supervisor or a colleague when you have completed the journaling.

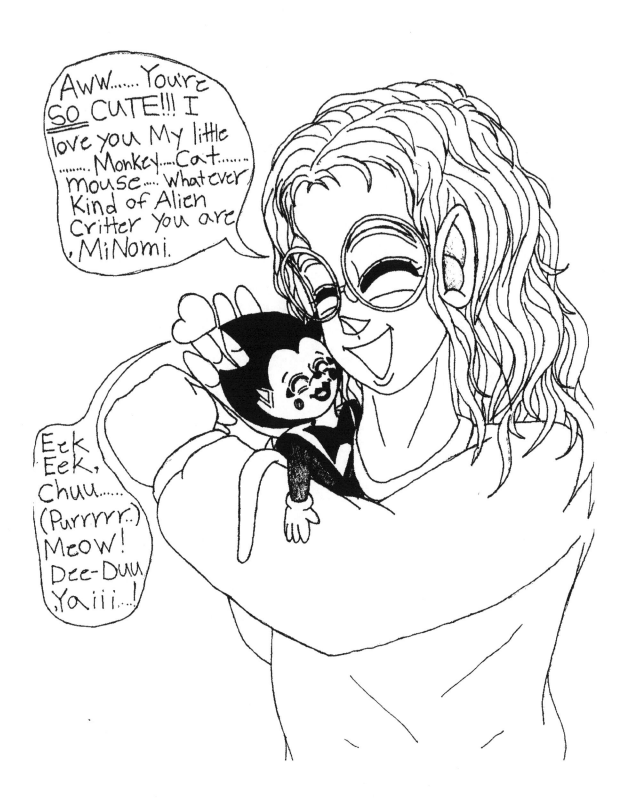

Chapter 10

Positive Emotions

When in 2011 Dr. Martin Seligman, one of the founders of positive psychology, amended his original authentic happiness theory of positive psychology to that of well-being theory, positive emotion was added and highlighted as a core feature (2011).

This is not surprising. After all, we generally feel better, happier, and more relaxed when we are experiencing positive emotions as opposed to those that are negative or filled with anxiety. When we are in the company of a loved one, a friend, or an acquaintance, and that individual is happy and content, with a smile on his or her face, we tend to feel happy and smile as well. And we all know from experience that this is far superior to feelings of fear, worry, anxiety, sadness, stress, or negativity.

The epidemic of physician ill-being and the increasing rates of depression and suicide in the population as a whole tell us that we, as physicians and as human beings, have a long road to travel in terms of understanding and appreciating the importance of positive emotions in positive health and overall human well-being. This chapter will explore positive emotions and their contribution to positive health, effective medical practice, and overall flourishing.

A LOOK AT POSITIVE AFFECTIVITY

Positive affectivity is the term used to denote the trait that reflects stable individual differences over time in positive emotional experience (Watson & Naragon, 2011). Positive affectivity has been found to be a moderately stable trait over time and across situations. Individuals with high levels of this trait experience frequent feelings of pleasant mood, enthusiasm, and high energy.

Positive and negative affectivities comprise the broad spectrum of emotional experience. That positive affectivity and negative affectivity are independent of one another is not surprising when one understands the evolutionary background of each one individually. Negative affect is a component of the withdrawal-oriented behavioral inhibition system. This system is designed to keep the organism out of danger by inhibiting behavior that might lead to pain, punishment, or other undesirable outcomes. Positive affect, in contrast, is a part of the approach-oriented behavioral facilitation system. This system directs the organism toward situations and experiences that are likely to yield pleasure and reward. The behavioral facilitation system is adaptive in that it facilitates the attainment of resources that are key to survival of the organism and the species. Such resources include food, water, shelter, sexual partners, and the cooperation of helpful others (Watson & Naragon, 2011).

The distinctively different evolutionary background and purposes of the negative and positive affect systems highlight the distinctiveness of their dimensions and variables. Therefore, negative and positive affectivity must be assessed and analyzed separately, as opposed to being regarded as extremes of one continuum. We see this in measurement scales such as the PANAS (Positive and Negative Affectivity Scale), which yield two different scores, one for positive and one for negative affectivity, as opposed to a single score along one continuum (Watson & Clark, 1994).

Positive affectivity is a trait that is strongly influenced by genetics. The literature involving pure measures of positive affectivity reveals heritability estimates in the .40 to .50 range (Watson & Naragon, 2011). In addition, twin and adoption studies indicate that the common rearing environment essentially has no effect on the development of positive affectivity. These genotypic differences appear to manifest primarily in the area of the resting prefrontal cortex. Happy individuals appear to manifest greater resting activity in the left prefrontal cortex (whereas dysphoric individuals display greater resting activity in the right frontal area). The left prefrontal activity, in turn, is then linked to the mesolimbic dopaminergic system, the behavioral facilitation system, and the subjective experience of positive mood.

Although objective demographic factors are relatively weak predictors of happiness and positive affectivity, positive affectivity is consistently moderately correlated with various indicators of social behavior, such as the number of close friends an individual has, frequency of contact with friends and relatives, the opportunity to make new acquaintances, involvement in social organizations, and the overall level of social activity. In addition, positive affectivity is consistently linked to those people who describe themselves as "spiritual" or "religious." This latter fact may be due to the sense of meaning and purpose implicit in religious belief, as well as the social behavior and supportive relationships offered by many organized religious groups.

POSITIVE EMOTIONS, AS OPPOSED TO POSITIVE AFFECTIVITY

Contrary to positive affectivity, positive emotions include pleasant or desirable situational responses, ranging from interest and contentment to love and joy. Whereas positive affectivity refers to positive feelings over a sustained span of time, positive emotions include positive subjective feelings, heightened cognition and facial expressions, cardiovascular and hormonal changes, and other changes that occur over a relatively short period of time. Why, you may well wonder, would these relatively brief positive emotions be of such great importance to thriving and flourishing?

Because positive emotions do not generally occur in the context of life-threatening situations, they do not evoke or require a specific or focused immediate response. Actually, the opposite generally occurs. Positive emotions lead to broadened and more flexible responses, and a greater array of thoughts and action possibilities come to mind (Fredrickson & Cohn, 2008). For example, joy might create the urge to play, which involves exploration and learning. Love creates urges to explore, learn about, and savor. These broadening thought-action sequences build personal resources that, in turn, have long-term benefits long after the positive emotion itself is gone. These personal resources, in fact, remain as resources that can be used by the individual to deal with future challenges and negative emotional states long after the initial positive emotional experience has ended.

This benefit of positive emotions is part of a theory of positive emotions known as the broaden-and-build theory, which was put forth and described by Dr. Barbara Fredrickson (Fredrickson, 2001; Fredrickson & Joiner, 2002). This well-known theory of positive psychology can be broken down into the broaden hypothesis and the build hypothesis.

The broaden hypothesis, stated simply, is that positive emotions broaden perception, thoughts, and actions. For example, induced positive emotions broaden visual search patterns under experimental conditions, leading to increased attention to peripheral stimuli (Fredrickson & Cohn, 2008). Positive emotions broaden cognition by producing patterns of thought that are flexible, inclusive, creative, and receptive to new information. Flexibility and openness are important attributes of positive emotions' cognitive effects, particularly in medical doctors, who constantly need to think flexibly and be open to new information regarding diagnosis and treatment for their patients.

Positive emotions also broaden social attention, leading to enhanced attention to others. Once again, this is a great asset for medical doctors, who must be professionally focused on the needs of their patients, among other important priorities.

The broadened mind-sets resulting from transient positive emotions encourage a broadened range of actions, which, over time, build enduring personal resources. Thus, even those lacking in genetic positive affectivity experience, grow, and flourish from even transient experiences of positive emotions.

The build hypothesis is the second portion of the broaden-and-build theory. This part of the theory emphasizes the huge permanent growth and acquisition of personal resources that occur over time as a result of the broadened range of actions induced by transient positive emotions. A review of this literature by Lyubomirsky and associates found that positive emotions lead to positive outcomes, ranging from increased satisfaction at work and in relationships to improved physical health and effective problem solving (Lyubomirsky, King, & Diener, 2005).

One way to directly test the build hypothesis is to randomly assign subjects to experience enhanced daily positive emotions through training in loving-kindness meditation, a practice that focuses on the deliberate generation of the positive emotions of compassion and love. The control group consisted of those subjects assigned to a waiting list. After just three weeks of practice, those in the meditating group began reporting higher daily levels of various positive emotions when compared to the control group. After eight weeks of practice, meditators demonstrated an increase in physical wellness, agency for achieving important goals, increased ability to savor positive experiences, an increased quality of close relationships, increased hope, and an increase in overall life satisfaction (Fredrickson, Cohn, Coffey, Pek, & Finkel, 2008).

Further research on positive emotions demonstrates that those who experience higher levels of positive emotions tend to resist and avoid illness and disease more successfully, live longer lives, and experience less pain and disability related to chronic health conditions than those who are lacking in positive emotional experiences. This is likely related to the neutralizing effects of positive emotions on the stressful experience of illness or other threats to the individual. These individuals tend to exhibit more resiliencies, recover quickly, and bounce back. As a physician, consider the number of hospitalized patients who are depressed and discouraged, and consider the negative impact this has on healing, recovery, length of stay, and other parameters. If we focused on creating positive emotional experiences for patients in the hospital, recovery times might greatly decrease, along with pain and disability.

While the physiological changes that accompany stress, illness, and negative emotions are beneficial for decisive, immediate action in a threatening situation, they are detrimental to long-term health. Therefore, it is advantageous for the body to properly regulate and control the stress response. Positive emotions have been shown to be an effective tool in regulation, neutralizing the body's neurochemical stress response once the threat is past. In one study, participants were exposed to an anxiety-provoking experience and then shown an emotional film clip while their biological and physiological stress responses were being monitored. Those who were shown a positive emotional film clip recovered more quickly than those viewing either a neutral or a negative film clip (Fredrickson, Mancuso, Branigan, & Tugade, 2000). None of the film clips had any biological effect at all in the absence of the initial anxiety-provoking stressor. From this we can conclude that the impact of positive emotions on the cardiovascular system is primarily as a neutralizer and a reverser of the negative effects of stress.

This study and many others like it demonstrate that individuals who are resilient tend to recover more quickly, and they do so through the generation of positive emotions during the recovery process (Fredrickson & Cohn, 2008). On the other hand, those who remain stressed, activated, and in a state of preparation to react accumulate physiological and psychological wear and tear and are more vulnerable to morbidity and ill-being.

Unfortunately, we health-care professionals see this phenomenon all around us. With 40 to 60 percent of the medical profession suffering from burnout and ill-being (see chapter 1), all one need do is to walk through the halls of any average hospital to see intense individuals, many with their heads down, in stressed isolation, rapidly moving to put out the next fire. In many cases, we are those individuals.

Chapter 1 of this book highlights the negative cultural and situational realities of medicine today that contribute to this reality. However, even in situations in which individuals experience prolonged negative emotions, studies have shown that when these individuals also experience positive emotions along with the negative ones, they demonstrate greater psychological well-being a year or more later. At least a portion of the explanation for this is that positive emotions are associated with the ability to take a longer view of a situation and develop positive goals for the future (Moskowitz, Folkman, & Acree, 2003). In other words, resilient physicians are not in denial of, nor are they devoid of, stress and negative emotions. However, they have found and created opportunities to feel positive emotions, which neutralize many of the effects of a stress-filled, narrow mind-set. This form of psychological resilience is associated with the ability to distinguish many finely differentiated positive emotions, thereby making it easier and even possible to find positive moments without denying the seriousness of the negative situation. These results contradict frequent criticisms that positive emotions are not useful or are inappropriate in negative situations. Even adults dealing with suicidal thoughts or disclosure of childhood sexual abuse demonstrated better coping when positivity accompanied their painful feelings (Fredrickson & Cohn, 2008). While research on pessimism and depression recognizes a self-reinforcing downward spiral, the evidence is strong that positive emotions contribute to an upward spiral of increasing resources, life successes, and flourishing.

The creation of positivity

Dr. Tom Smith was an extremely busy and popular obstetrician/gynecologist, who was well-liked by his physician colleagues, by hospital staff, and particularly by his patients. He was pleasant and cooperative with everyone. He was awarded many times for his excellent teaching and mentoring of residents and medical students. His children were grown, and he was now a grandfather. He was in a stable marriage with his second wife. I was quite surprised when he asked to speak with me and began telling me that he was feeling depressed and burned out. I asked him to tell me about his typical day.

He typically awakens between four and four thirty in the morning and cannot return to sleep. Therefore, he gets up and goes in to work at about five o'clock, and works until six or seven o'clock. He might have to stay later if there is a meeting he must attend in the evening. Once he gets home, he has dinner with his wife, and then he finishes up work from the day that he had to take home. To get his work done, he often must skip things that he enjoys, such as spending time with his wife, playing the violin, or pleasure reading. Finally, when he is too exhausted to do any more work, he goes to bed, and repeats the process the next day.

When I questioned him about the volume of his work, he told me that he never says no to a new patient and that there are often so many patients who need to see him in one day that he cannot complete the paperwork and must take it home to finish later that evening. Although he loves his work, he feels that it has consumed his life and that there is no longer any joy or anything to which he can look forward.

Unfortunately, this is not an atypical presenting story for a burned-out physician.

It is obvious from the above scenario that some individuals are quite lacking in positivity, or have structured their lives to allow for a dearth of positive emotions. But how much is actually enough? Research has suggested that a ratio of at least three to one positive to negative emotions will allow for a flourishing existence, creativity, and increased resilience, although the mathematical basis of this theory has recently been questioned (Fredrickson, 2013).

The positivity ratio is derived from the combined work of Dr. Marcial Losada and Dr. Barbara Fredrickson. Losada worked from a quantitative and statistical perspective, studying high-performance teams. High-performance teams maintained a ratio of positive-to-negative statements of at least three to one, even through challenges and stresses. They remained open to new ideas, asking questions, and focusing outward, staying united as a team (Losada & Heaphy, 2004).

The positivity ratio has been tested in other settings of individual and group thriving. For example, John Gottman (Gottman & Silver, 1999; Ryan, Gottman, Murray, Carrere, & Swanson, 2000), an expert in the science of successful marriage, found several ways to compute the positivity ratio of marriage. Doing similar comparative work with flourishing and broken marriages as had been done previously with individuals, he found marked variation in positivity ratios. Among flourishing marriages, positivity ratios were about five to one, whereas languishing and failed marriages had positivity ratios lower than one to one!

The benefits of a high positivity ratio do not indicate that a state of being free of negativity is possible or even healthy. Negativity is part of reality and is also a necessary ingredient in a flourishing life. For example, healthy engagement in conflict in a marriage can be productive when it leads to greater mutual understanding. Letting go of uncomfortable or dissonant feelings in a team setting is critical, as it leads to greater trust and a more united team purpose. Individual anger often leads to remedial actions to resolve the negative situation. Without negativity, it is easy to lose touch with reality. As Fredrickson notes, the ratio of positivity to negativity can be seen as a balance between levity and gravity. Levity is that unseen force that lifts you skyward, whereas gravity is the opposing force that pulls you earthward. When properly combined, these two opposing forces can leave you buoyant, dynamic, realistic, and ready for anything. Appropriate negativity delivers the promise of gravity. It grounds you in reality. Heartfelt positivity, by contrast, provides the lift that makes you buoyant and ready to flourish (Fredrickson, 2009).

When we look at the case of Dr. Tom Smith (above), it is easy to recognize that he lacks a preponderance of positive emotions in his life. To truly feel positivity in your heart requires you to slow down the pace of your life. Those of us who, like Dr. Smith, live a fast-paced life have a constant focus on what is going on outside of ourselves. Dr. Smith's focus was predominantly on his patients, on being well-liked and respected by others, and on keeping up with the out-of-control growth of his practice. Over time, this outward, external focus and constant tension lead to emotional exhaustion and a numbing of one's heart and feelings. This, in turn, eliminates the potential for experiencing any positivity or joy.

Only by helping Dr. Smith recognize his own self-destructive patterns and by helping him slow down the pace of his life were we able to awaken his heart so that he could begin to experience more positive emotions. All genuine positive emotions come from the heart. Most burned-out and unhappy professionals must recognize this need to *slow down* the pace of life in order to open the heart and begin to build positivity.

Methods of building and creating positive emotions

As has been stated earlier in this chapter, even those who did not inherit a genetic tendency for positive affectivity can learn from and practice activities to induce positive emotions. For example, a key way to increase positivity is to find positive meaning and purpose in your day-to-day work and life circumstances (see chapter 8 for an entire chapter devoted to meaning and purpose). Look for the positive meaning in your circumstances and accentuate it. Reframe unpleasant circumstances in a more positive way. Will you see the cup as half empty or half full? The goal is not to eliminate or to sugarcoat negativity. The goal is, rather, to bring out the positive that can be found in even the most negative of situations through the meaning and goodness you find in that situation. Having a positive meaning for your life as a whole makes it easier to see the positivity in a particular negative situation you might encounter.

For example, an experience of note in my life occurred when I was a single parent of two autistic teens and I became severely ill. For two years the illness robbed me of my ability to walk, work, take care of my children, and enjoy all of my favorite activities, as the doctors searched for a diagnosis. Once I finally got an accurate diagnosis and treatment, I regained enough function to return to work, but sustained permanent losses to my physical functioning. All of the things I loved to do, such as running, dancing, skiing, and playing with my children, were taken away. I could not even walk unassisted. Although this was a difficult and challenging time in my life, I consider it a gift and an overall blessing for a very important reason. The reason is that prior to my illness, I was doing everything for my autistic children. Once I became ill and stopped doing everything for them, they began to function more independently. In fact, each of them underwent tremendous growth, which continues to this day, and which, I believe, would never have happened had I not become ill. My illness was a blessing for them. To this day, I think of my illness as a gift to their growth and well-being.

Another strategy for increasing positive emotions is savoring. Although many people think of savoring only in the context of sensory experiences, such as savoring an excellent meal, savoring consists of turning a positive event into an even more richly positive experience by intensively focusing on that which is good in it. People who savor extract more positivity from life and everyday experiences. It is a mental habit that allows one to extract more goodness before, during, and after a pleasant event. When you savor, you willfully generate, intensify, and prolong your deeply felt enjoyment of an event or circumstance. As with any other positive emotion, savoring involves slowing down your pace of activities and mindfully attending to the details of your current experience and your enjoyment of it.

Counting your blessings is a useful tool for creating positive emotions. When, at the end of the day, we take the time to write down three blessings that occurred during the day, we learn to appreciate the kindness of another, to see the blessing behind otherwise ordinary daily events, and to appreciate the beauty we experience during the day. Some people find it useful to record their blessings in a gratitude journal, so that gratitude and blessings can be reviewed from time to time.

Performing acts of kindness for others creates positive emotions. Individuals who flourish are more attuned to kindness, more focused on the well-being of others, and more alert to opportunities to contribute to the positivity of others. Kindness and positivity foster each other, creating what Frederickson refers to as "upward spirals" of positivity (Fredrickson & Joiner, 2002; Fredrickson, 2009). Simply recognizing your own acts of kindness initiates an upward spiral of positive emotions. Studies show that if you intentionally boost your kindness, you will also increase your positivity. Interestingly, the patterns one uses to perform acts of kindness make a difference in the degree of associated benefit. To derive maximal benefit, perform several large acts of kindness on a single day each week, as opposed to spreading them out or doing one small act each day. This prevents the acts of kindness from feeling routine or ordinary. For example, one might create a "kindness day" each week or set aside several hours once each week to do special volunteer work helping others. This will give a huge boost to your positive emotions.

There are numerous other techniques for creating more positive emotions. One easily accessible example is using and acting on your highest character strengths. As we reviewed in chapter 6, using your signature strengths and using them in new ways create positive emotions and feelings of well-being. A technique reviewed in chapter 9 is connecting with others and actively pursuing positive relationships.

Connecting with nature is yet another method of boosting positive emotions. Individuals who spend twenty or more minutes outside when the weather is nice demonstrate a measurable increase in positivity over those who do not. Further, they demonstrate more expansive and open thinking, in addition to increased working memory span. The fascination with and being in the vastness of nature seem to contribute to this increase in positivity and openness. Further to this point, studies show that individuals can put themselves on healing trajectories simply by spending time outdoors.[13]

Loving-kindness meditation (metta)

Earlier in this chapter, one or two studies were referenced in which positive emotions were created under study conditions through loving-kindness meditation. *Metta* (Sujiva, 1998) is a word derived from the ancient language known as Pali. Pali is the scriptural language for Theraveda Buddhism. Metta refers to kindness, which has a special quality of love and care associated with it. Metta is an unconditional well-wishing for the safety, happiness, good health, and comfort of any living being, including oneself. It is loving-kindness. Although people practice and teach loving-kindness in a variety of ways, loving-kindness is something that is cultivated and grown over time. This requires a heart and mind that are open to loving-kindness and provide a fertile environment for it to develop.

Loving-kindness is something that all humans possess. It is common to all human beings. What varies among beings is the number and severity of obstructions and mental or emotional blockages that stand between us and prevent access to our pure loving-kindness. By learning to see through or remove these blockages and obstructions, we can learn to gain access to our natural loving-kindness within each of our hearts.

Loving-kindness is unconditional. Thus, when we wish goodness and wellness to ourselves and to other beings, it is done without the expectation of anything in return.

Loving-kindness is expressed as a series of four phrases that first we must wish and apply to ourselves. These wishes—to be free from danger, mental suffering, and physical suffering, and to joyfully care for the self—may not be completely true for each of us. Too many of us face emotional and physical challenges. However, in metta, we may wish for them to be true at some point in the future, without expectation, but with openness and joy. Because this can be difficult when we, ourselves, are suffering, this is why in loving-kindness we need to start with ourselves. Only if you feel genuine loving-kindness for yourself can you truly have loving-kindness for others. In addition, if you develop loving-kindness for yourself, this is the only certain way to attain a heart filled with loving-kindness. When you feel that loving-kindness in your own heart, you can understand the pure quality of it. This cannot reliably come from any external source.

Loving-kindness development is a form of concentration or tranquility meditation, which means that concentration is of utmost importance during its practice. One simply repeats and concentrates on each of the following four phrases, focusing on their meaning.

The first phrase is: "May I be safe from inner and outer harm." Inner harm refers to that suffering that we bring to ourselves through fear, worry, anger, impatience, or other needs of the bounded self. Outer harm, by contrast, refers to external and physical danger. Even if this phrase does not feel entirely comfortable for you, or some obstruction comes up in your mind as you say it, you can keep lovingly reciting this phrase until you begin to feel it in your heart, and it begins to have meaning for you. Loving-kindness is a long-term practice at which one must persist until the true and complete meaning comes through in your heart for each phrase.

The second phrase for developing loving-kindness toward the self is: "May I be free from mental suffering." This line asks for happiness and peace, which are the positive mental states that result when we are, indeed, free from mental suffering.

The third phrase is as follows: "May I be free from physical suffering." This third line refers to our body and our physical condition. We are asking to be healthy and strong.

The final, fourth phrase states: "May I take care of myself, happily." This fourth phrase asks for comfort in life, and for joyful and positive outcomes as we lovingly care for ourselves.

These four phrases contain the natural wishes that all human beings have in their own hearts toward themselves and toward other beings.

While you are learning and reciting the first line, over and over, you may also say the other lines to give your mind some variety and to be aware of all other aspects of loving-kindness.

Comfort is important during loving-kindness meditation for several reasons. Pain can provide a distraction from the heart's pure focus on loving-kindness. In loving-kindness meditation, it is helpful to ignore distractions and bring your mind back to its focus on the phrase at hand. In loving-kindness meditation, distractions are ignored while the mind is gently brought back to loving-kindness. In addition, when we feel pain, it often creates negative feelings to arise in the mind, which can block loving-kindness. Therefore, one should relax and sit comfortably when doing loving-kindness meditation and change position to a more comfortable position if one notices discomfort. However, it is important to keep one's mind and body alert.

There are instances in which one says, "May I be safe from inner and outer harm," and yet that individual does not feel happy or at peace. Therefore, the individual can repeat the phrase "May I be happy and peaceful," and attempt to incorporate that as a heartfelt reality. Or one asks to be free from physical harm, but one is sick or weak. Then you might recite, "May I be healthy and strong." As you keep repeating this, the mind will become focused, and then calm and still. As a result, you will feel happier, calmer, and perhaps a greater sense of physical well-being. This, in turn, increases the happiness and peace you feel inside your heart.

Once one becomes an accomplished practitioner of loving-kindness meditation, achieving these four states of loving-kindness toward oneself in one's heart becomes an easily accomplished goal during meditation. Therefore, the four wishes become a present-moment experience for you. "I am feeling at peace, I am feeling healthy and strong in this moment, and everything around me is unfolding as it should." Loving-kindness, peace, and tranquility continue to build in your heart and mind. Once we feel them securely and plentifully within ourselves, we can begin to move to the next step and share them with others.

There are five different categories of individuals toward whom we can develop loving-kindness in order to make it strong within us. These categories include: oneself, a respected individual, a dear friend, a neutral person, and a hostile person. Once you have become secure and comfortable in developing loving-kindness within yourself, the second level is to share it with another within the second category. These include teachers, respected elders, wisdom figures, or someone who has offered you valuable guidance. This should be a living person to whom you have no physical or sexual attraction. Because these are individuals whom you greatly admire, your loving-kindness should flow easily to anyone in this category of individuals, and it feels natural to want to share your loving-kindness with them.

The third category of individual we learn to develop loving-kindness toward is a dear friend. This is an individual with whom you share great closeness, with whom you can share your secrets, in whom you have great trust. If there is no one like that in your life, a good friend is a next-best choice. Once again, it is someone who is living, to whom your loving-kindness flows with ease.

After you develop loving-kindness fully for yourself, and then for your respected elder and a dear friend, you next select a neutral individual. Specifically, this is someone whom you know but who is unfamiliar to you in the sense of knowing little about his or her character. For example, you might choose a teller who works at your bank, a mail deliverer you see pass by daily, or an individual you pass on the street each day in your daily routine. Developing loving-kindness toward this individual is a bit more of a challenge. It is difficult to develop unconditional well-wishing in your heart for someone you don't even know. However, if you can develop loving-kindness toward a neutral person similar to that which you have for yourself, a respected person, and a dear friend, your loving-kindness is growing and becoming stronger.

Finally, when your loving-kindness is well-developed and strong, you are able to share it with a hostile person. Although this is an individual for whom you carry feelings of anger or frustration, the strong practice of loving-kindness has you reciting the four positive phrases toward this individual, and not attaching to any negative mental state that may come to mind as you continue to recite the loving-kindness and good wishes. This often takes time and does not come easily. However, the important point is that if your loving-kindness is strong, you can share it with anyone at any time, which, in turn, creates great positive emotions. Ultimately, it is the feeling of loving-kindness that is most important, not the words themselves. However, it is the continuing deep focus on the phrases and the wishes contained therein that builds the positive feelings of loving-kindness in one's heart. Loving-kindness is best learned and practiced with a group in your local area led by an individual who is certified in the practice and teaching of it. However, once it is internalized and mastered, I feel it is a very positive and helpful tool for physicians and others who tend to work in high-pressure and high-stress situations with their fellow human beings, where caring and sensitivity can make the difference between a life saved and a life lost.

Group discussion questions

- This chapter points out that resilient physicians are neither in denial of nor devoid of stress or negative emotions. However, they have found, built in, and created opportunities to feel positive emotions that well exceed the negative emotions. Identify and discuss what these opportunities might be and what they might look like. How might each of them fit in with your current lifestyle?
- Referring back to the story of Dr. Tom Smith, what might he do to allow for more positivity in his daily life? What changes might he make at work? What might he do at home? Examine his reluctance to say "no" to a new patient. What is implicit in this story regarding the need to develop and set priorities?
- Referring to and using the principles of the broaden-and-build theory of positive emotions, explain why it is essential for medical students, house staff, doctors, and all hospital personnel to maintain a healthy positivity ratio. How might this relate to missed diagnoses, medical errors, and poor communication with patients?
- Why is it difficult for an overworked professional or student to experience positivity?

Individual exercises

- Add to your health habits journal a page or column that is headed "My Blessings." Two days each week, make a habit of thinking of some of the small, often underappreciated things or events you routinely encounter in your day-to-day life that are actually hidden treasures or great blessings. For example, at the bus stop you notice a lovely display of flowers. It has been there all the time, but until today, you have been too busy to notice its beauty. When you get home from work, there is always a hot cup of tea waiting for you thanks to your spouse, but you never took the time to say thanks or to appreciate how lucky you are to have a supportive spouse. Two days each week, perhaps Monday and Thursday, write about three blessings that you have experienced since your last entry.

- Savor moments of positivity. Once each week, take the time to think of an extremely positive event in your life. Alternate between events that occurred in the past and events that are occurring in the present. Think of the event in great detail, savoring and appreciating all the wonderful things about it. Make a creative entry in your health habits journal that allows you to continue to savor the event through words, drawings, photos, or whatever enhances your savoring of the joyful experience.

- Focus on creating high-quality connections. According to Jane Dutton at the University of Michigan, connecting with others in a high-quality manner is a life-giving process (2003). It recharges your energy and vitality and creates positive physiological changes. The four ways to build high-quality connections include respectful engagement (be present, attentive, and affirming), support of what the other person is doing (helping him or her to succeed), belief that you can depend on this person to meet your expectations (trust), and allowing time to goof off with no particular outcomes in mind (play). Engaging with others in one or more of these ways produces endless sources of genuine positivity both at work and at home. The big challenge is to build high-quality connections where none existed prior to now. Think of the wonderful gift you are giving, both to yourself and to others. Pick one individual with whom you work closely. Using Dutton's four-pronged approach above, brainstorm and implement a plan to improve the quality of that connection. What was the result?

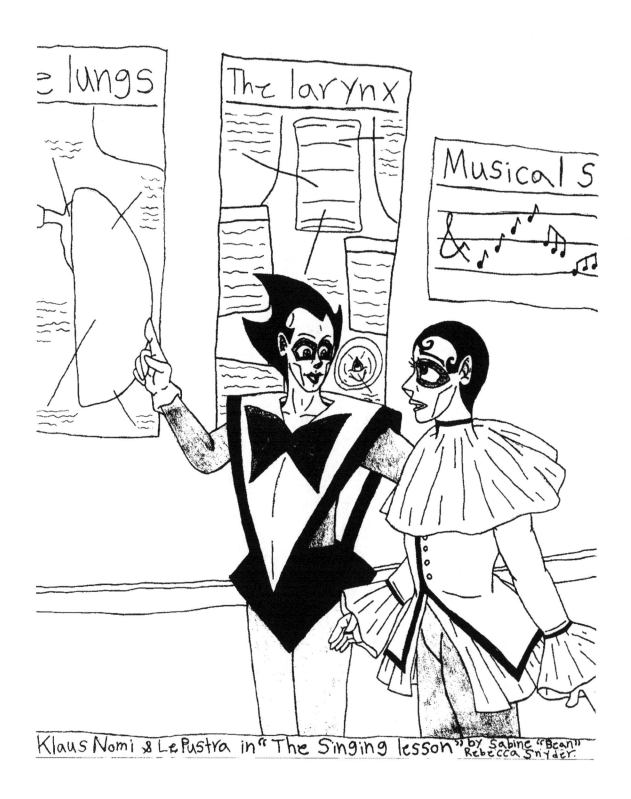

Klaus Nomi & LePustra in "The Singing lesson" by Sabine "Bean" Rebecca Snyder.

Chapter 11

Professionalism

One might question the relevance of professionalism in a book focused on positive health. However, the connection is easy to understand once explained. Experts in medicine continue to approach the field as a science of disease. However, health care is both a science of human health and well-being and an art, involving complex human interaction. This human interaction must be solidly anchored in an in-depth understanding of ethics, values, and human behavior. Without a deep understanding of these key factors, doctor-patient communication suffers, diagnoses are missed, medical errors are made, and satisfaction for the patient and the physician is low. Sadly, with all of the efforts toward health-care reform taking place, the role of professionalism and values remains absent from public discussion and from physician education.

The most productive way to see the role of professionalism in health care may be to view it as a multidimensional competency. Viewing professionalism as a competency presents it as a skill that can be taught and continually strengthened through assessment and education. Thus, from entrance into medical school and throughout his or her career, the physician is taught critical thinking, skill building, and deliberate practice, which, in turn, help the physician to grow positive skills, in contrast with a negative approach in which nothing is taught and doctors are punished (e.g., legally) for the skills that they lack.

The sophisticated competencies that are included under the umbrella of professionalism are profoundly influenced by the organizational and environmental contexts of current medical practice. Although these forces need to support professionalism, all too often, they foster unprofessional behavior (see chapter 1). Professionalism must be a combined effort of individual physicians, the medical education establishment, health-care delivery system leaders, and policy makers.

In this chapter, several key competencies that are involved in professionalism and also affect positive health and human understanding will be reviewed. This list of competencies includes emotional intelligence, compassion, self-regulation, empathy, and communication skills. These are competencies that are crucial not only for a healthy doctor-patient relationship but also for any flourishing professional. To be clear, this chapter is intended to be neither a comprehensive review of professionalism nor an instruction guide in mastering these competencies. Absent from this chapter are topics such as positive ethics and moral judgment, which are equally important. Professionalism and the key competencies therein need to be introduced in the first year of medical training, with education, exposure, and mentoring continuing throughout one's medical career to achieve mastery. However, because they are, as yet, unrecognized as important topics in any medical-school curriculum in the United States, this chapter highlights the importance of this subject matter in the successful career of doctors, with the hope that doctors will seek further knowledge until such time that it is readily available in medical-school curricula and through continuing medical education (CME) courses.

EMOTIONAL INTELLIGENCE

Emotional intelligence includes the skills of perceiving emotions, using emotions to facilitate thinking, understanding emotions, and managing emotions. Almost all models of emotional intelligence fit within four domains: self-awareness, self-management, social awareness, and relationship management.

Emotional intelligence resides in brain areas that are distinct from those of intellectual abilities. This is the reason why many highly intelligent professionals need to develop expertise in emotional-intelligence skills through education and training. Brain areas such as the right amygdala, the right somatosensory cortex, the right insular cortex, the anterior cingulate, and the ventromedial area of the prefrontal cortex are crucial in the function of emotional intelligence. For example, individuals with lesions or injuries to the right amygdala (midbrain) show a loss of emotional self-awareness (i.e., the ability to be aware of and understand one's own feelings). Injury to the right somatosensory cortex, on the other hand, creates a deficiency in self-awareness and a loss of awareness of the emotions of others. It is important to note that self-awareness—the ability to feel and understand one's own emotions—is critical in the ability to understand and empathize with the emotions of others.

The right insular cortex is another part of the brain that is crucial for empathy. This area is a node for brain circuitry that senses our entire bodily state and tells us how we are feeling (Goleman, 2011). Tuning into how we feel on a personal level is a key ingredient in how we sense and understand the feelings of others.

The anterior cingulate contributes to emotional intelligence through its ability to regulate impulse control. It is activated when strong feelings and distressing emotions come into play in a given situation. The ventromedial area of the prefrontal cortex allows us to solve personal and interpersonal problems, manage our impulses, effectively express our feelings, and relate well with others.

It is the balance between the logical prefrontal cortex and the emotional centers in the midbrain (e.g., the amygdala) that allows for positive behavioral regulation and emotionally intelligent action. Self-mastery requires self-awareness plus self-regulation, both of which are key components of emotional intelligence. These components include an awareness of our internal states and the management of those states. A person who is rushed, overloaded, and overwhelmed has no time to focus awareness on oneself and one's internal states. Competencies such as managing emotions, the drive to achieve goals, adaptability, and initiative—all based on one's own ability to self-manage—become elusive under such negative conditions.

The prefrontal cortex guides us when we are at our best, exerting cognitive control; regulating attention; and facilitating decision making, voluntary action, reasoning, and mental flexibility in response to a challenge. Because the amygdala is a trigger for emotional distress, anger, impulse, and fear, leading us to act in ways we might later regret, dominance of the prefrontal cortex in behavioral regulation is particularly important in professional circumstances and in dealing with loved ones. This struggle for balance between the functions of the prefrontal cortex and the functions of the amygdala, therefore, becomes the basis of self-mastery.

According to Schwartz (Schwartz & McCarthy, 2010), the five top triggers of amygdala-generated responses in the workplace setting are as follows: (1) condescension and lack of respect, (2) being treated unfairly, (3) being unappreciated or underappreciated, (4) feeling as if you are not being listened to, and (5) being held to unrealistic deadlines. You will note from chapter 1 of this book that all five of these conditions are seen commonly in the medical workplace because of the medical culture as it now exists. Bringing professionalism and emotional intelligence training and awareness into the medical-student curricula and physician CME allows us to change this in two important ways. First, physicians who are aware of the benefits of emotional intelligence and the potential problems within the currently negative culture will be motivated to create changes in the culture of their hospital or medical system to a more open, supportive, and generative one. Second, each individual practitioner with increased awareness of how to exert internal controls over the negativity and react instead with positivity and creativity will contribute to a growing positive culture in medicine and health care.

Yet another part of the brain that is key in emotional intelligence is the *social brain*. When we look at the social brain, it is important to be aware of and understand mirror neurons. These are neurons that activate exactly what we "see" in another person, such as the other person's emotions, movements, and even intentions. This brain function explains why emotions are so contagious in a group of people. The implications of this finding (and the effect in a professional situation) are really quite remarkable, because it means that we are constantly affecting the brain states of others. To clarify, we help shape the feelings of those with whom we interact, particularly in a professional setting, for better or worse. In this sense, relationship skills are related to managing brain states in others and us. Such emotional contagion occurs whenever humans interact, be it in the form of a dyad, a group, a work team, or an organization (Goleman, 2011).

The team approach to teaching social and emotional intelligence has shown great promise. This method works through workgroups that are organized to achieve a common goal. High-level collaboration and effective communication skills, both important abilities for emotional intelligence, are developed through this team approach. Self-awareness (i.e., knowing one's own strengths and limitations) is also emphasized, as well as self-management skills (e.g., self-discipline in keeping your commitments to the team). In a team setting, empathy (i.e., tuning in to how your words and behavior affect others) and other interpersonal skills, such as communication, collaboration, and negotiation, can be more clearly viewed and demonstrated. Chapter 15 of this book, which deals with the spirited multidisciplinary team, reviews many of these processes in greater detail.

Therefore, just as intellectual skills are learned and developed, so too can we develop a repertoire of positive emotional skills. However, instead of mastering a body of factual information, emotional intelligence involves understanding one's own emotions and the emotions in others; it also includes the capacity to reason about emotions and use them to assist reasoning (Salovey, Caruso, & Mayer, 2012). Examples of the former includes perceiving emotions, understanding emotions, and managing emotions in a growth-enhancing manner. Using emotions to facilitate thought is the sole example of the latter.

More specifically, perceiving emotions refers to registering, attending to, and understanding emotional messages. Emotional messages are not always expressed directly through verbal exchanges; they often are shown through facial expression, tone of voice, nonverbal cues, or other expressions of one's emotional state. Consequently, an emotionally intelligent doctor must focus on all types of messages that the patient is sending to fully and accurately understand the patient's physical and emotional status. Likewise, the doctor should be highly aware of any emotional messages that he or she may be sending to the patient and ensure that they are open and reassuring.

Using emotions to facilitate thought can, more specifically, be broken down into several components, all of which are important and useful. For example, when we are asked to understand and appreciate several different points of view in a discussion, we are able to do this by capitalizing on mood changes (of self and other) and our empathy with another person's experience. Generating emotions also facilitates judgment and memory. Problem solving and creativity are facilitated by one's ability to use emotions. We are aided in our ability to prioritize and redirect our thinking on the basis of the associated feelings of self and others.

Understanding emotions can be more clearly explained in terms of the abilities it entails. One ability is that which enables a person to label emotions with words, which, in turn, facilitates discussion of emotional issues. Another important aspect of understanding emotions is recognizing the relationships among emotions. Closely related to that is the ability to perceive the causes and consequences of emotions. Many doctors see this illustrated on a daily basis when they walk into a patient's examination room. If the doctor is calm and unhurried, has a smile, and takes a seat, we see an entirely different emotional response from a patient than if the doctor rushes in to the room, remains standing, hurriedly asks a few questions, and leaves. Understanding emotions also includes the ability to perceive emotional complexities and contradictory emotional states, as well as comprehending transitions from one emotional state to another.

Finally, emotional intelligence involves managing emotions. This skill includes the ability to manage emotions and to be open to feelings and emotions in oneself and in others, be they pleasant or unpleasant. This encompasses one's ability to monitor and reflect on emotions and the ability to engage, prolong, or detach from an emotional state when any one of those responses is appropriate or helpful.

The four-branch model of emotional intelligence described previously is the basis for the Mayer-Salovey-Caruso Emotional Intelligence Test (MSCEIT, v2.0) (Mayer, Salovey, & Caruso, 2002). This assessment of emotional intelligence is used for both research and practice situations. It involves the assessment of eight skills, two for each of the four branches of emotional intelligence. Branch 1, perceiving emotions, is measured through (1) the identification of emotions on faces and (2) the identification of emotions conveyed by landscapes and designs. Branch 2, using emotions to facilitate thought, is measured by (1) a sensations task in which emotions are compared with tactile and sensory stimuli and (2) a task in which participants identify emotions that would best facilitate a type of thought. Branch 3, understanding emotions, is measured through (1) changes, that is, which emotion would likely change into another (e.g., frustration into aggression); and (2) blends, which asks participants to identify which emotions might lead to a third complex feeling state. Branch 4, managing emotions, measures (1) emotional management, or how hypothetical scenarios would affect maintaining or changing emotions; and (2) emotional relations, which involves the management of emotions in others (Salovey, Caruso, & Mayer, 2012).

The MSCEIT produces an overall score in addition to scores at each of the branch levels and scores at each individual measurement (eight in all). Although emotional intelligence is significantly different from intelligence quotient (IQ), it is interesting that individuals who score high on the MSCEIT tend to have higher grades in school than individuals with lower scores (Salovey, Caruso, & Mayer, 2012, p. 452). Those with high scores are also less likely to engage in bullying or violent behavior or take illicit drugs.

Individuals with higher scores on the MSCEIT tend to report more positive interactions and relationships with other people as well.

Based on this knowledge and insight about emotional intelligence and the emotional nature of the interactions that doctors experience daily with patients, the patients' families, the caregiving team, and their colleagues, it is almost unthinkable that training in emotional intelligence skills is not available on a broad scale for anyone working in the health-care profession. Several attempts have been instituted on a small scale, including Balint Groups for Family Practice residencies and Schwartz Rounds, which have begun on a monthly basis in about a hundred to 150 hospitals nationwide. Both of these programs have had successful beginnings in building emotional intelligence skills in doctors. However, building an emotional-intelligence curriculum in medical-school education, starting in year 1, is most important to prevent burnout and create a generation of healthy doctors who are able to give excellent, compassionate care to their patients.

COMPASSION

Compassion is the desire to relieve a person from his or her suffering, even under the least appealing circumstances (Vaillant, 2008). It is a process that first involves connecting with another person through empathetic understanding and then taking action to relieve that person's suffering. Compassion is an emotion that is vital to the effective practice of medicine and similar professions, such as nursing, social service, and other helping professions. In spite of this need, it seems that, as medicine becomes increasingly technological, patients long for doctors with empathy and compassion.

Often it is what we fear the most that activates the highest level of compassion when we see it in others. Compassion is both private and social. It is interesting to note that people who are suffering and receive our compassion have little awareness of the feelings that they evoke in others. For example, children who have been raised in poverty know of no other life but their own. Likewise, an individual with a disability learns to live out each day with adaptations to his or her life due to that disability. Neither person tends to view this existence as suffering. It is simply life as they know it.

At its core, compassion is a process of connecting with another human being through the process of identification. The process of identification in humans begins with infancy, when the infant begins to mirror the facial expressions and bodily movements of the mother. The child is also able to mirror the emotional state of the parents, which allows identification to continue as the child grows into the domain of feelings. As children reach their teens, identification continues with the peer group, with the child switching away from the parents.

Even individuals from widely diverse circumstances and backgrounds share humanity with one another. This is the reason why we are able to identify with people from vastly different nations and cultures. We identify with others through our knowledge of the common human condition.

The more one knows about another and understands that person, the less likely one is to assign blame for his or her misfortunes. An example of this behavior is the young resident physician in the emergency room in chapter 1 who incorrectly assumed that the young unconscious man in dirty clothes was an alcoholic living on the street and that he was intoxicated. Had the doctor taken a more compassionate and open-minded stance, he might have correctly diagnosed the malignant brain tumor in the head of the CEO's son.

People (and doctors) differ in the depth and intensity of their compassion. The difference seems to lie in the varying degree of ability to identify with the suffering of others. Such identification cannot occur if one is preoccupied with the self or self-related issues such as ill-being or burnout. Therefore, a physician practicing positive health and thriving has a far greater likelihood of mastering identification and compassion skills, and can, in turn, build a rapport and meaningful communication with his or her patients.

Clearly, one important aspect of compassion is identification and the ability to see what might cause distress in oneself through the plight of another. Yet there is another equally important aspect of compassion, which is that the knowledge that another person is suffering moves the compassionate person to take action to relieve the suffering. When referring to suffering, I am speaking of a state of severe distress associated with events that threaten the integrity or well-being of a human being (Cassell, 2009). Suffering is, by nature, a lonely, isolated experience due to its highly personal and individual nature. This loneliness and isolation further add to the suffering. This problem is just one of the many reasons why a compassionate caregiver can be a true gift and a blessing for a sick patient.

Compassion is not simply a desirable trait for physicians. It is called for in item I of the American Medical Association's *Principles of Medical Ethics* (American Medical Association, 2001). This statement reads: "A physician shall be dedicated to providing competent medical care, with compassion and respect for human dignity and rights." Most people believe that compassion should be an inherent part of medicine and that physicians and caregivers should be compassionate (Barber, 1976).

Because compassion evokes the desire to take action against suffering, it motivates positive behaviors in caregivers to relieve the suffering of the patient and to reduce the internal tension caused by the emotion. When a doctor truly listens to a patient recount the story of his or her illness, along with all the pain and the associated difficulties, compassion is aroused, a type of fusion occurs, and the doctor begins to listen, observe, and intuit with greater intensity. This process, in turn, encourages the flow of information from the patient, which enables the doctor to make a better and more accurate diagnosis.

Physicians should understand the importance and the methods of delivering compassionate care, of restoring hope for the patient and maintaining the ability to treat the sick, even when the physician is personally threatened by feelings of hopelessness. "Even when physicians know these things, unfortunately, their knowledge is usually untaught, unvoiced and wordless ... This body of information is too vital to the proper care of the sick to remain the tacit (and spotty) possession of only some physicians. It should be part of medical education. Who knows enough to teach it, however, even if a place were to be made in the medical curriculum? The kind of knowledge of human behavior ... is in the domain of positive psychology ... It must continue to be studied scientifically and taught systematically. It is crucial to medicine's progress." (Cassell, 2009, p. 402).

How can medical schools adapt their curricula to ensure that physicians are compassionate providers of medical care? A curriculum of positive health, professionalism, resilience, and emotional awareness throughout medical training, beginning in year 1, is vital. Building emotional awareness and skills, along with cognitive medical skills, is crucial to success as a physician and a long, flourishing life.

HEALTHY SELF-REGULATION

In exploring the healthy self-regulation of behavior and emotions, we must consider the motivation or the "why" of behavior. This question must be asked because the motivational orientations that guide behavior have important consequences for healthy behavior regulation and psychological well-being. This concept is the basis of a theory first described by Deci and Ryan and known as the self-determination theory (Deci & Ryan, 2000). This theory describes autonomously motivated behavior as that which is self-endorsed and volitional, that is, self-determined. On the other hand, behavior that lacks autonomy is motivated by real or perceived controls, restrictions, and pressures that arise from either the social context or internal forces. The relative autonomy of behavior has important consequences for the quality of the experience, the quality of one's performance, and self-regulation, and it affects every domain of behavior, including health, work, education, and interpersonal experiences.

The self-determination theory also distinguishes intrinsically motivated behavior from that which is extrinsically motivated (Deci & Ryan, 2000). Intrinsic motivation represents a natural inclination toward creativity, exploration, interesting activity, and mastery. Activities are intrinsically motivated only when they are done solely for the interest and enjoyment that they provide. Intrinsic motivation is associated with enhanced task performance and higher psychological well-being.

Extrinsically motivated activities, on the other hand, are those that are done as a means to an external end. There are several levels of extrinsic motivation, which vary in the degree to which they are autonomous or self-determined (Ryan & Deci, 2000a). More specifically, these four levels, ranging from least autonomous to most autonomous, include external regulation, introjected regulation, identified regulation, and integrated regulation.

At the external-regulation level of extrinsic motivation, behaviors are performed either to obtain a reward or to avoid punishment. In other words, one is solely complying with external demands. This situation creates feelings of being controlled by forces or pressures outside of the self. It is a common experience among medical students and house officers. This is the level of extrinsic motivation that is the least self-determined and the least autonomous.

With introjected regulation—the next step closer to autonomous regulation—the locus of causality remains at the external level. However, the behavior is performed to meet demands or rewards that have become introjected (incorporated unconsciously into one's own psyche) and are, therefore, not completely external. Hence, the behavior is performed to attain introjected ego rewards or pride or to avoid guilt, anxiety, or disapproval from oneself or others. Introjected regulation tends to be associated with a greater degree of stress and anxiety, which, in turn, creates self-handicapping and a lack of persistence with difficult tasks. This condition exists because, although the ego has some involvement, the locus of motivation remains largely external.

Identified regulation is the third category of extrinsic motivation, with higher autonomy than external and introjected regulation. At this level, the locus of causality becomes somewhat internal. That is, the behavior in question is consciously valued and embraced as personally important. The behavior feels more volitional and, therefore, is associated with greater persistence, performance, and more positive effect.

Integrated regulation is the fourth and most autonomous form of extrinsic motivation. At this level, the behavior and values involved have become completely internalized and are, therefore, congruent with and synthesized into one's own value system. Thus, this behavior has an internal locus of causality and is self-endorsed. However, because the behaviors are performed to obtain a separately distinguishable outcome, rather than as an end in themselves, they are still regarded as extrinsic.

This model has great relevance to a common phenomenon in hospitals that has been mislabeled *the difficult physician* or the *acting-out* physician. In many hospital situations with a hierarchical organizational structure (see chapter 15), physicians and the frontline multidisciplinary care team are disempowered and regulated by administrators who do not understand their specific problems. They operate at a level of external regulation, unable to solve their problems creatively, work effectively, and self-regulate. With a more horizontal organizational structure, in which the frontline physician and multidisciplinary team are empowered to participate in decision making and problem solving, physicians are able to operate at a more autonomous level of motivation and are, therefore, more easily self-regulated, as opposed to acting out frustrations.

According to the self-determination theory, as children grow, most of their socialized behavior is regulated in a more autonomous fashion as they integrate behavioral regulation into the self (Brown & Ryan, Fostering healthy self-regulation from within and without: A self-determination theory perspective, 2004). In very early childhood, behavior is intrinsically motivated. However, as the child grows, the ratio of intrinsic to extrinsic motivation begins to shift toward extrinsic activities. We spend less time pursuing what interests us and more time focusing on goals and responsibilities that are required by our environment. Because these imposed activities are all external, the key issue becomes how to foster internalization and integration of the value and regulation of these important activities, such as schoolwork, good nutrition, exercise, and finishing tasks in a timely fashion, to name a few. This task is, initially, the job of the parents, and if they are successful, children learn positive self-regulation skills. Later, the same task gets taken over by teachers, bosses, and doctors, as well as others. Internalization is most likely to occur in an environment in which relating and feeling connected is at a high level. The greater the degree of internalization and integration of regulation into the self, the more self-determined the behavior is felt to be. Within the self-determination theory, the connection between autonomy support through positive relationships is viewed as a lifelong dynamic (Brown & Ryan, Fostering healthy self-regulation from within and without: A self-determination theory perspective, 2004). For example, more autonomous extrinsic motivation in an academic setting is associated with greater academic support, engagement and performance, higher-quality learning, and greater psychological well-being.

Intrinsic motivation represents a distinctly autonomous form of functioning in which behavior is performed strictly for its own sake and is completely self-endorsed. Intrinsic motivation is facilitated in circumstances that support its free expression and is aided by a sense of competence in the performer. Therefore, any setting in which external rewards are used to control or motivate behavior tend to undermine intrinsic motivation. Threats, deadlines, demands, imposed goals, and external evaluations also undermine intrinsic motivation. Obviously, we tend to see a lot of such external control in medical school and in the existing medical culture. Such settings tend to undermine healthy self-regulation.

This scenario does not have to be the case. The provision of choice and opportunities for self-direction, as well as acknowledgment of perspectives and feelings, all create a greater sense of autonomy and enhance intrinsic motivation. Because intrinsic motivation occurs more frequently in supportive contexts in which instructors convey respect and caring, the person who is being motivated is free to invest in interests and challenges presented in the learning environment (Ryan & Deci, 2000b). The same holds true for the doctor-patient relationship. When the doctor conveys respect and caring, the patient is better able to internalize the instructions and explanations that the doctor shares with him or her. An atmosphere of put-downs or other negativity rapidly undermines autonomy, thereby making effective learning difficult. In short, internalization is highly dependent on an atmosphere of autonomy support. The greater the external controls over an individual's behavior, be it a medical student, a doctor, a patient, an employee, or a child, the greater the likelihood for that individual to be externally regulated in actions and behavior. Consequently, the individual fails to develop a sense of value or personal investment in the behavior and, instead, is solely dependent on external control. This external control undermines self-motivation, autonomy, and acting on one's own values and desires. For physicians, the external control presents a high-risk situation for the development of frustration, burnout, and ill-being. An example of such a scenario is the patient who does not follow the prescribed diet or medication regimen—perhaps because of lack of instruction or a disengaged physician—who is mislabeled as noncompliant.

Integrated regulation, on the other hand, is facilitated by a perceived sense of choice and freedom from social controls to think, feel, or act in a particular way (Ryan & Deci, 2000b). Integrated regulation is also facilitated by a clear explanation of the meaning behind an extrinsic action, so that the person to be motivated clearly understands what is being asked of him or her. With a clear understanding, the individual can begin more readily to endorse the values, perceptions, and overt behaviors as his or her own, which is an essential first step toward identified or integrated behavioral regulation. Once the behavior and values are internalized, they become self-endorsed and highly autonomous, leading to cooperation and high performance.

The role of supportive conditions in the patient-care setting has been examined in situations in which issues of adherence to treatment are of great concern. Patients who were more likely to express feelings such as "My doctor listens to how I would like to do things" showed greater compliance with medication regimens, as opposed to patients who regarded their physicians as controlling and poor listeners (Williams, Rodin, Ryan, Grolnick, & Deci, 1998). Longitudinal research has demonstrated that autonomy support from counselors in a health program for smokers was predictive of declines in smoking frequency and higher quit rates—even among those smokers lacking the intent to quit at program outset (Williams, et al., 2002).

Brown and Ryan (2004) emphasize an additional point regarding self-regulation that is highly relevant to busy, overworked physicians. They point out that the internal resources centered in consciousness and awareness play a role in fostering more autonomous regulation. This ability also involves attention and the capacity to bring consciousness to bear on events and experiences as they unfold in real time. The power of awareness and attention in this regard lies in raising the consciousness of information that is necessary for healthy self-regulation and wise decision making. The more consciously aware an individual is of what is occurring both internally and in the environment, the more likely that the individual's behavior will be healthy, adaptive, and consistent with his or her values. Under normal circumstances, we are consciously aware of only a small fraction of our perceptions and actions. When we are extremely busy, burned out, or on overload, we are even less aware. (This phenomenon is reviewed and explained in chapter 7 in the discussion regarding thinking traps and resilient thinking.) This lack of awareness obviously can hinder the optimal regulation of one's behavior, often accounting for the phenomenon that has been variously mislabeled as *the acting-out physician* or *the sociopathic physician*.

Mindfulness is an extremely useful tool in these circumstances. Consciousness and focused attention, when brought to bear on a present reality or situation through mindfulness, can add an element of self-direction and self-regulation to behavior that was formerly unconsciously regulated. Mindfulness allows us to do this by creating a mental distance between the self and the contents of the consciousness, one's behavior, and the environment. Taking this observant stance allows for increased self-awareness, as well as the ability to take time to choose the form, direction, and additional specifics of action— in other words, to act in a more autonomous manner. Self-awareness (i.e., knowledge of one's own feelings, needs, and values) is an important facilitator of self-determined behavioral regulation. Although automatic processes may activate behavior, mindfulness of motives and the range of possible actions that flow from them can lead to redirection of these processes (Ryan & Deci, 2004). Mindfulness allows behavior to be directed toward self-endorsed ends. Further, it encourages the adoption of higher goals and values that reflect healthy self-regulation. Mindfulness is a highly valuable tool to effect healthy self-regulation in physicians and other overworked professionals.

EMPATHY

The term *empathy* has its origins in the German word *einfühlung*, which means "feeling within." It also comes from two Greek roots: *em* and *pathos*, which mean "feeling into." Empathy is the ability to step into the situation of another person, including the effort to understand his or her feelings, emotions, and perspectives and then to use that understanding to guide our actions and responses (Batson, Ahmad, & Lishner, 2009). A core skill in social awareness, empathy allows us to sense what others are thinking and feeling and, thus, is an essential building block of a compassionate response. Anatomically speaking, when we empathize with another, our mirror neurons mimic the other person's state. The anterior area of the insula reads that pattern and identifies the state for us. Therefore, at the brain level, reading emotions in others actually involves the ability to first read and identify those emotions in oneself (Singer, Critchley, & Preuschoff, 2009).

Empathy is consistent with the full spectrum of emotions, including empathetic joy at another's good fortune. However, when an empathetic emotion is evoked for another felt to be in need, this response tends to also evoke altruism, which is a motivational state with the ultimate goal of improving or increasing the welfare of another. Therefore, empathy is not only the result of perceiving another as being in need and adopting the perspective of the other person. It also includes valuing the welfare and well-being of that other person.

Whereas human nature was formerly understood as primarily self-interested and self-oriented, evidence shows that we are wired for empathy and social cooperation (Eisenberg & Miller, 1987). We are emotionally primed for empathy by strong attachment relationships in the first two years of life. This growth is then nurtured throughout life under positive circumstances. Curiosity expands our empathy as we grow, particularly when we meet and talk to people outside of our usual social circle. This action enables us to encounter and appreciate lives and views that are different from our own. By making an ongoing effort to meet and talk to new people on a regular basis, we further cultivate our curiosity and expand our potential for empathy. To be truly empathetic, one must first be an excellent listener and both hear and appreciate exactly what is occurring within the other person at that moment. An empathetic bond that is built on mutual understanding can then be created.

The empathy-altruism hypothesis states that feeling empathetic emotion for someone in need evokes altruistic motivation to relieve that need (Batson, 2014). The greater the empathy felt for one in need, the greater the altruistic motivation to see the need relieved, and the greater the helping behavior. So how do we account for the withdrawn, cold behavior in the burned-out doctor or the physician suffering from some other form of ill-being? People suffering from burnout or ill-being often avoid or deny their empathetic feelings. They are aware of the extreme effort involved in helping and their own perceived inability to possibly be helpful (Maslach, 1982). They therefore emotionally withdraw from all such interactions.

Research conducted specifically in the medical setting has found empathy to be very valuable in many ways, particularly with regard to patient care. In situations in which physicians are more empathetic, patient satisfaction is higher. Empathy has been linked to prosocial behavior, decreased malpractice litigation, increased competence in performing histories and physicals, improved moral reasoning, greater physician satisfaction, improved therapeutic relationships, and positive clinical outcomes (Hojat, et al., 2002). Physician empathy in the clinical context is a multidimensional concept involving perspective taking, compassionate care, and the ability to "stand in the patient's shoes." Empathy can be improved and successfully taught, but to be most effective, that teaching should begin in year 1 of medical school and continue through a doctor's clinical career. One important tool in mastering empathy is improved listening skills. Doctors are often in such a hurry that they rarely afford the patient the opportunity to talk beyond a one-word response to a directed question. The ability to ask open-ended questions and then actively and effectively listen to the patient's answers is an essential doctoring skill and step 1 in the development of empathy. Empathy is positively related to successful job performance and job satisfaction, which makes it even more confusing as to why it would be undervalued and under-taught in the medical setting.

COMMUNICATION SKILLS

Nearly one half of all adults in the United States have difficulty understanding what their doctor tells them about why they are sick and how to comply with their treatment regimen, according to the Institute of Medicine (Nielsen-Bohlman, Panzer, & Kindig, 2004). The fact is that most physicians overestimate what their patients are able to understand. In a study of patients with limited health literacy, participants lacked understanding of words regularly used by physicians, such as *bowel*, *colon*, and *screening test* (Davis, et al., 2001).

Communication skills are essential skills for physicians to master for several reasons. Two of the most important purposes are: (1) the ability to communicate with and relate effectively to patients, and (2) the ability to communicate with and work effectively with the health-care team and other care providers involved with a common patient or situation. Effective communication has the potential to generate understanding, spread knowledge, overcome isolation, enable coordination, and improve problem solving. However, when it is ineffective, communication can be disruptive, distracting, misleading, and even destructive. Positive communication practices bring people together through the development of mutual understanding. When communication is respectful, it emphasizes trust, honesty, self-respect, and the willingness to trust and respect others. Positive communication is a helpful tool in the maintenance of healthy relationships through social support, which leads to an increase in happiness and well-being of the other person and acts as a protector against stress. Comforting communication channels interpersonal warmth. Positive communication is constructive; it tends to make a situation better and is often solution-focused, future-oriented, and collaborative.

Clear communication is one of the major keys to outstanding service (as in servant leadership), both one-on-one and in the health-care team setting. Excellent communication has, as its core, the realities of what is occurring interpersonally or with the team versus the melodrama that individuals or team members often create about the team, customers, patients, or a specific project. Unfortunately, the emotionally charged melodrama tends to focus on irrelevant factors and causes communication to become muddled. Communication focused on facts, situations, or specific behavior, however, makes a huge positive difference in getting one's message across clearly, particularly in a high-stress health-care setting.

Problems can occur when individuals withhold communication. People can withhold communication for a variety of reasons. Often it happens due to negative feelings that a person feels awkward or forbidden to express. This inhibition creates a feeling of incompleteness in one's communication. Emotions that often accompany feelings of incompleteness are general upset, being overwhelmed, confusion, agitation, or alienation from the team or dyad. Withheld communication diminishes team effectiveness and undermines trust in relationships between doctor and patient. Therefore, allowing the time and "space" for open and complete communication is essential. The specifics of this concept within the health-care team are discussed in more detail in chapter 15, "The Spirited Multidisciplinary Health-Care Team," under Phase 5.

A common health-care situation in which clear and complete, reality-based communication often suffers is in hand-off procedures. This situation occurs when a patient is moved from one location (e.g., the operating room) to another (e.g., to the recovery room) at change of shift, when one group of professionals hands off care to another, or when residents or doctors rotate on and off a given service and hand off care to another physician. Without complete, clear, and thorough communication accompanying the handoff, the risk of medical errors increases greatly and patient care suffers.

In terms of improving communication skills with patients, active listening is key. It is important to allow the patient to tell his or her story without interruption and without breaking in with one's own conclusions or questions. The doctor must listen with an open mind or risk missing important clues to the actual diagnosis. Active listening can be difficult for a physician, particularly when certain symptoms and clues are associated with specific diagnoses. However, it is important to keep an open mind and allow the patient to fully complete his or her story prior to drawing any conclusions so as to avoid a misdiagnosis. Trust and rapport established early in the doctor-patient relationship will facilitate more difficult conversations in the future, when the patient might become critically ill or is at the end of life.

When communicating a new and difficult diagnosis and treatment to a patient, it is important to acknowledge the patient's emotions and anxiety about the new diagnosis. Reassuring the patient that this type of reaction is common may be helpful. Encouraging him or her to have a family member, friend, or significant other along to listen to your explanation of the diagnosis and treatment options can be an asset to the patient whose anxiety might result in forgetfulness or poor registration of information. Patients often vary in the amount and detail of information that they want to—or are ready to—hear. Before initiating explanations, it is often helpful to assess the level of information wanted or needed by the patient. For example, the doctor might begin by asking the patient, "What is your understanding of this diagnosis?" The doctor might also ask, "What information can I provide that would be helpful to you?"

Using multiple modes of communication when explaining diagnoses or medical issues to patients can be most helpful. For example, the use of drawings, anatomical models, or diagrams as you speak, or sending the patient home with a written summation of what was covered, can be helpful. After you have explained something to the patient, asking the patient to repeat to you what he or she has heard and understood will ensure that an accurate message was received. It is also important to take time to answer any remaining questions the patient might have.

Obviously, dealing with emotions is an important aspect of facilitating communication with patients. Because many physicians are uncomfortable with dealing with their own emotions and, in turn, patients' emotions, this problem can interfere with the doctor's access to key patient information. For example, a patient who is fearful may be silent and not ask any questions. A simple awareness and acknowledgment of the patient's silence and the underlying emotions by the doctor could be the key to opening communication. With a simple and gentle statement, "You seem anxious," observed by the doctor, the patient is given an important and much-needed opening to discuss his or her feelings. The doctor can then acknowledge the appropriateness of these feelings, which will put the patient at ease and assure the patient that you are there to support him or her through the experience. This support by the physician increases the patient's level of comfort and trust and greatly facilitates further communication.

Unfortunately, because doctors are trained to be oriented solely about the diagnosis—not in emotional awareness, communication skills, or other professional skills—they often miss the unspoken emotions behind the medical questions posed by the patient. For example, Mr. Smith asks Dr. Jones, "Is my tumor getting bigger?" When Dr. Jones answers with a simple statement, "Yes, it is one centimeter larger" and then moves on to a different topic, he has missed the unspoken fear and anxiety within the patient that also needs to be addressed to promote healing and recovery (as we have learned throughout this book from the study of positive health). It is not unusual for patients to ask questions when they are seeking emotional support as opposed to actual medical facts. Doctors who excel in communication skills are also skillful in acknowledging and addressing both the medical and emotional needs of their patients.

When the opportunity does arise for a physician to be engaged in a conversation with a patient regarding emotions and feelings, it is important for the doctor to be empathetic and supportive and encourage the patient to be complete in his or her expression of emotions. This approach can be accomplished through brief supportive statements that encourage the patient to elaborate on the feelings that he or she has introduced.

One of the primary barriers to open patient communication is if the patient feels rushed or was previously rushed or ignored by the physician. Physicians can add to the problem if they give nonverbal cues to their patients indicating that they feel time pressure. In such cases, patients may try to protect their doctors. A helpful way for a physician to avoid this situation is to enter the patient's room and sit down near the patient, giving full attention to what the patient has to say. This approach includes not allowing distractions by pagers, office personnel, or others while you are speaking to the patient. These distractions can and should be handled outside of the patient examination room. Even if you are a busy physician and on a schedule of seeing patients every fifteen minutes, the same approach is possible, and you can allow your patients to speak without interruption, ask questions, provide teaching, and deal with emotional issues. In one study, patients who were allowed to speak without interruption for as long as they wished spoke for only an average of one minute, forty seconds (Marvel, Epstein, Flowers, & Beckman, 1999). Having to see a patient every fifteen minutes is clearly not ideal, but the advantages of having an open doctor-patient communication are clear. Excellent physician communication consistently leads to increased patient adherence to treatment regimens and improved patient outcomes (Svensson, Kjellgren, Ahlner, & Säljö, 2000). Everyone benefits, including physicians, patients, and the entire health-care system, and health-care dollars are saved as well.

Discussion topics

1) Emotional awareness (process recordings): Emotional awareness often begins by looking at simple exchanges that occurred between yourself and another individual and trying to increase your awareness of the emotions and motivations behind what was said. This technique was introduced to me in my first year of clinical training as a registered nurse. After a discussion with a patient, I would record the discussion, line by line, and leave a column next to each line to fill in the emotions and motivations that were likely occurring in both the patient and myself at that time. Although this method was difficult at first, with time and the help of an advisor, it greatly increased my emotional awareness.

Divide into groups of three: Person A, Person B, and Person C. Person B should initiate a three-minute discussion with Person A about a recent life event that was very difficult, with Person A responding and further discussion occurring back and forth. Person C will be the timekeeper and the objective observer of the discussion by recording what is said during the three-minute exchange. When three minutes are up, the conversation stops. Persons A and B then each create a process recording on their own of the conversation, including what was said and the emotions and motivations behind each statement. (Allow ten minutes.)

When all process recordings are complete, each group of three meets together. Person A and Person B each present their interpretation of the conversation, allowing their conversation partner and observer, Person C, to clarify any misinterpretations, points of confusion, or forgotten highlights. This is an incredibly helpful learning tool regarding awareness of one's own and others' emotions.

When you have completed that exercise, switch roles, with Persons B and C being the discussants and Person A becoming the objective recorder and timekeeper. This time, Person C should initiate a three-minute discussion with Person B regarding a recent joyous or successful event that occurred in his or her life. Follow the same procedure.

Once you have mastered this tool, I recommend its use in the clinical situation as a tool to help you understand both your own and your patients' emotions, particularly in difficult situations. Reviewing what you have written with a respected advisor or colleague may shed light on a situation that, until now, had been difficult to understand.

2) Enhancing communication in groups: On the next page is a model that distinguishes between the awareness of self and others in group or team communications. It is a model for understanding how communications can be improved through fostering authenticity (i.e., expanding the public area in the diagram). This model demonstrates how information flows within a team or group. Along the *x*-axis is information that we gain through feedback from others in the group, and along the *y*-axis is information that we disclose about ourselves or the team to others. When the team practices open communication with one another, the boundary along the *x*-axis moves to the right, increasing the information known to each team member, increasing the public area, and decreasing the blind and unknown areas. When we, as individual team members, authentically disclose our perceptions and feelings to the team, the boundary along the *y*-axis moves downward, further increasing the public area and eliminating the closed area. From Heermann (1997).

Table 11-1. Johari's Window: Blind, closed, and unknown areas confound communication in the team.

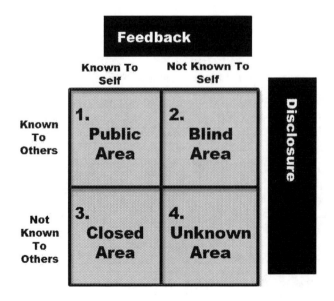

Gather in groups of four people or in your work team. Begin by having all individuals take five minutes to write down three closed topics that they have not disclosed to their colleagues, and three items of constructive feedback that they would like to give to colleagues but have withheld. Once that task is accomplished, gather together and first go around the circle, allowing each person to reveal his or her three topics that, heretofore, had been kept closed. Then, go around the circle once again, with each person offering his or her constructive feedback. Once everyone has spoken, allow time for open discussion regarding the process of making these disclosures, what occurred for them during the process, what was helpful and what could have been more helpful, and how this tool can help in improving group/team communication in the future.

3) Emotional intelligence: The team approach to teaching social and emotional intelligence has shown great promise. Using information from the exercise you completed above (number 2) with your team, answer the following questions:
   A) What new awareness have you developed regarding your own strengths and limitations?
   B) What have you learned about your empathy skills (tuning in to how your words and behavior affect others)?
   C) State two positive goals you can work toward to improve your emotional-intelligence skills.

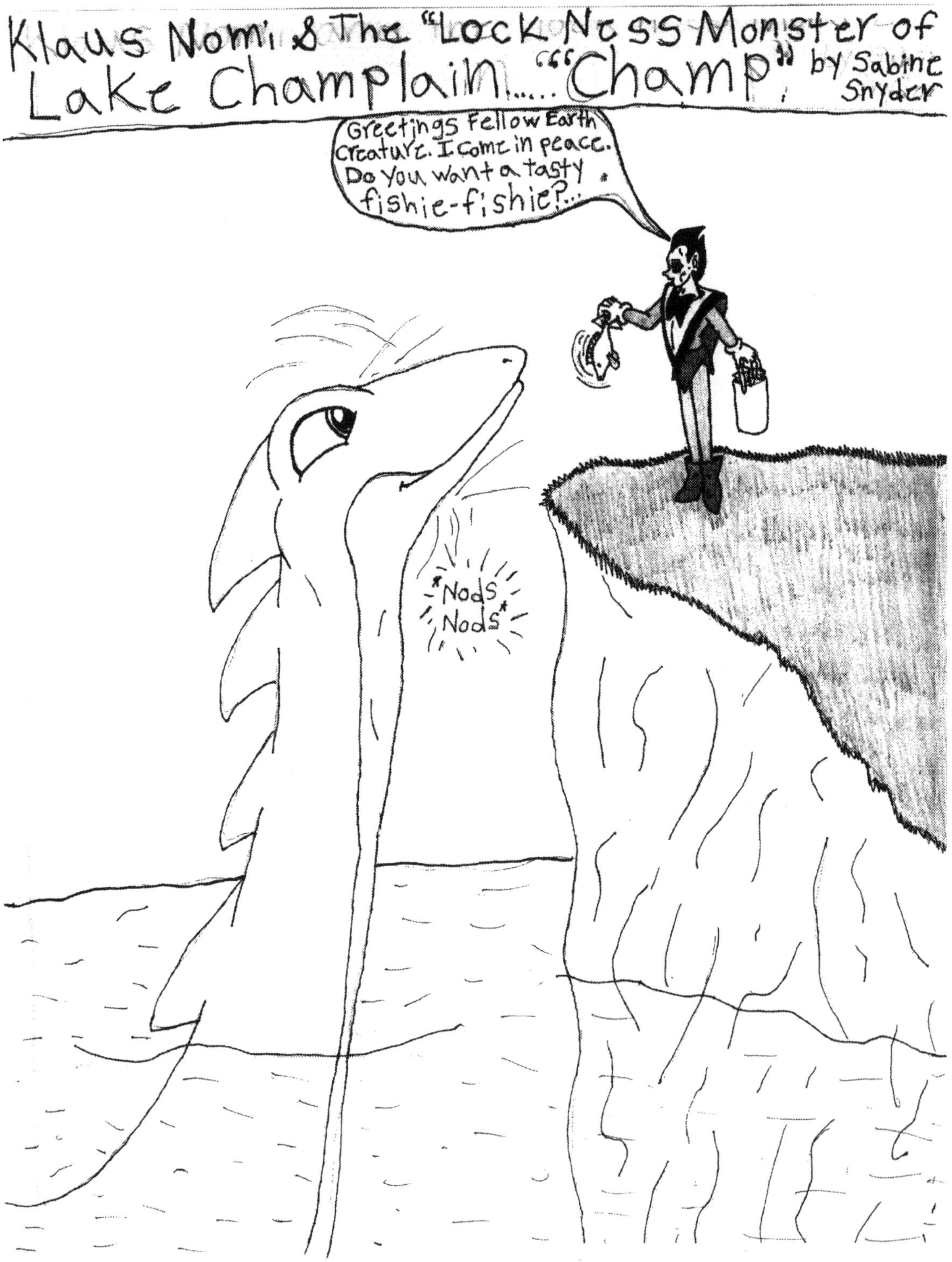
Klaus Nomi & The "Lock Ness Monster of Lake Champlain....."Champ" by Sabine Snyder
Greetings Fellow Earth Creature. I come in peace. Do you want a tasty fishie-fishie?...
Nods Nods

Chapter 12

Posttraumatic and Post-Ecstatic Growth in Medicine

Guest Author: Judith Mangelsdorf, MA, MEd, MAPP

Victor Frankl, a Holocaust survivor and neurologist, wrote in his best-known book *Man's Search for Meaning* (1946; 1985, p. 148): "I know that without the suffering, the growth that I have achieved would have been impossible." This notion, expressed by a doctor who had not only survived years in concentration camps but also had treated hundreds of patients during this time, shall lead us through this chapter addressing trauma in medicine.

While being imprisoned for three years in different concentration camps, Victor Frankl saw many people die. Only very few of the thousands of people entering a concentration camp survived the devastating conditions of their imprisonment, leading Frankl to ask the inevitable question: What was special about them? The answer that Frankl found was the cornerstone of his later work that made him famous as a physician, psychologist, and inspiring person.

This chapter provides an introduction to the concepts of posttraumatic and post-ecstatic growth—where they originate, how they are facilitated, and what role they can play in a lifetime of development. It will focus specifically on theories and examples that can also be applied to the life and clinical routine of medical personnel. Some of these examples show opportunities for growth, while others illustrate where processes can go wrong, leading to post-traumatic stress disorder (PTSD) and breakdown. First, this chapter aims to convey an understanding of what doctors can do, learn, or change to be able to grow from both traumatic and ecstatic experiences in their private and professional lives. Second, it will focus on the trauma of severe illness that patients experience and on the question of how doctors can support their patients in posttraumatic growth. Finally, the concept of post-ecstatic growth will be discussed, highlighting the fact that growth can also stem from life's peak experiences.

Marsha W. Snyder, MD., MAPP.

TRAUMA AND TRANSITIONS

In considering trauma, most people think of extremely negative and unpredictable events, including a serious car accident, war, or severe illness. All of these events are potentially traumatic; however, there are people who experience them without suffering psychologically for long, while others develop severe psychological problems after facing less-threatening events. One explanation of why events with varying degrees of severity are experienced as either traumatic or not traumatic was provided by the neuroscientist Gerald Huether (2010). Huether suggested that, depending on previous experiences and their neuronal representation, the novelty and unfamiliarity of an event is a key factor for the psychological impact of an experience. An unfamiliar first-time experience will be more likely to lead to psychological disruption. Thus, for some people, a certain experience may result in severe traumatization, whereas the same experience may have no lasting impact on others.

Table 12-1. Social Readjustment Scale

Items 1–10 (Holmes & Rahe, 1967)

Rank	Life Event
1	death of a spouse
2	divorce
3	marital separation
4	imprisonment
5	death of a close family member
6	personal injury or illness
7	marriage
8	dismissal from work
9	marital reconciliation
10	retirement

At the same time, there are life events with a higher risk of causing traumatization. To investigate whether stressful life events lead to illnesses, Holmes and Rahe (1967) examined 5,000 medical records of patients, comparing their stressful life events and medical data on their illnesses. In analyzing these data, they developed a list of life events and asked their participants to rate the necessary readjustment period following the event in comparison with the event of marriage. Based on this methodology, Holmes and Rahe were able to determine which events were perceived as severe and difficult to adapt to. They found that patients who experienced a greater number of highly stressful life events were more likely to suffer from illnesses (table 12-1).

The ranking of stressful events indicated that, for a majority of people, the death of a spouse is the most severe event, followed by other important events such as the death of a close family member (rank 5) and personal injury or illness (rank 6). Although the level of readjustment needed is only a proxy parameter for potential traumatization, these findings suggest that stressful events that are common in a clinical setting, including major illness, injury, and death, represent potentially traumatic life events for patients and their families. It is also plausible that physicians who are faced with such events on a daily basis might not be immune to the traumatizing effect that they can have.

The various reactions that different individuals show after facing a traumatic event can be categorized into one of four components: resiliency (McFarlane & Yehuda, 1996, 2007), recovery (Bonanno, 2005), PTSD (Foa, Keane, Friedman, & Cohen, 2008), and posttraumatic growth (PTG) (Tedeschi & Calhoun, 1996). This section will focus on the definitions and distinguishing features of the four constructs. In addition, interactions and connections among these psychological processes will be briefly explained. Figure 12-1 shows the different dynamics of personal development after trauma. Each of the four graphs represents the development of psychological function (i.e., the ability to pursue one's psychological goals and maintain one's psychological well-being) in a prototype pattern for resiliency, recovery, PTSD, and PTG.

Figure 12-1. Prototype pattern for resiliency, recovery, PTSD, and PTG

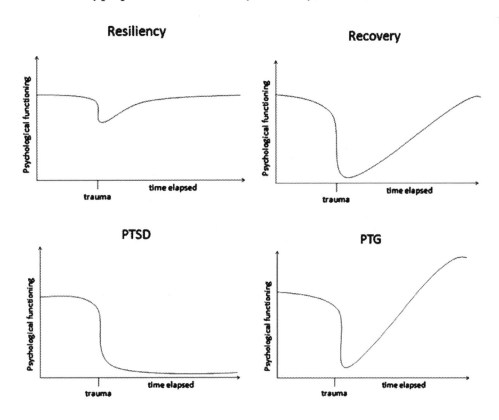

Marsha W. Snyder, MD., MAPP.

Resiliency

Resiliency is the most common response to trauma (McFarlane & Yehuda, 1996, 2007; Bonanno, 2005). Often resiliency is referred to as the ability to persist in the face of adversity and to bounce back from highly stressful experiences (Reivich, Seligman, & McBride, 2011; Tugade & Fredrickson, 2004). It is characterized by a rather mild and brief experience of psychological distress, which allows individuals to maintain a high level of psychological functioning even while coping with stressful life events (Bonanno, 2005). Typically, as indicated in the figure above, resilient individuals show a mild psychological impairment as a reaction to a traumatic event and quickly bounce back to their original level of psychological functioning.

Example: A young clinician—let's call him "Dr. Irving" for purposes of this discussion— who specialized in pediatric heart surgery is taking care of a new patient. The patient's name is Mathew, and he closely resembles Dr. Irving's five-year-old son, Adam. Dr. Irving is very fond of Mathew. The surgery that Mathew needs is a standard procedure that Dr. Irving has performed countless times—always with a positive outcome. The chances look good, and he is sure that there will not be any problems. Dr. Irving performs the surgery to the best of his ability and goes home in high spirits. The next day, before he even enters his office, Dr. Irving makes a detour down the hallway to check on Mathew. Opening the door, Dr. Irving finds the patient's bed empty. Concerned, he asks his colleague (who was on night shift) about Mathew, only to find out that Mathew had died during the night after suffering complications that may have resulted from the surgery.

Example of resiliency: Dr. Irving is shocked for a moment. This event was the first time that a patient of his had died. He takes his colleague out for a coffee to talk about what went wrong and what could be done differently next time. Dr. Irving is sad that he was not able to save this child's life, but he also keeps in mind that he treated many other patients successfully. After the coffee break, Dr. Irving continues his shift. He takes a moment to call his partner and talk about what happened and discuss his fears that he may be responsible for Mathew's death. He decides not to go to a party that he was invited to and walks home instead and takes some personal time for himself. After calling the parents of the child to express his sympathy, Dr. Irving finds some peace. A few more days pass, in which Dr. Irving feels sad and his thoughts circle around Mathew's death, but after a weekend in the mountains with his family, he is back to normal again.

Recovery

A second trajectory that people may follow after facing a traumatizing situation is recovery. Individuals who follow the pattern of recovery after trauma show a moderate to severe immediate reaction and then often experience a disruption of psychological functioning (Bonanno, 2005). They recover gradually, and it takes them a long time to eventually find their way back to their pre-trauma level of functioning. Resilience and recovery can be distinguished by two key dimensions. First, individuals who recover from trauma need more time to readjust than resilient individuals. Second, the process of recovery indicates a higher level of experienced distress and a more severe decline of psychological functioning (Bonanno, 2005).

Example of recovery: When he opens the door, Dr. Irving is shocked. How could this be possible? He walks into the empty room, sits down on the bed, and starts to cry. His colleague from the night shift finds him in the patient room and starts talking to him about the night. When Dr. Irving learns that his mistake could have been responsible for the child's death, he begins to doubt his own abilities. He is paralyzed and barely listens to the rest of the story that his coworker is telling him. After excusing himself, he returns home, unable to eat, sleep, or talk. He cannot block out the thought that it could have been his own son dying there. The following months challenge him and his family. He is haunted by a feeling of dread whenever he enters the hospital, and he spends hours thinking of his own failure. After a while, he starts feeling better, but his despair affects him and his family. Slowly, there are more and more moments in which Dr. Irving is able to acknowledge that there were many other children whom he was able to help and that he is, in fact, a good clinician and is needed at his workplace. After months of recovery, Dr. Irving fully returns to his normal life as a father and physician.

Post-traumatic stress disorder

Post-traumatic stress disorder is a severe psychological condition that may follow exposure to a traumatic event. It is characterized by several symptoms that severely restrict the quality of psychological functioning in affected individuals. Such symptoms include reliving the traumatic experience; high arousal; emotional numbing; and avoiding people, thoughts, places, and memories that are connected to the traumatic event (Foa, Keane, Friedman, & Cohen, 2008). Figure 12-1 illustrates that individuals suffering from PTSD experience a severe decline of psychological functioning and extremely slow or no recovery from that level. Like individuals following the recovery pattern, PTSD patients also suffer a dramatic decline of psychological function as a consequence of a traumatic event. However, instead of recovering, they stay at a severely limited level of psychological function for a long period of time.

Example of PTSD: After learning of the death of his patient, Dr. Irving is paralyzed and in deep shock. He calls his partner, leaves the hospital immediately, and does not return for months. During the first weeks, Dr. Irving is unable to sleep or eat properly. Every night, he wakes up with nightmares, living through visions of his own son's death as a result of his insufficient work. He cannot answer the phone when Mathew's parents try to call him. Driving to the supermarket, Dr. Irving takes a different road to avoid seeing the hospital, because he cannot stand being confronted with anything reminding him of Mathew's death. For a long time, nothing really matters to him anymore. Dr. Irving has lost his confidence and stays home as much as he can. Whenever his partner or one of his friends tries to talk to him about the surgery, he turns away and mentally submerges in his feelings of numbness and loss.

Posttraumatic growth

The last trajectory of development after trauma is posttraumatic growth (PTG) (Tedeschi & Calhoun, 1996). The phenomenon of posttraumatic growth is the focus of this chapter; it is also known as stress-related growth, adversarial growth, benefit finding, or perceived benefit (Affleck & Tennen, 1996; Helgeson, Reynolds, & Tomich, 2006; Park, Cohen, & Murch, 1996). It describes the phenomenon in which people experience positive changes in their lives as an outcome of a traumatic experience. Posttraumatic growth is the only one of the four trajectories described in which individuals manage to realize a higher level of psychological functioning after successfully coping with trauma. Figure 12-1 indicates that immediate recovery sets in after the rapid decline of psychological functioning, but it might also be preceded by an initial period of psychological malfunctioning. Individuals who experience PTG report having closer social relationships, a deeper sense of meaning, more spirituality, enhanced personal strengths, a greater appreciation of life, and more openness to new experiences.

Example: Dr. Irving suffers for weeks after Mathew's death, but several months after the surgery, he realizes that his family, friends, and even his coworkers supported him in a way that he would never have expected. He still suffers from the feelings of guilt, but at the same time, he comes to feel something else: gratitude. Dr. Irving is thankful that his own children are healthy, and he realizes that many of the things that he had worried about in his life, such as earning more money or dealing with annoying neighbors, just are not important enough to waste time on. Questioning himself and his work again and again, Dr. Irving talks to Mathew's parents and finds out that there was a shortcoming in his professional expertise. He realizes that he had never learned how to talk to parents about the potential death of their child. He decides to ask Mathew's parents for help. The three of them meet and talk about Mathew, his death, and the information and insights the parents would have wished for. Dr. Irving returns to his workplace. He isn't quite the same person as before. He is still an excellent clinician, but he has also gained existential insights about life and how he can communicate with the parents of the next child he will try to save.

The relationship of the four patterns

The four trajectories described above are, of course, not completely separable from one another. For several years, the bell-curve theory was widespread and advocated the idea that the reaction to traumatic events can be understood as a bell-curve distribution (Seligman, 2010). Figure 12-2 shows an illustration of the bell-curve theory.

Figure 12-2. Bell-curve theory of psychological reactions to traumatic experiences

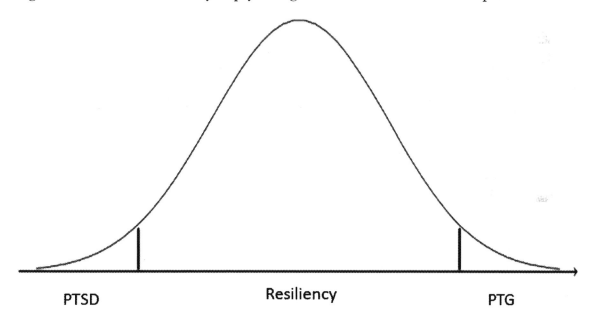

PTSD   Resiliency   PTG

People at the left-hand side of the bell curve would suffer from PTSD; people in the middle of the bell curve would be resilient, while individuals experiencing PTG would be found at the right-hand side of the distribution. This understanding of PTG indicated that PTG and PTSD are highly distinguishable experiences, and that people suffering from PTSD are not the same as those individuals who experience posttraumatic growth. An increasing body of research, however, suggests that PTSD symptoms can be accompanied by PTG processes (Park, Cohen, & Murch, 1996; Larner & Blow, 2011; Schorr & Roemer, 2002). That theory means that people who suffer from PTSD symptoms may also experience growth as a result of the trauma. Figure 12-3 shows PTG as an immediate reaction to trauma. However, it is also possible that posttraumatic growth follows a period of extensive suffering from PTSD, as indicated in figure 12-4.

Figure 12-3. PTG as immediate reaction to trauma

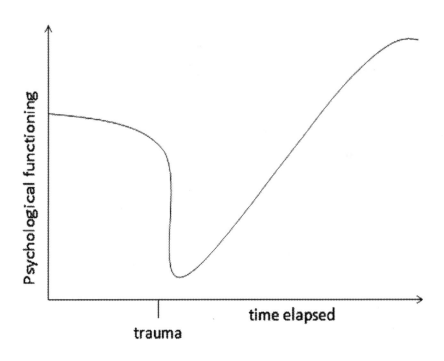

Figure 12-4. PTG following a period of PTSD

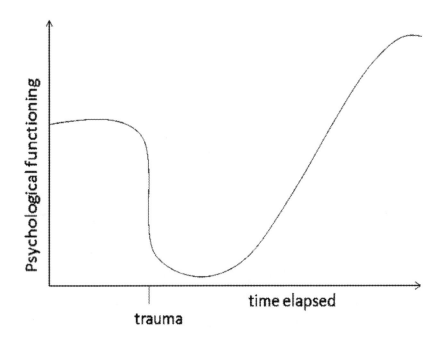

A second, often misunderstood, interaction exists between posttraumatic growth and resiliency. Although both concepts indicate desirable outcomes, they usually don't occur simultaneously (Levine, Laufer, Stein, Hamama-Raz, & Solomon, 2009). Resilient people experience trauma without a shattering of their world assumptions, which allows them to return to their normal life and level of psychological functioning quickly (Larner & Blow, 2011). However, because of the small impact of the traumatic event on their life, there are also only small benefits. Resiliency prevents individuals from suffering from PTSD, but it is also inversely related to posttraumatic growth, thus preventing them from experiencing potentially positive outcomes as well (Levine, Laufer, Stein, Hamama-Raz, & Solomon, 2009).

Traumatic experiences and previous traumatization

The way people react to a certain traumatic situation depends on a variety of factors, including their gender (Vishnevsky, Cann, Calhoun, Tedeschi, & Demakis, 2010), the level of traumatization (Butler, et al., 2005), and the frequency of previous traumas (Breslau, Chilcoat, Kessler, & Davis, 1999). Previous exposure to trauma of any kind is associated with a higher risk of PTSD when facing a new, potentially traumatic event (Breslau, Chilcoat, Kessler, & Davis, 1999). This effect increases if there were multiple traumatic events.

One of the key factors in understanding the impact of previous traumatization may lie in the success of coping with it. Whereas previous traumatization that was accompanied by PTSD without successful coping mechanisms may lead to a higher vulnerability to suffer from PTSD again, successful coping could be a facilitator of resiliency.

Medical professionals, such as emergency ambulance personnel, are likely to face potentially traumatic events (Shakespeare-Finch, Smith, Gow, Embelton, & Baird, 2003). A challenging risk factor that could be examined in clinical work, therefore, is frequent exposure to highly stressful situations that increase the chances for suffering from PTSD.

Example: In the PTSD scenario, Dr. Irving withdraws from his job and his private life. He avoids any kind of situation or interaction that might have reminded him of the surgery. When he finally returns to his workplace, he is able to block out his bad memories. However, the next time that he faces a similar event, he suffers again. Worse yet, new and old memories mix with fears and accelerate the cycle of traumatic experience.

In the PTG scenario, Dr. Irving learns that he can rely on his social network. He finds new means of communication and increases his skills to talk to the families of his patients. Because of his previous experience, Dr. Irving communicates differently when he informs his patients about the potential risks of an impending surgery. Even after an unsuccessful surgery, he is able to cope with the situation differently, because he used his first traumatic experience to learn and grow.

Marsha W. Snyder, MD., MAPP.

Fostering resiliency and posttraumatic growth

Resiliency can be seen as the immune system of the mind. A variety of factors contribute to resiliency and posttraumatic growth, in the same way that there are different possibilities to boost the immune system. However, there are some factors of critical importance that will be discussed in the following section, including creating meaning from traumatic experiences, raising hope and optimism, building on social relationships, creating positive emotions, and most importantly, taking personal initiative to grow. The aim of this section is to highlight opportunities that can foster growth both in others and in oneself.

Meaning making

"He who has a why to live, can bear almost any 'how.'"—Friedrich Nietzsche

This chapter opened with a focus on Viktor Frankl's observations about the Holocaust survivors. What he observed during his time in the concentration camps was the critical importance of finding meaning in life. He was watching fellow inmates die within days after they had given up on life in the unbearable conditions of the concentration camps. Those who survived, including Frankl himself, were able to endure these hardships not only because of chance, but also because they were able to find meaning in their destiny.

The role of meaning making as a coping strategy has been emphasized strongly in research on posttraumatic growth (Larner & Blow, 2011; Park & Ai, 2006). One of the core ideas of the concept of meaning making is that individuals will have a better and more positive outcome after traumatic experiences if they are able to incorporate their experience into their existing global system of meaning (Larner & Blow, 2011).

Victor Frankl (1946; 1985) describes the search for meaning as a crucial and salient human need that is especially critical in times of adversity. He founded a therapeutic school called logotherapy, which helps clients to find and recognize meaning in their life and the circumstances in which they live. Finding something meaningful in traumatic experiences may be of great importance in facilitating posttraumatic growth.

In the PTG example, Dr. Irving transforms the experience of loss into an opportunity to advance to a new level of professional performance. By talking to Mathew's parents about better ways to communicate, Dr. Irving is able to enhance his skills, which allows him to follow his purpose of helping severely ill children and their families. The traumatic experience, then, becomes an important developmental step for him and his professional work. Through this path, Dr. Irving turns his traumatic experience into a meaningful and important event for his personal development.

One of the key factors associated with PTSD is a disruption of core beliefs (LoSavio, et al., 2011). Every individual holds core beliefs about the world, such as "I am safe walking the streets at night," or "My parents always want the best for me," or "I am a good clinician." Through experience, such as robbery, abuse, or the death of patients, these beliefs can be challenged or disrupted. The disruption of one's core assumptions forces individuals to change their cognition to accommodate these stressful experiences (LoSavio, et al., 2011). Although this process can be seen as a threat to the psychological system, the reestablishment and rearrangement of one's core assumptions can also be an opportunity for growth (Cann, et al., 2010).

Group discussion

Many stories of people who created meaning from adversity include the idea of using traumatic experiences and the learned insights to help others with comparable experiences. Often people decide to volunteer for an NGO, work in a certain field, or dedicate their life to a special idea as the result of this process.

- Take a moment to think about a person you know (personally or from the media) who created meaning from the negative experiences he or she had. What happened to this person, and how did he or she transform the traumatic experience?
- If you have the chance, take some time to talk to people who passionately dedicated their life to something larger than themselves. How many people report that finding their calling was connected to a major life event?

Hope

Traumatizing events are often experienced as hitting bottom in one's life. At the same time, facing life's low points has one inherent positive aspect: from there, it can only get better. Hope is a major facilitator for posttraumatic growth, enabling people to continue their life and maintain a high level of psychological functioning by preventing depression (Ai, Cascio, Santangelo, & Evans-Campbell, 2005). At the same time, finding hope for a better future or recovery can be a challenge while one is facing a threatening event.

Chris Feudtner (2005), a physician who specialized in palliative care, provides a framework that suggests that hope can be understood from three different perspectives. Hope is either a goal-directed, cognitive process (hoping for a certain outcome), a cognitive and emotional heuristic that influences how people select their goals (generally being hopeful), or a subjective experience (having hope).

Because hope influences how individuals select their goals (Feudtner, 2005), raising hope can directly affect decision-making processes in medical settings, such as deciding for or against a certain course of treatment. If we understand hope as a goal-directed process, there is one crucial question that we need to ask individuals who are in a difficult situation to understand their personal goals: "What is it that you hope for?" This question not only fosters a positive and trusting relationship between physician and patient, but it also helps the physician to clarify the patient's inner goals and values.

Especially in clinical settings, patients tend to have unrealistic goals, such as saying, "I hope that my paralyzed child will walk again," or "I hope that I will survive even though the doctors say that there is no chance." These unrealistic wishes seem to be naïve; however, it is important not to dismiss them and destroy the hope that they present. Hope itself has tremendous physiological benefits, such as decreasing stress, and therefore, it can directly influence the healing process (Feudtner, 2005). Furthermore, allowing people to maintain unrealistic hope opens the opportunity to ask for smaller goals that are hoped for, which may be reachable.

Example: Conversation between Dr. Irving (DI) and Mathew's mother (MA).

DI: Ms. Anderson, I know that you are desperate. Believe me, I often thought about my own son these days, and how awful it must be to lose a child.… There is something I wanted to ask you. [He pauses.]

Is there something, and I mean anything, that you hope for right now?

MA: There is nothing I can hope for anymore. The only thing that I could think of is waking up tomorrow morning and finding out that all this was only a nightmare.

DI: I understand that the whole situation must feel like a nightmare for you, and I admire that you said yes when I asked you. If you would come to talk with me during this difficult time … I think I would hope for the same, if I were in your shoes … [He pauses again.]

Is there anything else that you hope for now?

MA: Hmm … I hope that my son will not be forgotten. He had such a short life, and I want him to remain in this world somehow.

The example above illustrates two critical points: First, Dr. Irving does not dismiss Ms. Anderson's illusionary hope; he acknowledges it. Second, allowing her to hold on to her hope opens space for her to think about other things that she hopes for that are more realistic. The conversation continued, with Dr. Irving and Ms. Anderson discussing the possibilities of how to remember Mathew. This interaction supports Matthew's mother in her attempt to find out what small things she hopes for and allows her to become more active and less helpless in coping with the death of her son.

Group discussion

Pair up in groups of three people, each with an assigned role—patient, physician, or observer.

Think about a situation that you have experienced or heard of in a hospital or clinical setting in which people were desperate or confronted with trauma. Explain the situation briefly to the other group members. Afterward, practice the doctor-patient interaction of actively fostering hope in the patient.

Patient: Try to put yourself in the shoes of the patient and react in this way to the questions and suggestions that you hear from the doctor.

Physician: Talk to the desperate patient. Try to raise hope in your patient by finding out what your patient hopes for and how it could be realized.

Observer: Write down what went well, which interactions did not work, and why you think these interactions succeeded or failed to raise hope.

After the discussion, the observer gives feedback to the physician first. The patient provides the second piece of feedback. In the next two rounds, roles change until everyone has participated in every role.

Optimism

"Everything will be okay in the end; if it's not okay, then it's not the end." —Paulo Coelho

Although hope includes a specific goal (Feudtner, 2005), optimism is the dispositional or situational expectation of positive outcomes (Segerstrom, Taylor, Kemeny, & Fahey, 1998). Optimism can be seen as a booster of the physical and mental immune system. An optimistic mind-set has a great impact on health-related factors (Seligman & Csikszentmihalyi, 2000), including higher natural killer-cell cytotoxicity and a greater number of helper T cells (Segerstrom, Taylor, Kemeny, & Fahey, 1998), which strengthens the immune system. At the same time, optimism is associated with an individual's perceived capability to meet the demands of a traumatic event (Benight & Bandura, 2004), boosting the immune system of the psyche.

It is possible to distinguish between dispositional and situational optimism (Segerstrom, Taylor, Kemeny, & Fahey, 1998). Dispositional optimism is a tendency to expect positive outcomes in general. In contrast, situational optimism is the specific expectation of a positive outcome in a certain domain or as the consequence of a specific event. This distinction is of crucial importance, especially in clinical settings, in which the interactions between doctors and patients are usually rather brief. Whereas building up dispositional optimism is a time-consuming process, situational optimism can be sparked even in very short conversations.

Group discussion

Despite the far-reaching positive consequences of optimism, critics often point out that optimism fosters unrealistic expectations of the future; therefore, what is the right way to behave for a clinician? Should doctors raise unrealistic but optimistic expectations in their patients, even if it may lead to disappointment, or should they provide medical facts only and a realistic outlook?

In an informative discussion of different treatment options, should doctors paint an optimistic picture, or should they emphasize the possible risks involved in the treatment options?

A new approach that addresses the dilemma between optimistic and realistic outlooks is the concept of realistic optimism (Schneider, 2001). This concept maintains that reality is not an objective truth. Schneider (2001) refers to this lack of accuracy as "the fuzzy nature of reality," emphasizing that our perception of reality depends on the reference points we use to interpret it, such as our previous experiences.

Example: Let us compare two possible scenarios in which Dr. Irving talks to the families of his young patients.

In the first situation, Dr. Irving talks to the family before Mathew's surgery. Because of the experiences that the doctor has had up until then, he talks about the surgeries that he conducted successfully and the many lives he saved. Dr. Irving also talks about the risk factors involved in Mathew's case, but because of the reference points in his previous experience, Dr. Irving draws a positive and realistic picture of the possible outcome.

In the second situation, a different family comes to Dr. Irving's office to talk about their child, immediately after Mathew's death. In this situation, Dr. Irving is very aware of the risks and emphasizes the possible complications. He might also refer to past surgeries that went well, but not without mentioning that the surgery could be fatal. Because he has a new reference point, Dr. Irving now draws a rather pessimistic but also realistic picture of the outcome.

What is evident in these two examples is that Dr. Irving is giving a realistic assessment of the situation in both conversations. The chances of surviving this specific surgery, as reported by the available evidence, has not changed. However, while the first family will leave the room with a feeling of optimism, the second family will leave accompanied by the fear of the sudden death of their child.

The concept of realistic optimism offers a third point of view between harsh reality and unrealistic optimism. It indicates that there are a variety of optimistic outlooks that people can be given that are not necessarily unrealistic (Schneider, 2001). As illustrated above, the picture that we draw in giving an outlook into the future depends on past experience and one's personal focus. Most people tend to focus more on negative rather than positive information (Rozin & Royzman, 2001). This phenomenon, called negativity bias, might be one of the key inhibitors in raising optimism and hope in others.

Research on the impact of optimism on mental and physical health has shown that optimism is associated with a broad range of beneficial aspects, including longevity (Peterson, Seligman, Yurko, Martin, & Friedman, 1998), less frequent episodes of physical illness (Scheier & Carver, 1992), less psychological distress (Carver, et al., 1993), and—important—resiliency (Larner & Blow, 2011). Considering these beneficial consequences of a more positive explanation of facts, raising realistic optimism might be an important skill for clinicians.

Group discussion: Communicating bad news

Split up in pairs. Following is a list of diagnoses that need to be communicated to patients or family members. Write down alternative ways to present the given information: first, in a realistic but optimistic way; second, from a realistic but pessimistic perspective. After you have finished writing, choose a role (either patient or physician) and test some of the examples that you have developed in interaction with your partner. Discuss how your interactions between positive and negative outlooks differed in both roles.

1) A seventy-five-year-old woman has been diagnosed with metastasizing breast cancer. According to recent studies, about 25 percent of persons in her age group die within six months after diagnosis, 50 percent live for another year, and 25 percent survive up to two years or more.
2) A twenty-five-year-old man is paralyzed after a serious car accident. Most people with comparable injuries will never walk again.
3) A four-year-old girl has been diagnosed with acute leukemia. About half of the children with her condition survive, depending on participation in different courses of treatment.

The communication task above highlights critical moments in the interaction between patient and clinician. Most physicians experience the process of delivering bad news to the patient as inhumane and damaging (Baile, et al., 2000). However, the relationship between doctor and patient and the way in which potentially traumatic news is delivered influence the patient's ability to absorb and cope with the information (Slavin, O'Malley, Koocher, & Foster, 1982).

Good social relationships and delivery of bad news

Social support is one of the key environmental resources that helps to successfully overcome life crises (Prati & Pietrantoni, 2009). By facilitating coping processes and successful adaption to challenging events, close relationships can contribute to personal growth (Prati & Pietrantoni, 2009). While Tedeschi and Calhoun's primary model of posttraumatic growth (1996) included closer social relationships as an outcome variable, it has also been shown that individuals who are surrounded by supportive friends and family members are more likely to experience growth after trauma (Schroevers, Helgeson, Sanderman, & Ranchor, 2010). Thus, social relationships can be seen as an outcome variable as well as a predictor of posttraumatic growth.

One of the first rules of immediate intervention after trauma is to ensure social support personally or—if that is not possible—through others. For many traumatized patients, not being left alone is important to help them cope. In the later process of recovery, having a constant medical contact person also facilitates readjustment.

One of the challenges of the doctor-patient relationship lies in the inevitable task to deliver bad news that might shatter the patient's life. In the following section, main aspects of how to break bad news to the patient based on a good patient-physician relationship will be introduced. Baile and associates (2000) created a six-step protocol on how to deliver bad news to patients. They defined four key objectives of the critical conversation: (a) gathering information about the patient's knowledge, (b) providing medical information, (c) giving support, and (d) engaging the patient's collaboration in developing a treatment plan. Baile and associates (2000) provide the following six-step protocol to break down the delivery of bad news:

S - Setting up the interview (mental preparation, setting up the room)

P - Perception (assessing the patient's perception of his or her medical condition)

I - Invitation (obtaining the patient's invitation to provide full information or only the answers to certain questions or to talk again at another time)

K - Knowledge (providing knowledge and medical information to the patient in the framework set out by the invitation)

E - Emotions (addressing the patient's emotions)

S - Strategy and summary (discussing treatment options)

Baile and associates (2000) point out that the complexity of the topic and the emotionally loaded interaction can lead to severe miscommunications. To avoid misunderstandings and mental overload, it is important for the physician and the patient to decide together whether they wish to talk about medical information and a possible treatment plan right away or if they prefer to continue the discussion at another time. Being confronted with life-shattering news can lead to psychological shock that could prevent the patient from processing further information. In these situations, it can be more helpful to organize support first—before discussing medical facts and future treatments.

The protocol introduced is a helpful, broad guideline for delivering bad news. Simultaneously, from a growth perspective, there are additional aspects that should also be taken into account. There should be three additional goals of the interview to reduce the emotional impact and foster growth: giving hope, raising optimism, and emphasizing the patient's personal resources and strengths.

Most people are actively engaged in community work or an activity, such as sports, the arts, or religion, or they have family or close friends. However, under psychological shock, most people are not able to draw from these resources. Working out a plan for how to make use of these personal resources in the face of trauma might open up discussion with the patient about treatment. Simultaneously, it will enhance the doctor-patient relationship in a unique way in accompanying patients through the process of healing or—in cases of terminal illness—good dying.

Group discussion

Although the SPIKES protocol provides a guideline on which aspects should be covered, it is also important to know how to address its key issues.

Step 1: Split up in groups of four people. Each group will deal with a unique case example dealing with bad news in a clinical situation. In each group, one person is responsible for two of the six aspects of the SPIKES protocol (SP, IK, ES). The fourth person covers personal resources (R). Individually, each of you can think about questions that can be asked to address each key aspect and write them down. You should also think about important details that need to be taken into account in this particular situation.

Step 2: Afterward, meet in a large group. What do each of these situations and the strategies you developed have in common? How are they different?. After sharing ideas, come up with the strategies the group feels are most ideal and appropriate.

Positive emotions

One key facilitator of growth is the prevalence of positive emotions. These emotions provide the neuronal activation for changes in the brain that are related to a broadening of thought-action repertoires. Fredrickson's broaden-and-build theory of positive emotions (2004) provides a framework that explains the impact of positive life events and emotions on human development. The theory postulates that positive emotions promote the discovery of novel and creative actions, ideas, and social bonds. These new discoveries build social and psychological resources that can be drawn on in times of adversity and increase the chances of successful coping (Fredrickson & Branigan, 2005). In Fredrickson's framework of positive emotions, psychological peak experiences lead to increased resiliency and psychosocial growth through creating positive affect. In this sense, positive emotions are not only a momentarily pleasant experience, but also show long-term effects on an individual's cognitive and socio-emotional development.

As discussed in the section about meaning making, the broadening of one's thought repertoire by assigning meaning to past events is a crucial facilitator for growth after negative life events (Larner & Blow, 2011). One core component of psychological therapies is the focus on the transformation of meanings that clients assign to traumatic experiences (Larner & Blow, 2011). In this way, posttraumatic growth relies on the broadening of thought repertoires. Many people experience positive emotions, life energy, human functioning, and deep inner happiness after overcoming difficult challenges in their lives. Csikszentmihalyi (1990) offers a possible explanation for these findings. He describes two states of the human mind: teleonomy (order) and entropy (chaos). In this framework, building new cognitive scripts and personal growth are connected with shifting from entropy to teleonomy, which is associated with emotional equilibrium.

Csikszentmihalyi's theoretical suggestion that growth occurs through shifting between entropy and teleonomy is supported by research on the role of emotionality and posttraumatic growth. Norlander, Schedvin, and Archer (2005) asked people about the frequency in which they experienced positive and negative emotions in the last two weeks and measured their perceived level of posttraumatic growth. They classified the participants into four groups: self-destructive (high on negative and low on positive emotions), low affective (low on negative and low on positive emotions), self-actualizing (low on negative and high on positive emotions), and high affective (high on negative and high on positive emotions). Table 12-2 shows the four different groups of emotionality.

Positive Emotions Negative Emotions	Low	High
Low	Low affective	Self-actualizing
High	Self-destructive	High affective

Table 12-2. Types of emotionality (Norlander, Schedvin, & Archer, 2005)

Norlander and associates (2005) found that people who were low on positive emotions were least likely to show posttraumatic growth independently from the frequency with which they experienced negative emotions. People who reported experiencing positive emotions on a regular basis but rarely experienced negative emotions were more likely to grow after trauma than the groups who reported being low on positive emotions. However, the category showing the greatest posttraumatic-growth results was the high affective group. People who experienced both positive and negative emotions regularly also reported the highest level of posttraumatic growth. The findings of Norlander and colleagues (2005) emphasize the importance of facilitating positive emotions in times of adversity.

Individual Exercise: The vade mecum

One of the critical points of trauma and highly negative events is that they undermine people's sense of what might help them feel better.

Please take a moment and think about a highly stressful event in your own life that you managed successfully. Take a piece of paper and write down everything you or others did that helped you cope with it or simply cheered you up. Also add other activities that come to mind that might help you feel better when you really feel down. Collect at least ten activities and continue the list every time something new comes to your mind.

Store the list in a place where you can find it quickly when you need it. When you feel down, take the list out. Even if you do not feel like doing anything with it, choose at least three of the activities that you wrote down earlier and put them into practice.

Personal growth initiative

Posttraumatic growth and resiliency are often perceived as developments that happen automatically after a traumatic life event based on personal disposition. This perception may stem from the idea that even young children who cannot draw from the same resources as adults can show resiliency to challenging life events (Masten, 2001). However, a person's reaction to challenging life circumstances is not only a process that occurs according to chance and personal characteristics. It is also connected to one's personal initiative to achieve growth.

An individual's personal motivation and active behavior to overcome trauma is a central facilitator for posttraumatic growth. Robitschek and colleagues (2012) identified two major groups of clients in psychotherapy: those who are ready to actively use counseling for self-improvement and those who are naïve about their individual growth process. Individuals who actively use their life experiences to improve themselves show four key skills: readiness for self-change, planfulness on how to implement self-changes, usage of resources that promote self-change, and intentional behavior to realize these changes (Thoen & Robitschek, 2013). Robitschek's work highlights the importance of motivation and personal initiative for overcoming trauma. It is evident that resources, such as a strong social network, cannot unfold their positive effect of helping a person to overcome challenging circumstances if they are not actively pursued.

Marsha W. Snyder, MD., MAPP.

How to work with traumatized patients and help them to foster growth

One of the crucial insights gained from research on trauma and potential growth is that timing plays an important role. As indicated in figure 12-1 of this chapter, traumatization is a dynamic process that changes over time. In the very beginning, there is a steep decline in psychological functioning, accompanied by high arousal, which has severe consequences for an individual's coping ability. Figure 12-2 shows the most vulnerable phase of traumatization, which is shortly after occurrence of the event. Often, traumatized patients in the acute phase of trauma need basic support, including adequate sleep and rest, eating food they like, spending time outdoors, feeling safe, and receiving emotional and social support. The sudden disruption in psychological functioning often prevents people from sensing things that might make them feel better. One of the best options in supporting patients during this time is to take care of their well-being and to help them reduce their arousal. These basic needs are universal in all four trajectories that may follow after a traumatic event. Demands that exceed the care of basic needs might be harmful during this vulnerable phase. Therefore, complex efforts such as making patients see benefits in their situation or asking them to acknowledge that life is a gift should be initiated carefully and only if the patient is ready to take these concepts on.

Group discussion

Split up in groups of three to five people. Assign each group a task group: A, B, or C. After completing the tasks, rejoin and discuss your results.

The very strict schedule and organization of most hospitals often prevent patients from psychological recovery. Based on your own hospital experiences and the needs described above, which changes in the clinical schedule or interventions would you suggest for …

Group A: … patients who have experienced a serious car accident?

Group B: … patients who were diagnosed with breast cancer for the first time and just had their first surgery?

Group C: … relatives who were just informed that one of their close family members has died.

Were different interventions suggested across groups A, B, and C? Can these interventions also be applied to the other respective groups?

Post-ecstatic growth

This chapter has primarily addressed traumatic events and the key components that are necessary to transform threatening situations into growth. We now turn to a different transformational process, which has not yet been discussed: the phenomenon of post-ecstatic growth (Roepke, 2013).

The idea of stress-related growth has a long history. Benjamin Franklin's famous notion "No pain, no gain" highlights the assumption that personal development is necessarily connected to adversity. Transformational processes, however, do not only appear after the worst experiences individuals encounter; they also occur because of highly positive events, such as the birth of a child or achievement of a crucial long-term goal.

Post-ecstatic growth is the positive, multidimensional development that can result from highly positive life events. The upward spiral of positive experiences can catalyze growth processes that occur in different areas of the self, including meaning in life, self-esteem, or social bonds (Roepke, 2013).

One of the main reasons why traumatic experiences have such a tremendous influence on people's lives is that they disrupt one's assumptions about the world (LoSavio, et al., 2011; Cann, et al., 2010). Similarly, observing highly moral behavior, such as a stranger risking his life to save the life of someone else, can be highly inspirational and, therefore, facilitate growth as well (Keltner & Haidt, 2003). The inspire and rewire hypothesis builds a theoretical framework for the phenomenon of post-ecstatic growth, emphasizing that deeper social relationships and moral growth can occur after highly positive life events (Keltner & Haidt, 2003).

In a first pioneering study, Roepke (2013) asked undergraduate students about their best experience in life and how this event changed them as a person. Four different factors were reported as outcomes of life's best experiences: new meaning and purpose in life, an increased spiritual development, and higher self-esteem. The findings indicate that highly positive experiences can catalyze multidimensional growth and lead to changes comparable to those that are based on adversarial events.

Although life-threatening medical conditions, such as severe illnesses and even death, are inevitable parts of the day-to-day life of many clinicians, truly positive events are also frequent experiences. Managing the delivery of a baby, successfully completing a challenging surgery, or creating an environment that allows patients to die peacefully are only a few examples of the wide range of highly positive experiences that can occur in the medical field. These kinds of events are not only extraordinary moments in life, but they can also provide opportunities for growth if actively considered and learned from.

Positive life events can work as a buffer for stressful adversarial events, prevent depression, and diminish physical symptoms (Cohen & Hoberman, 1983). In many cases, however, the chance to thrive and build resilience is left unused. One of the reasons for not savoring the good may lie in the negativity bias previously mentioned (Rozin & Royzman, 2001). Because individuals pay more attention to negative events and information, failure often plays a more important role than success, even though savoring positive events would be highly adaptive. Thus, a critical question is presented: How can people grow from life's best moments?

Fostering post-ecstatic growth

In every person's life there are opportunities to experience post-ecstatic growth, including personal successes, falling in love, or having a baby. However, for some people, these experiences pass by without having a lasting positive impact. To make the most of life's best moments, there are different ways to seize these opportunities for growth. In the following sections, five ways are explained in detail.

Common factors. Some of the factors contributing to post-ecstatic growth equal those that facilitate posttraumatic growth and are described above. Positive and negative events may pass without resulting in growth. One of the reasons why lasting effects may not occur after positive events is a lack of personal initiative, which is necessary for self-improvement. Robitschek's concept of personal growth initiative (2012) emphasizes two of the most important elements of personal development: a person's readiness for self-change and active behavior.

Another common factor contributing to both posttraumatic and post-ecstatic growth is meaning. In the section on posttraumatic growth, the importance of meaning making was emphasized. Individuals who are able to draw meaning from a traumatic event and who are able to integrate that experience into their existing global system of meaning are more likely to develop posttraumatic growth (Larner & Blow, 2011). The same seems to be true for highly positive life events. Experiences that align with an individual's meaning in life correlate with post-ecstatic growth (Roepke, 2013).

Savoring and social relationships. One of the most effective ways to place emphasis on a positive life event is to savor it actively. Bryant (Bryant, 2003) defines savoring as the action of mindful engagement in behaviors and thoughts that deepen the effect of positive experiences. According to Bryant's work, savoring can enhance meaning, engagement, and gratitude; facilitate mindfulness; and increase positive emotions. There are three temporal forms of savoring: anticipating (looking forward to a positive event), savoring the current moment (intensifying and prolonging enjoyment of present experiences), and reminiscing (looking back to rekindle positive feelings) (Bryant & Veroff, 2007). Savoring is a highly individualized process that can include a variety of activities. One of the most common and effective savoring strategies is sharing positive experiences and memories with others.

Supportive relationships are a crucial moderator for growth after major life events. Many individuals experience positive change after a good event by using a strategy of capitalization and savoring (Bryant & Veroff, 2007). Simultaneously, sharing good experiences improves the relationship with those who participate in them (Gable, Reis, Impett, & Asher, 2004). Gable and colleagues (Gable, Gonzaga, & Strachman, 2006) introduced a communication technique called active-constructive responding (ACR), which includes asking questions about the event, showing interest, and celebrating each other's joy, which in turn can be catalyzed for growth. Active-constructive responding is a proactive approach to enhance positive relationships and thereby amplify the beneficial effects of positive life events.

Learning from best practices. One of the unique opportunities to acknowledge and emphasize success and incorporate new knowledge is learning from best practices. In medicine and psychotherapy, frequent team meetings, supervision, and intervision processes are used to discuss the best treatment options for challenging cases. Problems and failures are addressed, while smooth and successful treatments or therapies are often neglected. Despite the fact that this procedure is highly adaptive for difficult cases, it disregards one of the biggest resources of development: learning from best practices.

Grol and Grimshaw (2003) pointed out that, in medicine, the widespread procedures to introduce new scientific evidence into existing routine daily practice often results in inappropriate, unnecessary, and harmful care. As an alternative (or complementary) approach, discussing successful treatments and therapies in team settings might have highly positive consequences for patients and doctors alike. This different perspective improves patient care on more than one level: Although the information about best-practice experiences can present additional or superior options for treating other patients, sharing personal success stories and positive experiences can foster resiliency (Cohen & Hoberman, 1983) and personal growth in medical personnel.

Group discussion: Discussing best practices

Split up into groups of five people for this exercise. The first step should be done individually; the second step is the group.

Step 1: Think about an experience with a successful treatment or therapy that you or someone you know had. What happened and why did it work well? Pay attention to details of the process that might not be obvious, such as including family members or spending extra time talking to the patient. What was your key takeaway?

Step 2: Present your experience to the other group members.

As other group members share their experiences, use constructive responses to highlight the positive aspects of the experience.

Step 3: Write down the unexpected details that you observed. What new insights did you get from the story you heard? Discuss your insights in the group.

CONCLUSION: HOW TO GROW IN MEDICINE

In contrast with many other professions, working in medicine includes constant exposure to highly stressful experiences. Even though this frequent exposure can be a threat to psychological functioning, it might also be a unique chance to grow professionally and personally.

This chapter covered four different trajectories of development that can follow highly stressful life events: resiliency, recovery, post-traumatic stress disorder, and posttraumatic growth. Which of these reactions occurs depends on a variety of factors, such as previous exposure to trauma, coping strategies, and available resources. The emphasis here is on posttraumatic growth and highlighting factors and interventions that can contribute to positive psychological change after traumatic life events in medical settings. Additionally, the concept of post-ecstatic growth was introduced; emphasizing that both negative and positive experiences can contribute to psychological growth and resiliency.

Today's medical world places a stronger emphasis on technology rather than on personal encounter. Although the ongoing technical progress continues to provide new treatment options, it also leads to decreased social interactions. When we look at the facilitators of growth, however, there is one inevitable factor: social relationships. For most people, meaning making is embedded in contributing to the lives of others. Positive emotions are highly related to social interaction, and a close social network is one of the key factors contributing to physical and mental health. To reach the goal of delivering the best possible care to patients and to contribute to a physician's growth, there is no more important means than the human bond.

If one insight can be drawn from this chapter and from Victor Frankl's life, it is the understanding that every path in life can be turned into growth and that life's best and worst moments are unique opportunities to thrive.

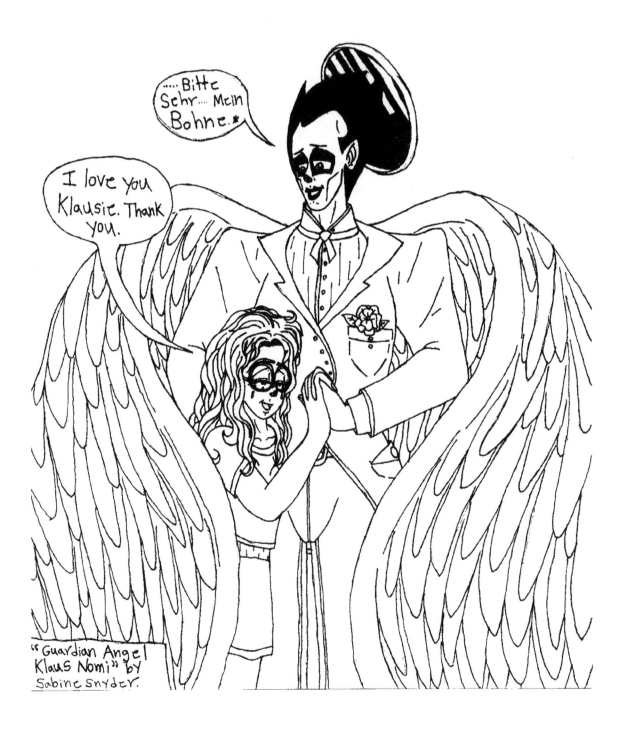

"Guardian Angel Klaus Nomi" by Sabine Snyder.

Chapter 13

Spirituality and Well-Being

Spirituality is a cultural reality today in the United States and throughout many cultures. Ninety percent of Americans state that they believe in God and engage in prayer on a regular basis. Eighty-four percent believe that either religion or spirituality is important to their lives (Pargament & Mahoney, 2009). In light of the trend toward spirituality and religious belief, the focus of this chapter is to discuss the ways in which spirituality can be understood as a natural part of life. Although spirituality is not taught to doctors as part of their medical-educational curriculum, it is clearly a part of life that is linked to well-being. Even if you, as a physician, do not include religion or spirituality in your life, the fact that 90 percent of Americans believe in God indicates that you are highly likely to encounter issues of spirituality through your patients, and you will need to understand its nature. Spirituality is pervasive in our culture, and with it come unique approaches to well-being.

Historically speaking, religion has been referred to in psychiatry and psychology only when describing a delusion or other aspect of a patient's illness. During the 1950s, thought on this topic began to change when Harvard psychologist Gordon Allport made the distinction between extrinsic religiosity (religion as a means to other ends) and intrinsic religiosity (religion as an end in itself) (Allport & Ross, 1967). The extrinsically religious tend to participate in institutionalized religion because it provides security, satisfies social needs, or confers status. The intrinsically religious, in contrast, internalize religious beliefs and bring their other needs into harmony with them (Peterson C., 2006, pp. 294-297).

It wasn't until 1975 that the American Psychological Association created a division devoted to the psychology of religion. Since then, research in this area has steadily grown, and large private foundations, such as the John Templeton Foundation and the Fetzer Institute, have facilitated that growth. Following the lead of the larger culture, psychologists began to distinguish between religiosity and spirituality. Religion subsumes traditional religion-based ways of experiencing the sacred and the transcendent. Spirituality is an ever-expanding term that not only includes one's religious experience but also one's compassionate experience with nature or humanity. Therefore, people may describe themselves as being spiritual because they feel elevated in nature or they have moral values, but they may not necessarily believe in God or worship in a congregation with like-minded people. It is possible that the concepts of religion and spirituality may overlap and occur within the same person.

Professed religiousness in young people in the United States is associated with a tendency to avoid all manner of antisocial activities. Children and adolescents who score high on measures of religiousness show greater emotional self-regulation, engage in fewer acts of aggression, have better academic records, and are less likely to use drugs and alcohol (Peterson C., 2006, p. 295).

Pargament defines spirituality as a search for the sacred (Pargament & Mahoney, 2009). The term *search* implies a process involving great effort to discover and then hold onto the sacred. The *sacred* includes concepts of God, the Divine, and transcendent reality, despite the fact that these concepts cannot be proven as scientifically true. A third aspect of this definition of spirituality includes transforming the sacred when necessary. These pathways involving the sacred can either be individually constructed or a part of well-established tradition. They include personal ends (e.g., meaning in life), social ends (e.g., closeness with others), and sacred ends in themselves (e.g., living according to a sacred set of values) (Pargament, 2002).

Describing a person as *spiritual* indicates that he or she is trying to find, know, experience, or relate to whatever he or she perceives to be sacred. This search for the sacred is a dynamic process rather than a fixed one. Spiritual persons often consider themselves to be on a lifelong journey to develop, maintain, and further their relationship with God.

There are many different spiritual pathways that can be followed to foster one's relationship with the sacred. Many include social organizations, which range from traditional religious institutions to less traditional spiritual groups and gatherings (e.g., meditation centers). The pathways involve systems of belief—traditional or nontraditional—that are shared by the members of the group. Additional pathways include prayer, reading of sacred or spiritual texts, yoga, music and other art forms based on the sacred, and other established traditions and practices that are unique to that respective group (Pargament & Mahoney, 2009).

Using the lens of spirituality to develop a deeper understanding of human flourishing provides unique and interesting insights. Most people engage in a form of spiritual practice, which can give rise to bold and unique ways of thinking from these religious and spiritual mind-sets. For example, the fact that 90 percent of Americans believe in God and engage in some form of prayer shows that spirituality is an important social element in itself and that most humans derive something positive from participating in spirituality throughout their lives. Furthermore, randomized controlled studies demonstrate an association between religious coping mechanisms and a lower six-month mortality rate in open-heart surgery patients, as well as better overall physical health and well-being (Pargament & Mahoney, 2009). Hence, the benefit of spirituality affects humans positively at the neurochemical and the biological level. This concept may bear fruit in many disciplines related to human flourishing, including medicine, positive psychology and positive health, religion, and sociology if pursued and studied in greater depth.

Pargament and Mahoney conclude in their empiric work that whether spirituality is helpful or harmful depends on its degree of integration (2009). At best, spirituality is responsive to life's situations, nurtured by the larger social context, capable of flexibility and continuity, and oriented toward a life-enhancing destination. This knowledge helps us to better understand the outcomes of our spiritual search, which are most commonly connected with thriving. Generally speaking, the search for the sacred is associated with beneficial outcomes, such as a greater sense of connection with the sacred, using spiritual methods of coping, and experiencing better health and well-being. Spirituality, at its best, includes pathways that are broad and deep. It is responsive to life's common problems and everyday needs, and it exists in harmony with and nurtures the larger social context. Spirituality is flexible, ongoing, and oriented toward a sacred destination; it encompasses the full range of human potential, together with a powerful guiding vision.

A poorly integrated spiritual system, on the other hand, that is exclusionary, is not supportive of the social system, and does not support individual values, can quickly lead to chaos and decline. For example, exclusively harsh and punitive views of God can interfere with one's ability to enjoy the pleasures of life, with multiple negative consequences.

Studies have shown that a deeply internalized sense of spirituality is associated with mental-health benefits (Pargament & Mahoney, 2009). Individuals who feel a secure attachment to God report less psychological distress than those who describe a weaker attachment.

What is unique and remarkable about the insights that we can derive from spirituality and how it relates to human flourishing come from its bold mind-sets. For example, Ricard (2011), in his reflection on the Dalai Lama, discusses the meaning of enduring happiness from the Buddhist perspective. He describes happiness as a way of being, and a skill that can be cultivated. Happiness is an enduring trait that arises from a state of mental balance, which in turn, is an unfiltered awareness of the true nature of reality. Happiness has everything to do with our mind and our inner thoughts and little to do with what is happening external to us. The goal is to live a meaningful and constructive life and to free oneself from mental states that cause suffering for oneself or others—to find a state of inner peace. It is obvious that the Buddhist philosophy of happiness and well-being represents a major departure from what we experience on a day-to-day basis in capitalist society in America today.

To take this idea a step further, the work of Karen Armstrong (2010) is another potent example written from the spiritual perspective. She created and launched a Charter for Compassion written by leading faith-based leaders to restore compassion to the heart of religious and moral life in 2009. Armstrong is a strong advocate for the Buddhist-based belief that compassion is natural to humans and enables us to love all beings equally and impartially. This ability, however, requires setting the needs of the selfish ego aside and treating every human being with sanctity and justice. It also includes a positive appreciation of cultural and religious diversity. More specifically, compassion asks us to look into our own heart and determine what gives us pain and then refuse to inflict that pain on anyone else, including those who are considered our enemies. Armstrong then developed a twelve-step program that was modeled after Alcoholics Anonymous to help us overcome our addiction to egoism and nurture our compassion.

Although Armstrong's book is viewed as controversial by many, there is much to learn about spirituality and human flourishing from her ideas. Her theory of compassion is filled with positive emotion, engagement, and relationships, and it places a high emphasis on meaning and purpose. The goal of compassion, as conceived by Armstrong, is a major accomplishment if achieved. Armstrong's theory presents a novel approach for those of us who are oriented toward Western thinking and introduces many new ideas for growth and flourishing. There is a great deal of value that can be applied to the health-care setting, in which compassion is of the utmost importance but often gets lost in the fray of a system that promotes stressed-out, overburdened doctors.

It is obvious from the engagement of most individuals in a spiritual life, as well as from the many bold ideas of love and compassion that come from spiritual thought, that the wisdom and insights of spirituality continue to help us develop our understanding of human flourishing and bear great relevance to our practice of positive health and thriving.

Spirituality offers a unique set of resources for well-being and living by providing methods by which to understand and deal with aspects of our lives that are beyond our control. These aspects include events such as birth, death, accidents, unexpected transitions, and illness, many of which physicians encounter on a daily basis. The language of the sacred—faith, mystery, grace, transformation, and sacrifice—differs greatly within medical and psychological language. However, the integration of spirituality into the medical setting, between patients and practitioners, will greatly facilitate the achievement of hope, meaning, and positive, flourishing health. Psycho-spiritual interventions are becoming more common in hospital settings, and the body of research in this area continues to grow.

For a long period of time, the subject of religion was included infrequently in psychiatric and psychological literature except as it related to disease. However, due largely to the influence of Pargament and others like him, who addressed spirituality from a place of empirical rigor and great respect, a positive turn in the field of spirituality has occurred, and we can look for new insights into what drives human flourishing through their findings.

Pargament's empirical studies (2002) considered the correlates and consequences of religious beliefs and behavior. From these data, he was able to draw five important conclusions:

1) Only a religion that is internalized, intrinsically motivated, and built on the belief in a greater meaning in life, that has a secure relationship with God and has a sense of spiritual connectedness with others, has positive implications for well-being.

2) There are advantages and disadvantages to even the most controversial forms of religion, such as fundamentalism. For example, fundamentalism is tied to rigid thinking and greater prejudice; however, it also provides an unambiguous sense of right and wrong, a set of clear rules for living, and optimism.

3) Religion is particularly helpful to socially marginalized groups (e.g., the elderly, the poor, ethnic minorities, women) and those who embed religion fully into their lives.

4) Religious belief and practice is especially valuable in stressful situations that push individuals to the limits of their personal and social resources (e.g., death, extreme illness, poverty).

5) The efficacy of religion is tied to the degree to which it is integrated in an individual's life and supported by his or her larger social context.

Pargament's empirically based conclusions both reinforce current knowledge of well-being and raise new questions. Conclusion 1, which reinforces meaning in life and positive relationships; conclusion 2, which reinforces positive emotions, positive relationships, and meaning; and conclusion 5, which highlights that beliefs must be practiced and socially supported to be effective, all seem to reinforce current knowledge and theory of well-being. However, conclusions 3 and 4 raise new questions. Regarding conclusion 3, the obvious question is: Why would religion be particularly helpful to socially marginalized people? A knee-jerk response would be that the benefits of religion for these groups on social and positive relationships are obvious. Perhaps there is an additional, positive impact of spirituality, however, that can be easily noticed in socially marginalized groups, but is, as yet, unidentified. The same phenomenon may exist for people in stressful situations who are pushed to their limits (conclusion 4), or it might represent still another positive impact of spirituality yet to be identified. Only by further scientific study of these phenomena can we continue to bolster the contribution of spirituality to the science of human flourishing.

Spirituality, perhaps because it is pervasive and represents unique ways of thinking, tends to raise as many questions as it answers. It is these very questions, however, that, when explored, can aid the scientific study of human flourishing. One example is Karen Armstrong's concept of brain evolution and compassion—specifically mirror neurons in the frontal region of the brain, which light up on a brain scan when the emotion of empathy is invoked (Armstrong, 2010). Armstrong contends that, because empathy is hardwired in our brains, it helps us to transcend our ancient reptilian instincts (fleeing, feeding, fighting, and reproduction). When we have direct contact with other human beings and we learn to develop and enhance our skills of empathy, then compassion becomes easier and more automatic. That is, our ability to be empathetic with our enemy will, through his own mirror neurons, facilitate an empathetic response in kind and avoid conflict. This concept raises compelling questions in that we live in a time in which increasing conflict exists, yet far less direct communication occurs. Do mirror neurons have efficacy in technological forms of communication (e.g., social media, cell phones, Skype)? What are the implications of Armstrong's concept on an international level? What is the impact of this concept in the doctor-patient encounter? What are the implications for telemedicine? Could further scientific study of this phenomenon affect world peace? This impact of mirror neurons as described by Armstrong would certainly increase flourishing in all human beings!

His Holiness the Dalai Lama is a spiritual leader whose life is a lesson plan in the cultivation of human well-being. In the eyes of the Dalai Lama, the search for well-being involves purging hatred, compulsive desire, and ignorance and in their place cultivating benevolence, altruistic love, and compassion. Self-centeredness is a major source of discontent, and the pursuit of extrinsic, materialistic values is detrimental to our well-being (Ricard, 2011). One's major focus should be serving others, not the self. Positive emotions are those that strengthen our inner peace and seek the good in others.

The Dalai Lama exemplifies many ways to cultivate spirituality into well-being. He practices religion based upon PERMA (positive emotions, engagement, positive relationships, meaning and purpose, and accomplishment) (Seligman, 2011), with very strong emphasis on meaning and purpose and serving and loving others. The Dalai Lama attracts all people, both religious and secular, to him because of his genuine warmth and caring. He is simple and humble, but always giving, accepting, inclusive, selfless, and loving. He takes responsibility for the well-being of others, loves unconditionally, radiates spiritual warmth, and incorporates his way of being into his daily life with consistency.

The Dalai Lama is open and authentic about the struggles that he has experienced, including religious persecution. Because struggles are inherent in coming to terms with one's own spirituality, we experience elevation from learning of his struggles and how he was able to overcome them, and we arrive at peace and happiness. The Dalai Lama's ability to see and accept the world as it is, with eyes wide-open and with heightened awareness, to deeply understand the human condition, and to choose selfless love and unselfish service as his only path provides inspiration and hope for the cultivation of human flourishing in every man, woman, and child.

As you may recall from chapter 6, several of the character strengths and virtues include those that are based on or linked with the spiritual. These virtues include faith, hope, charity, gratitude, and forgiveness. Studies have found a relationship among religion, spirituality, and the character strength of gratitude (Emmons & Mishra, Why gratitude enhances wellbeing: What we know, what we need to know, 2011). Those who measure high on indexes of gratitude tend to be religiously or spiritually minded. In addition, those with high gratitude toward God experience a decrease in the effects of stress on their health, particularly in later life. This stress-buffering effect of theocentric gratitude is particularly pronounced in women. Furthermore, gratitude motivates moral behavior, that is, action undertaken to benefit another.

GROUP DISCUSSION

Jane Doe, a fifty-five-year-old single female, is admitted to the hospital for a work-up of abdominal pain and weight loss. When you enter the room to take her history, her first words are, "I would really like to speak to a chaplain." What is the most appropriate and therapeutic way to respond?

- How might Karen Armstrong's theory of mirror neurons and empathy affect the doctor-patient relationship? How might a highly empathetic doctor affect the subsequent doctor-patient interaction? Cooperation? Trust?
- What is the impact of gratitude on overall physical and emotional health? How does gratitude help to prevent burnout?

INDIVIDUAL EXPLORATION

One's spiritual beliefs are often deep and quite personal. How, as a physician, can you support the spirituality of a patient whose religious or cultural teachings are different from your own?

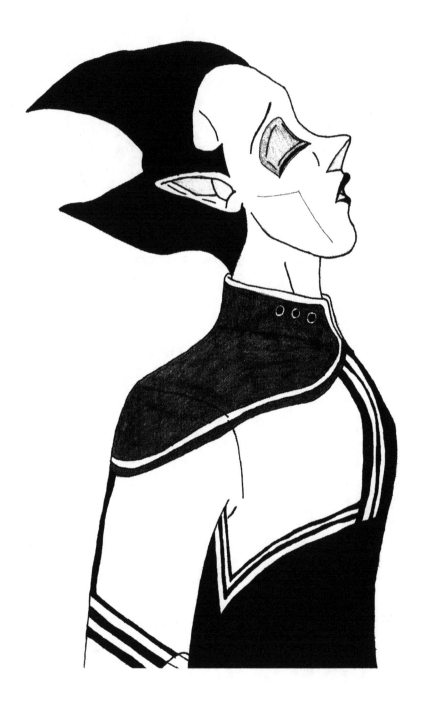

246

Chapter 14

Mindfulness-Based Strengths Practice for Physicians: Integrating Core Areas to Promote Positive Health

Guest Author: Ryan M. Niemiec, PsyD

This chapter reviews the research and practice around mindfulness and character strengths and the integration of these two popular areas of positive psychology. The importance of these applied areas in promoting positive health among physicians and medical students is reviewed. Practical tips for boosting physician well-being and applying these concepts in a medical setting are discussed. A comprehensive program, Mindfulness-Based Strengths Practice, is offered as an example of a program that can boost well-being among medical professionals.

MINDFULNESS

Mindfulness has captured the attention of the general public as well as practitioners around the world. Formalized programs are being developed and used with significant success in clinics and hospitals worldwide. That fact alone is a call for physicians and medical staff to at least understand the concepts, terminology, research, and best practices. However, there is even more reason to invest in the study. The science of mindfulness has exploded dramatically in recent years (Brown, Ryan, & Creswell, 2007; Sears, Tirch, & Denton, 2011), during which time, research literature has increased twenty-fold since the year 2000 (Black, 2010).

What is mindfulness?

Several conceptualizations of mindfulness have been proposed by educators, researchers, and practitioners. To bring unity to the construct being studied, a number of scientists gathered to discuss and create a consensual, operational definition of the construct (Bishop, et al., 2004). These scientists have proposed a two-component model of mindfulness:

> The first component involves the self-regulation of attention so that it is maintained on immediate experience, thereby allowing for increased recognition of mental events in the present moment. The second component involves adopting a particular orientation toward one's experiences in the present moment, an orientation that is characterized by curiosity, openness, and acceptance (p. 232).

In short, mindfulness involves the self-regulation of attention, along with an attitude of curiosity, openness, and acceptance. This approach to attention provides a counterbalance to the natural tendency of the human mind to wander, and it promotes the phenomenon of metacognition (i.e., thinking about our thinking). As metacognition builds, one is able to more easily see the complexity and automaticity of thought, as well as the vicious, negative circles that can result (Teasdale, 1999). A useful factor involved in the success of mindfulness is what is termed *decentering*, which refers to the act of viewing thoughts and other psychological phenomena as transient, mental events that pass through our awareness (Segal, Williams, & Teasdale, 2002).

Mindfulness in medicine

The use of mindfulness in medicine rose substantially in popularity in the latter decades of the past century due to the pioneering research and practice of Jon Kabat-Zinn at the University of Massachusetts Medical School. His research led to the creation of the program Mindfulness-Based Stress Reduction, which is now used by hundreds of hospitals and clinics around the world. Kabat-Zinn (1990) demystified the then-esoteric concept of mindfulness and trained patients to face their symptoms and illnesses directly, regardless of how severe. Kabat-Zinn taught mindfulness to help his patients gain better control of their serious chronic conditions.

Subsequently, research and meta-analyses have abounded, with both showing clear evidence that meditation has a positive effect on well-being (Sedlmeier, et al., 2012). Other meta-analyses have found that mindfulness has an impact on a broad range of people in helping them to cope with clinical and nonclinical problems resulting from cancer, heart disease, and other chronic conditions (Grossman, Niemann, Schmidt, & Walach, 2004). Medical patients are finding greater relief from vexing diagnoses such as diabetes (Gregg, Callaghan, Hayes, & Glenn-Lawson, 2007), rheumatoid arthritis (Pradhan, et al., 2007), cancer (Lerman, Jarski, Rea, Gellish, & Vicini, 2012; Speca,

Carlson, Goodey, & Angen, 2000), chronic pain (Kabat-Zinn, Lipworth, Burney, & Sellers, 1986; McCracken, Gauntlett-Gilbert, & Vowles, 2007), psoriasis (Kabat-Zinn, et al., 1998), irritable bowel syndrome (Gaylord, et al., 2011), fibromyalgia (Grossman, Tiefenthaler-Gilmer, Raysz, & Kesper, 2007), and debilitating stress related to severe medical conditions (Kabat-Zinn, 1990).

Many psychological disorders have been successfully treated through the use of mindfulness, for example, recurrent depression, chronic anxiety, borderline personality, substance abuse, binge-eating disorder, bipolar disorder, and insomnia, to name a few (Segal, Williams, & Teasdale, 2002; Grossman, Niemann, Schmidt, & Walach, 2004; Baer R., 2003; Baer R. A., 2006; Chiesa & Serretti, 2014; Lineham, 1993; Nyklicek, Vingerhoets, & Zeelenberg, 2010; Shapiro & Carlson, 2009). None of this treatment should come as a surprise, because the original purpose of mindfulness, which dates back 2,500 years to Buddhism, was to alleviate suffering.

A number of articles on the benefits of mindfulness have been published in *JAMA* (Krasner, et al., 2009; Ludwig & Kabat-Zinn, 2008; Sibinga & Wu, 2010). Krasner and associates (2009) reported that the practice of mindfulness among physicians led to improvements in burnout (emotional exhaustion), as well as improvements in several other areas, such as perspective taking, empathy, conscientiousness, and well-being (short-term and sustained). Physicians from John Hopkins University argue that mindfulness helps to reduce medical errors by reducing cognitive biases that physicians frequently display during diagnostic processes; therefore, it can help to recalibrate clinical decision-making processes (Sibinga & Wu, 2010). Pezzolesi and colleagues (Pezzolesi, Ghaleb, Kostrzewski, & Dhillon, 2013) also discuss mindfulness as a key approach for reducing medication errors, which can occur frequently because of individuals being forgetful, stressed, distracted, or overly engaged in multitasking.

In general, studies are showing that mindfulness is beneficial to the physical and psychological well-being of doctors, medical students, and other medical staff. In a study of participatory medicine that involved nearly two hundred patients and health-care providers during a four-year period, substantial benefits of mindfulness were found for multiple health status areas, including blood pressure, medication use, activity and energy levels, coping, and pain (Rogers, et al., 2013).

Mindfulness is an emerging approach for targeting physician and medical student burnout, stress, and compassion fatigue. One literature review found that fourteen medical schools formally teach mindfulness to students and residents, with the approaches ranging from extensive programs to full-day workshops, curricula integration, and lectures. Studies of these programs show that students experience less distress and greater quality of life as a result of extensive instruction in mindfulness (Dobkin & Hutchinson, 2013). In a study examining the long-term effects of mindfulness on burnout, mood, and empathy among primary care professionals, significant improvements were found, such as a reduction in burnout scores, improved mood and empathy, and higher mindfulness levels (Martin Asuero, Rodriguez Blanco, Pujol-Ribera, Berenquera, & Moix Queraltó, 2013). Another study of primary care physicians found a brief mindfulness intervention to significantly impact burnout scores, including emotional exhaustion, depersonalization, and accomplishment, as well as a favorable impact on stress, anxiety, and depression (Fortney, Luchterhand, Zakletskaia, Zgierska, & Rakel, 2013). No impact was found in this study for mindfulness on resilience or compassion.

In a study of Norwegian medical and psychology students, mindfulness training had a significant impact in reducing mental distress, increasing well-being, and decreasing study stress among female students (De Vibe, et al., 2013). Other studies found additional benefits for medical students, such as increased self-regulation and self-compassion (Bond, et al., 2013).

There is significant potential for mindfulness to directly affect the communication patterns and care delivered by physicians by promoting mindful listening and mindful speech. Beach and colleagues (2013) examined physician communication quality and patterns among those physicians who self-rated as high versus low in mindfulness. Those physicians who were high in mindfulness were more patient-centered in their communication, as shown by greater rapport building, more positive emotional tone, and discussion of psychosocial issues. Patients rated them higher on communication and reported greater satisfaction with their care.

Although these studies show optimistic results indicating the strong impact of mindfulness among physicians and medical students, it is important to note that many of these studies are only pilot, preliminary investigations, without benefit of a randomized, double-blind, controlled study.

Catch your AP-ASAP

The human mind is notorious for being anywhere but the present moment. Our minds wander from experiences in the past to future plans and various scenarios that may take place. This process pervades our daily life. Whenever we eat, walk, talk, drive, and work, our mind is usually elsewhere—thinking or reacting to things, rather than experiencing the present moment. This tendency is referred to as our mind functioning on *autopilot*. An important initial step in mindfulness practice is to notice that the mind has wandered away from the present moment. We can then return the focus back. You might remember this idea more easily by using the phrase, *Catch your AP-ASAP* (Catch your AutoPilot—As Soon As Possible).

Test it out yourself: Focus your attention on one constant stimulus in your current environment for ten minutes. This stimulus could be the edge of your desk, the sensations of your breath, or a candle flame. Whenever your mind wanders away from that stimulus, return your focus to your breath.

- What did you notice about this exercise?
- Were you able to "catch" your autopilot mind?
- Where did your mind tend to wander?
- Approximately how long did your mind truly stick with the stimulus and the stimulus alone? Research finds that our present moments last, on average, only three to four seconds (Stern, 2004).

Questions/exercises to consider (mindfulness)

- Why do you think mindfulness approaches are helpful for physician burnout?
- If you began a mindfulness practice—even five to ten minutes of mindful breathing each day—can you hypothesize whether the impact would be greater on your personal life or your professional life? Why?
- Although mindfulness should not be viewed as a panacea, make a list of the ways in which you could apply mindfulness in visits with your patients. What themes emerge from your list?
- Brief mindfulness exercises have a strong yet emerging research base. How might you integrate a mindfulness exercise into your daily medical practice?

CHARACTER STRENGTHS

As discussed in chapter 6, physicians now have at their fingertips a research-based, consensual nomenclature for understanding what is best in themselves and in their patients. The handbook *Character Strengths and Virtues* (Peterson & Seligman, 2004), outlining the Values in Action (VIA) Institute *Classification of Strengths and Virtues*, serves as the ideal complement to the *ICD-10* and *DSM-5* manuals. Indeed, it is important that physicians have a manual for what is best in human beings to complement the systems covering what is wrong with human beings.

The VIA classification has been found to be universal across cultures, nations, and belief systems (Peterson & Seligman, 2004; Biswas-Diener, From the equator to the North Pole: A study of character strengths, 2006; McGrath, 2014), and the VIA Survey is a validated measurement tool for assessing twenty-four strengths of character (see www.creatingpositivehealth.com, under heading of character strengths). The online VIA Survey has been quickly adopted by more than two million people across the globe (see chapter 6 for a review of the VIA Survey and an outline of VIA character strengths).

Core concepts

Character strengths are positive personality traits. They are the capacity to think, feel, and behave in ways that benefit oneself or others. There are many general principles that are important to consider in understanding or working with an individual's character strengths (Niemiec, VIA character strengths–research and practice: The first 10 years, 2012b). I will review a few of the salient ones.

Character strengths are multidimensional, with notable qualities that make up each strength. For example, kindness is more than just being kind; it involves dimensions of generosity, caring, nurturance, compassion, niceness, and altruism. The character strength of honesty involves dimensions of integrity and authenticity, and the character strength of zest has dimensions related to vigor, vitality, and enthusiasm.

Character strengths are plural (Peterson C., 2006), both in how we understand ourselves and how we express ourselves. Contrary to traditional approaches to character that are commonly found in athletic programs, schools, and political or religious entities, humans have a unique constellation of character strengths. In addition, humans rarely express just one strength at a time. In most circumstances, we humans express a combination of several strengths. When we are interacting with a patient as he or she shares problems, we are not only expressing kindness and empathy, but we are also displaying curiosity (asking questions, exploring), perspective (counseling, helping the patient to see the "big picture"), hope (presenting a degree of positivity and offering encouragement for a positive future), and creativity (offering the patient alternatives to a problem that he or she is having).

There is a golden mean when it comes to expressing our character strengths (Niemiec, 2014). The golden mean of character strengths can be defined as expressing the right combination of strengths, to the right degree, in the right situation. The character strength of love, for example, will likely be expressed differently with a family member (e.g., hugging/kissing), a work colleague (e.g., handshake), and a patient (e.g., expressing warmth and genuineness verbally). In addition, love will present differently when combined with curiosity, prudence, or judgment and critical thinking. The golden mean refers to finding that optimal balance in character-strength expression that is also contextually sensitive.

Character strengths are stable but can be developed (Peterson & Seligman, 2004; Borghans, Duckworth, Heckman, & ter Weel, 2008). A commonly held misconception is that character is immutable and unchanging. Character strengths are part of our personality, which is mostly stable over time; however, at the same time, our traits can shift through normative changes based on genetics and predictable changes in our social role (e.g., starting a family), deliberately chosen changes in our social role (e.g., joining the military), atypical life events (e.g., trauma), and deliberate interventions. In developing character strengths, the key is to create new habits that are established through practice over time, which allows us to break free from routines.

Three ideas are salient for medical practitioners to keep in mind when working with patients:

1. Never underestimate the value of strengths spotting.

   Every patient encounter presents an opportunity for strengths spotting. The approach can be quite simple—label the strength you see and offer a behavioral rationale that explains the strength. Express appreciation and value for the strength(s) that you observe. For example, a physician might offer this comment to a diabetic patient: "You used a strong amount of your strength of self-regulation by tracking your blood sugar and writing down your numbers this month." Or, "Nice work using your strength of perseverance to really stick with your new exercise program each day."

2. All twenty-four character strengths matter.

   It is important to remember that all of us, including our patients, have all twenty-four of these strengths within us to various degrees. Any of these strengths can become a focal point to build on and can be referred to in reference to meeting a medical or health goal.

3. Your signature strengths matter most.

   The practice of using one signature strength in a new way each day has been linked with significantly higher happiness and lower depression, with effects lasting as long as six months (Gander, Proyer, Ruch, & Wyss, 2012; Mitchell, Stanimirovic, Klein, & Vella-Brodrick, 2009; Mongrain & Anselmo-Matthews, 2012; Peterson & Peterson, 2009; Rust, Diessner, & Reade, 2009; Seligman, Steen, Park, & Peterson, 2005).

(Signature strengths are those strengths that are highest in your patients' strengths profiles and are most likely to be energizing and easy for them to express widely. When you comment on or reference these strengths in some way, you are acknowledging the patient's core identity.)

One physician who has studied strengths framed it this way: "Character strengths offer me a paradigm shift in how I view my patients and their suffering. I now view my patients in a completely different way."

Marsha W. Snyder, MD., MAPP.

Research

In less than a decade, more than 150 scientific studies have emerged that reveal positive outcomes and correlates with character strengths. For a review of the recent research, see www.viacharacter.org/www/en-us/research/summaries.aspx. For a review of hundreds of scholarly articles and books relating to each of the twenty-four character strengths, see Peterson and Seligman (2004).

Character strengths have been connected with several positive outcomes, such as work satisfaction, self-esteem, life meaning, achievement, and engagement at school or work. Studies show a potential causal link between strengths and well-being in that a focus on particular strengths highly correlated with happiness (e.g., zest, hope) and led to increased well-being (Proyer, Ruch, & Buschor, 2013).

Good connections also exist between character strengths and positive health outcomes. Studies show that character strengths are connected with not only good mental health but also good physical health (Leontopoulou & Triliva, 2012; Proctor, Maltby, & Linley, 2009). Preliminary work has been done on the impact of character strengths on recovery from physical illness (Peterson, Park, & Seligman, 2006), and links have been found with healthy sexuality among adolescents (Ma, et al., 2008). A recent study showed that greater endorsement of character strengths was associated with a number of healthy behaviors, such as feeling healthy, leading an active way of life, pursuing enjoyable activities, healthy eating, monitoring one's food intake, and physical fitness (Proyer, Gander, Wellenzohn, & Ruch, 2013). All twenty-four character strengths (except humility and spirituality) were associated with multiple healthy behaviors. Whereas the strength of self-regulation had the highest associations overall, the strengths of curiosity, appreciation of beauty and excellence, gratitude, hope, and humor also showed strong connections with healthy behaviors. Previous studies have found similar results with various specific character strengths—for example, the practice of gratitude has been linked with vitality and fewer physical symptoms (Emmons & McCullough, 2003).

Develop the skill of strengths spotting

Consider whether you find it easier to spot character strengths in action as they occur in you or as you observe others. Whichever you choose, start there and practice strengths spotting each day. Set up a cue that will remind you to do this exercise several times each day; some physicians set a phone alarm to sound off randomly once per hour. When you hear the alarm, pause and look for strengths in what you are doing or what you are observing in others. Write down your observations—the strength(s) that you spot and an explanation for the strength. After a week, shift your strengths-spotting focal point outward toward others or inward toward yourself.

Questions/exercises to consider (character strengths)

- What are your signature strengths? How could you use one of them more consciously in your daily medical practice?
- Might you be able to spot strengths in every single patient you see? This is likely to be true. With some intentionality, you will quickly spot patients who are brave as they face their illness, kind and humble as they ask about how you are doing although they are suffering greatly, zestful as they exude high levels of energy, honest as they report on how closely they adhered to their medication regimen, and grateful as they express appreciation for your help. For other patients, the strengths are not as obvious, but they are still present. For example, among those patients who are being stubborn or resistant, this behavior could be reframed as perseverant. Which label do you believe your patient would be more receptive to hearing and discussing?
- Appreciating the strengths of others is a deceivingly powerful approach. How would you express value to your medical colleagues for their unique character strengths? Speculate on the effect this might have.

THE INTEGRATION OF CHARACTER STRENGTHS AND MINDFULNESS

At this point, it should be clear that the use of mindfulness or character strengths alone can benefit one's clinical armamentarium and support the practice of medicine. What about bringing these powerful, intrinsic psychological processes together? What follow are the rationale and best practices for integration.

What did you notice about the scientific definition of mindfulness that was highlighted earlier? At the core of mindfulness are two character strengths: self-regulation (i.e., taking control of your attention) and curiosity (i.e., bringing an attitude of openness to the present moment). When we practice mindfulness, we are rehearsing these strengths.

The integration of mindfulness and character strengths promises a variety of benefits that have been detailed elsewhere (Niemiec, 2014). A few examples of these benefits are:

- a positive synergy of mutual benefit that can create a *virtuous circle* of positive impact. Mindful awareness boosts the use of strengths, which in turn, enlivens mindfulness.

- a greater awareness of the positive potential within us, and going a step further, the mindfulness aspect offers a pathway to develop and explore character strengths.
- increased self-awareness and potential for change activation by bringing one's character strengths more clearly into view. As Carlson's research (2013) found, mindfulness serves as a path to see oneself as one really is.
- the ability to respond appropriately and successfully in different contexts, that is, the integration of mindfulness and character strengths may promote psychological flexibility (Kashdan & Rottenberg, 2010) and help individuals to use greater practical wisdom in complex or conflicting situations (Schwartz & Sharpe, 2006).

There are two main ways to discuss the integration of mindfulness and character strengths: (1) bringing strengths use to our mindful living and mindfulness practice (referred to as *strong mindfulness*), and (2) bringing mindfulness practice and concepts to our strengths use (termed *mindful strengths use*).

Strong mindfulness

Strong mindfulness refers to bringing in character strengths to help in the practice of mindfulness. This approach helps individuals to overcome meditation barriers, enhance mindful living, and supercharge mindfulness practices (Niemiec, 2014; Niemiec, 2012a; Niemiec, Rashid, & Spinella, 2012).

One of the biggest challenges individuals face in developing a meditation practice is the challenge of the wandering mind, or what is often referred to as the *autopilot mind*. Mind wandering can compromise a number of cognitive skills, interfering with one's ability to integrate the present-moment experience into a general context, which may lead to additional problems (Smallwood, Mrazek, & Schooler, 2011). People are also less happy when their minds wander (Killingsworth & Gilbert, 2010). Mind wandering presents as a serious obstacle to those who want to start a mindfulness meditation practice—or any practice that involves self-regulation—such as relaxation and biofeedback, autogenic training, medical hypnosis, or other tools used to cope with medical conditions. Patients will frequently give up practicing these strategies because their mind wandering leads them to feel as if they are failing at the practice. Mind wandering and other obstacles—both physical and psychological—are a normal part of these practices and can be as varied as bodily discomfort and pain, difficulty with scheduling time to practice, experiencing distraction, and feeling unmotivated.

Character strengths can be deployed to assist with these obstacles. Individuals should consider their signature strengths and how they might be used to overcome or manage the obstacle. For example, perseverance could be used to stick with a practice, prudence might be used to become more planful in overcoming scheduling issues, and curiosity and bravery might be used to explore and directly face physical discomfort.

Strengths can also be used to enhance mindful living activities (Niemiec, 2012a). Mindful living refers to the practice of being tuned in and connected with daily activities, such as walking, eating, driving, speaking, working, listening, and bathing. Individuals might call forth their zest and appreciation of beauty while walking from examination room to examination room, their curiosity and kindness while listening to a patient, their hope and creativity when speaking to the patient, and their gratitude while eating.

In the end, character strengths are described as *supercharging* mindfulness because they bring the practice of mindfulness to the next level. To bring character strengths to meditation is to integrate a core part of oneself into the practice.

Application example (for you, the medical professional): Attending physician Dr. Elliott observed that a new resident had made a handful of medical errors during the last month. She pulled the resident aside to bring this problem to the resident's attention and to inquire further. The resident explained that he had been feeling distracted and stressed lately due to personal issues and stress in studying for his board examinations. They discussed his character strengths and the value of mindfulness practice. The topic of mindful walking came up as an area of interest, so they brainstormed ways to build this approach into the busy practice. The resident decided that he would practice mindful walking—even if just for a few steps—as he moved from examination room to examination room. He used perseverance to bring his attention back to the present moment, feeling his body move and the sensation of each foot making contact with the ground as he walked. On leaving an examination room, he would feel his in-breath and out-breath, and he would let go of the last patient encounter and become fully present in his body and mind. He walked slowly and with careful prudence, noticing each step. Often he would pause before the next room to ensure that he was fully centered before knocking and entering. This approach helped the resident to manage his stress and tension in the moment without having to take out additional time during the day.

Application example (for your patients): Dr. Samuels recognized the research base for applying mindfulness practices with his patients; however, with a busy primary care practice, he did not have time to spend offering long-winded meditations for each of his patients. In past years, he simply referred his patients to a counselor who used mindfulness techniques in treating medical and health problems, but Dr. Samuels found that very few patients actually followed through. Dr. Samuels then came upon the two- to three-minute character strengths breathing-space practice from Mindfulness-Based Strengths Practice (MBSP) and began working this approach into his patient visits. This method offered a powerful tool that patients could take with them after their appointment and practice each day. Because of the brevity of the exercise, Dr. Samuels was able to present this self-regulation tool to as many patients as he wished in a given day. An abridged script for the character strengths breathing space of Niemiec[42] follows.

This brief meditation is three steps, each involving use of one of your strengths. This first phase (strength of curiosity) involves bringing curiosity to your present moment. Take notice of your present moment. Open yourself to it. Observe the details. Take an interest in this moment. Notice what you can sense right now—be aware of sounds rising and falling, the contact your body makes with your seat. Allow your curiosity to explore the moment fully. Practice being curious about your thoughts and feelings, interested in whatever is in your presence right now. Simply notice these happenings in your present moment. If you find yourself getting caught up in one sensation or emotion, simply say, "What else? What else is happening in my present moment? What else is there to be curious about for me to take an interest in?"

Now, allow your attention to narrow to just one thing—your breath. This is the second phase (strength of self-regulation) of the breathing space, where the practice is to let go of all the happenings in your present moment with the exception of your breathing. Allow yourself to feel the fullness of your in-breath and the fullness of your out-breath. Feel the sensation of your breathing in your body. Concentrate just on your breath. When your mind wanders away from your breath, simply bring it back to the breath. Over and over, bring your focus back to your breath. Each time you bring your attention back to your breath, you are practicing self-regulation. This means you are "taking control" of your mind and attention. Always back to your breath.

While you continue to focus on your in-breath and out-breath, let's move into the final phase of the breathing space (strength of perspective). Allow your attention to expand to your body-as-a-whole. As you breathe, notice your wholeness, the oneness of your body and mind. Allow yourself to feel a sense of completeness or oneness. This can be viewed as using your strength of perspective—stepping back to see the wider view of your body/mind and your place in this present moment. This allows you to see and breathe with the bigger picture.

This character-strengths breathing space can be practiced during the patient visit and offered as a tool for the patient to take home and practice. As patients practice this particular meditation, they are not only developing their mindfulness but they are also cultivating three specific character strengths. These strengths in particular are core to meditation practice and thus help to nurture strong mindfulness.

Mindful strengths use

The use of mindfulness to facilitate character-strengths expression is referred to as mindful strengths use (Niemiec, 2014). Mindfulness serves as a doorway of awareness that helps individuals to see themselves more clearly and directs the use of strengths. In this way, mindfulness is a meta-process for working with strengths, helping individuals to tune into how they might be overusing or underusing strengths, find balanced expression, combat mindlessness about signature strengths, and assist in reappraising problems.

Consider a scenario in which you are running behind in your patient schedule for the day and you know that you must get to an event that starts immediately after your workday. The patient whom you are with begins to cry and asks for ten more minutes of your time to talk something through. Does this incident elicit your kindness and compassion strength to give the patient the extra time? Does your prudence (planfulness) strength strongly emerge, leading you to set a firm boundary? Do your judgment, critical thinking, and perspective strengths stand out while you try to find an alternate solution (e.g., asking a nurse to listen to the patient for a while so that you can move on with your schedule)? Or do other strengths emerge for you perhaps?

There is no one correct answer here, but often it is our signature strengths that dictate what we will decide during scenarios such as these that are considered *strengths collisions*. Mindful awareness of our strengths and the individual situation can help people strike a balance by aligning with the *golden mean* of character strengths. The golden mean refers to expression of the right combination of strengths to the right degree (amount/intensity) in the right situation (Niemiec, 2014; Aristotle, 2000; Biswas-Diener, Kashdan, & Minhas, 2011; Linley, 2008). Mindfulness is used to closely tune in to internal and contextual factors to express a balance with strengths.

Application example (for you, the medical professional): Choose one of your signature strengths. Examine it closely, mindfully, from many different angles. Give careful consideration to your use of it in the medical context. The questions below come from a worksheet used in the MBSP program; participants are asked to choose one strength and then answer the following questions:

- What does it mean to have or express this strength at work?
- What happens if you have too little of this strength (underuse) at work?
- What happens if you have too much of this strength (overuse) at work?
- In what situations and scenarios at work can you express this strength?
- What benefits does this strength bring to you and others at work?
- Describe this strength in six words without including the word itself.

Application example (for your patients): It is very common for patients to look at the rank-order of character strengths from the VIA Survey and immediately look to their bottom strengths. Often patients will respond with disappointment or self-criticism as they focus on a strength they wished was higher. There are a few important responses for physicians to consider in this situation:

1. Remind the patient that there are no weaknesses or deficits identified with this VIA Survey assessment. It is a measure of strengths. Those strengths that appear toward the bottom are considered to be lesser strengths (i.e., strengths that are not used as easily and are not as energizing for the individual as those strengths that are toward the top).
2. Those strengths at the top should be celebrated and explored and not mindlessly cast aside at the expense of lower strengths.
3. Mindfulness can be applied to those strengths that are lower in the profile. These strengths can be built up, although probably not to the level of a signature strength.
4. Ask the patient to consider how one or two of his or her signature strengths could be used to focus on the strength that the patient is concerned about. This approach involves listening to the patient's concern and interest (i.e., boosting a lower strength) while going ahead with what is likely to be successful and energizing (i.e., using a higher strength).

For example, patients high in curiosity might use that inquisitive strength to address their low kindness strength by spending time asking people questions and exploring their responses; they might address their low self-regulation by taking a curious, exploratory approach as they read about different approaches to diet and exercise and explore what might interest them the most.

Mindfulness-Based Strengths Practice (MBSP)

MBSP is a manualized, eight-week program that merges the science and best practices of character strengths and mindfulness to help individuals to flourish. Core aspects of the program involve boosting mindful strengths use and strong mindfulness. The crux of the program is self-awareness and self-discovery. Research on MBSP is in its infancy; however, pilot studies and qualitative reviews from MBSP groups spanning six countries reflect important benefits and positive outcomes, including increases in well-being, engagement, meaning, purpose, strengths use, mindfulness practice, flourishing, achievement, and positive relationships. The eight core topic areas and a brief description of each can be found in table 14-1.

Table 14-1. Mindfulness-Based Strengths Practice[42]

Session	Core Topic	Description
1	Mindfulness and autopilot	The autopilot mind is pervasive; everything starts with awareness.
2	Your signature strengths	Identify what is best in you; this exercise can unlock potential to engage more in work and relationships and reach higher personal potential.
3	Obstacles are opportunities.	The practice of mindfulness and of strengths exploration leads immediately to two things—obstacles and barriers to the practice, and a deeper awareness of the little things in life.
4	Strengthening mindfulness in everyday life	Mindfulness helps us attend to and nourish the best innermost qualities in ourselves and others; conscious use of strengths can help us deepen and maintain a mindfulness practice.
5	Valuing your relationships	How we relate to ourselves is an important element of self-growth. This has an immediate impact on how we connect with others.
6	Mindfulness of the golden mean	Mindfulness helps to focus on problems directly, and character strengths help to reframe and find different perspectives not immediately apparent.
Optional Retreat	MBSP half-day retreat	Mindful living and character strengths apply not only to good meditation practice, but also to daily conversation, eating, walking, sitting, and reflecting.
7	Authenticity and goodness	It takes character (e.g., courage) to be a more authentic "you," and it takes character (e.g., hope) to create a strong future that benefits both oneself and others.
8	Your engagement with life	Stick with those practices that have been working well and watch for the mind's tendency to revert back to automatic habits that are deficit-based, unproductive, or prioritize what's wrong in you and others. Engage in an approach that fosters awareness and celebration of what is strongest in you and others.

Shift from mindless to mindful

Mindlessness and frequent autopilot experiences are a normal part of the human experience. It is impossible—and no doubt unwise—to eliminate them completely. A first step, as noted earlier, is to become aware of the ubiquitous nature of our autopilot mind. An immediate second step that we can take is to return our attention to the present moment. An exercise used in MBSP that helps to take this idea to the next level is called *from mindless to mindful*.

Choose one regular activity in your medical practice that you are bothered by, causes you distress, or has a negative impact on your patients or medical colleagues (e.g., charting new-patient visits, using dictation, meeting with diabetics, treating children, consulting with a particular specialty, interacting with a pompous colleague). No doubt there are aspects of this activity that you perform on autopilot. As you reflect on this activity, consider those aspects of the scenario or individual that you are mindless to, the strengths in yourself that you are blind to, and moments when you become hypervigilant or overly sensitive. For the next week, as you engage in the situation or connect with this individual, practice two things: being mindful of yourself (i.e., your own thoughts, emotions, sensations, behaviors) and conscious of the character strengths that you might bring forth. Note that the target in this exercise is your own autopilot nature, *not* focusing on trying to change the individual or impact the results of the situation.

Individuals who practice this activity report making shifts toward cultivating virtue and making strength use more routine, as well as greater confidence in facing difficulties, stressors, and irritations.

Questions/exercises to consider (integration)

- Dr. Elliot has made a few errors in recent months in his diagnoses and charting. He has been challenged on these behaviors by his attending physician, who has told him that he needs to take immediate action or he will face serious consequences. Dr. Elliot took the VIA Survey and observes that his signature strengths are curiosity, fairness, forgiveness, teamwork, and love. How might he use these strengths with greater mindfulness in his medical practice? What is an optimal strengths-based approach that he might take with himself? If you were supervising Dr. Elliot, how would you follow up with him using a strengths-based approach?
- Dr. Jamison has been feeling less enthused about her work in the last year. She feels as though she is just going through the motions of her daily clinic routine, and she tries to get through her patients' visits as quickly as possible so that she can get home and be by herself. Dr. Jamison has some insight into this behavior and realizes that she is disengaged. She has recently learned that the use of character strengths can be one of the best pathways for reengaging with one's life and work. Her signature strengths are creativity, judgment, love of learning, humility, spirituality, and gratitude. What would you recommend to her? Is there a way that

she might use mindfulness and strengths to help her tap into her relationships? Be sure to hypothesize about the role of mindful strengths use.

- *Best possible self:* This research-based exercise is used in MBSP and is a way to link character strengths with mindful awareness of your goals. It involves three steps:

1. Select a time in the future (e.g., six months, one year, five years from now) and imagine that at that time you are strongly expressing your best possible self. Visualize the details clearly in a way in which you have worked hard and succeeded at accomplishing your personal or professional goals.
2. After you have a clear image, write about the details. Writing your best possible self down helps to create a logical structure for the future and can help you move from the realm of foggy ideas and fragmented thoughts to concrete, real possibilities.
3. Write about the *character strengths* that you observe in this image. Consider what character strengths you will need to deploy to make this best possible self a reality.

CONCLUSION

Mindfulness and character strengths are capacities in human beings that can be developed and turned to for increasing well-being and managing stress. The integration of mindfulness and character-strengths practices is an exciting and promising area for medical practitioners and students. There are deep applications not only for helping patients improve their coping and recovery from illness, but also future studies might also reveal these areas can serve as a force of prevention and healthy maintenance of good habits. The MBSP offers a rigorous program for promoting positive health, cultivating what is best in human beings, and capitalizing on what is already strong and present in order to create a flourishing life, a life of fulfillment, engagement, and meaning.

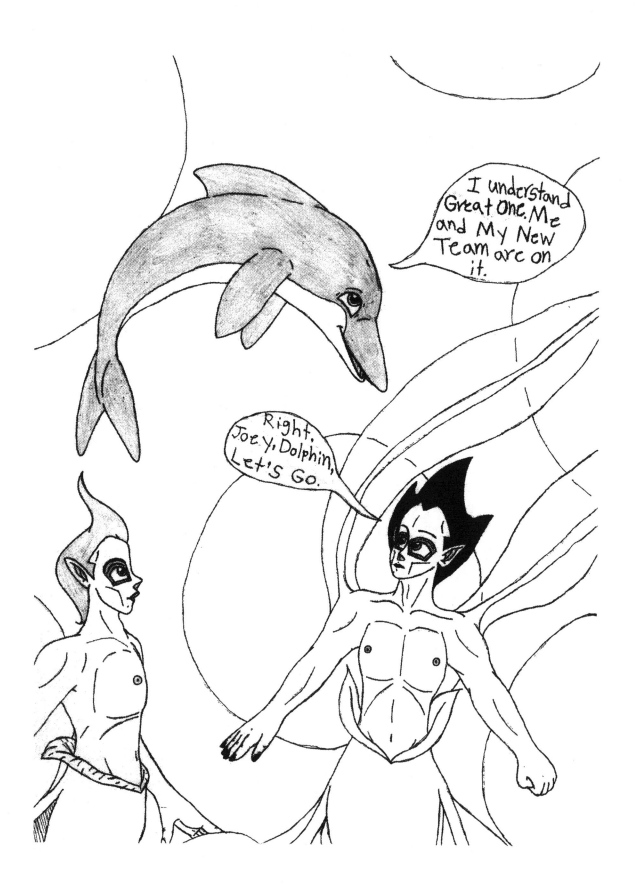

Chapter 15

The Spirited Multidisciplinary Health-Care Team

Coauthored by: Dr. Barry Heermann and Dr. Marsha W. Snyder

Anytime a diverse group of individuals comes together to work as a team, even in a professional setting, each individual member "sizes up" each of the other members of the team. Even the most open-minded and nonjudgmental people among us have automatic subjective reactions based upon our deeply held beliefs and our past experiences. Therefore, when we are introduced to an individual for the first time, we may feel automatically drawn to that person, or conversely, we may feel immediately uncomfortable with him or her. Of course, these initial reactions are then changed through our further ongoing social interactions and verbal exchanges with that particular individual.

As has been established in earlier chapters, health care often is a high-stress profession. When physicians and health-care workers become burned out, they lose focus on the tasks at hand and tend to withdraw from engagement with other people. Their frustration and anger can easily be projected onto their colleagues. This behavior results in relationships that lack professionalism and are divisive to a team, because the focus ultimately becomes the individual's personal conflict as opposed to the professional goals. It is at this point that communication breaks down and errors are most likely to occur.

In a healthy professional setting, each member of a team should have a common focus, that is, the mission of the team and the successful completion of the project at hand. In a health-care team, this common focus is the health and well-being of each patient and each team member, and the delivery of high-quality, compassionate, error-free, cost-effective care. To maintain professionalism, each member of the team must hold himself or herself, as well as the other members, accountable for retaining focus on the common goals of the team. Should tension arise within the team, it is a signal that the team needs to meet as a group to clarify the goals and the roles of each team member and work on team process and problem solving. This step will be discussed at length later in this chapter.

The longer a group of health-care professionals work together with the common goal of excellence in the care of patient health, the more united they are behind that goal and the more fluid their work together will be.

ACHIEVING SUCCESS

Teamwork and *health-care team* are often cited in a health-care institution's stated policies and values, but the reality is that most health networks are vertical organizations in which each discipline reports through separate discipline-specific hierarchies. A simplified example of one such organizational structure is shown in figure 15-1 below. In this scenario, the doctor comes to make rounds, and the nurses, social worker, residents, and others who follow the doctor around are often referred to as *the multidisciplinary team*. This is not the health-care team to which we refer.

Figure 15-1. The vertical organization and how it impacts the frontline multidisciplinary team

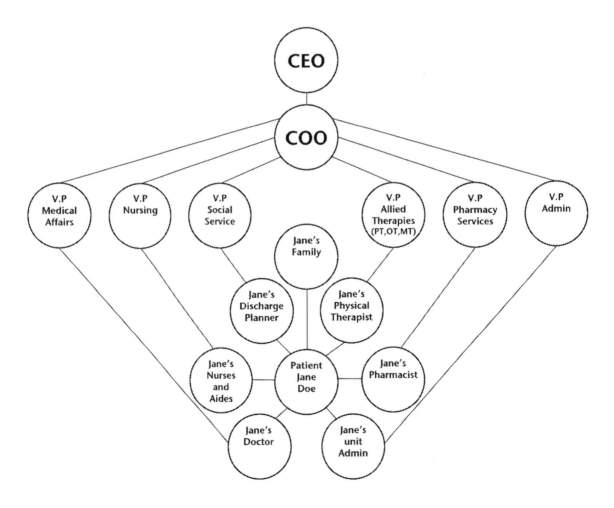

Organizations of the kind depicted in figure 15-1 are splintered by discipline, which creates several problems. Messages to the frontline caregivers are mixed and often do not address the needs of other frontline disciplines. With different hierarchies, there is an increased tendency to assign blame to other professional disciplines when problems arise. As a result, tension develops between disciplines, and little direct communication about the patients occurs. In addition, frontline workers are not engaged with one another and, therefore, are not empowered to problem solve at their professional level. Too often, problems are addressed in a punitive way by managers, who are remote and unaware of the frontline realities and issues of the team and the patients they serve.

The Joint Commission for the Accreditation of Healthcare Organizations (JCAHO) has noted that 60 percent of medication errors in the health-care setting can be attributed to impaired communication among doctors, nurses, pharmacists, and other frontline professionals (Timmons & O'Leary, 2004, p. 22). Most doctors and nurses work in a highly stressful working environment, which in turn, often leads to burnout. The interpersonal withdrawal that results from burnout further decreases communication among disciplines. Frustrations can seem overwhelming to the health-care professional, and the tendency for interdisciplinary blame and irritability to occur is quite high. This scenario fosters an absence of open conversation and teamwork, an absence of information, false assumptions, and an overall feeling of helplessness, which is a perfect breeding ground not only for disruptive behavior but also medical errors. Hence, success strategies are those that provide for and encourage teamwork, the alignment of goals, education, and training, and wide dissemination of information. The sections that follow will address these important areas individually and in greater depth. They are the key ingredients in eliminating medical errors and forming spirited, engaged multidisciplinary health-care teams.

Introducing teamwork into your organization

When health-care employees function in isolation and members of the true health-care team are administratively divided, there is no structure that facilitates open communication. The high-stress setting, coupled with increased demands and decreased available resources, creates an "every man for himself" mentality, with increased hostility and lack of trust. In the middle of all this chaos is a sick and suffering patient, who only wants to feel better.

As soon as the opportunity arises for individuals to work together—even if it is, for example, just two nurses working together on the same group of patients—an opportunity for dialogue and communication is created.

As noted above (Timmons & O'Leary, 2004), 60 percent of medication errors are attributed to miscommunication. Without the emphasis on teamwork, communication problems and medical errors will be unresolved issues.

Ideally, the health-care team should include all health-care professionals who participate in the care of a given group of patients. This team includes the attending physician in charge of the given group of patients, the nurses, social worker, occupational therapist, physical therapist, unit administrator, pharmacist, allied therapists, chaplains, and all other professionals who are involved in the direct care of any of these patients. The team should also include the patient and any family members who the patient wishes to include. With the increased use of hospitalists—as opposed to numerous private physicians taking care of their own hospitalized patients—the possibility of such teamwork in the hospital is enhanced.

Although the concept of including the patient and his or her family caregivers and supporters in the health-care team may seem new or unusual, there is widespread agreement that it is essential to ensure care that is patient-centered, compassionate, and cost-effective. This is the case with all patients. However, the involvement of caregivers is especially critical in caring for the elderly and the disabled (Gillick, 2013).

To facilitate the development of teams that establish optimal communication, there should be as much consistency as possible in the team membership. On an inpatient unit, for example, assigning nurses by doctor instead of by room number might help to achieve this goal. How might this be done? On a thirty-bed unit, consider dividing nursing personnel into two teams: team A and team B. Team A staff works exclusively with Drs. W. and X. Team B staff works exclusively with Drs. Y. and Z. The team A and B structure should be constant for all three shifts of nursing personnel.

Each doctor should ideally establish a consistent time for making daily rounds. At that time, the appropriate nursing team, allied therapists, pharmacy representative, and unit administrator will round together to assess the progress and determine the treatment plan for the next twenty-four hours for each patient. Input from all disciplines allows the plan to be comprehensive, accurate, and well-coordinated. At the same time, the patient and his or her family become active participants in the treatment team. Any questions and necessary clarifications can be posed and answered immediately so that mistakes caused by miscommunication are avoided.

As the team gets to know one another and works together, the work becomes more efficient. Difficulties within the team can be immediately addressed, which empowers the team to effectively problem solve together (see "Team Process and Phases of the Spiral" later in this chapter).

In addition to multidisciplinary teams on patient-care floors in hospitals, the concept applies to many other health-care settings and departments, both inpatient and outpatient.

With you as the physician leading the team, you are in an excellent position to suggest this structure and process in all settings in health care in which you count on a team to ensure outstanding care of your patients. For example, the operating room benefits greatly from open communication and planning within regular multidisciplinary teams. Because the operating room tends to be a high-stress setting, often involving life-and-death situations, miscommunication and acting out are likely to occur. As with inpatient units, each surgeon should, ideally, be assigned to a specific team of nurses, technicians, and anesthesiologists who are well instructed in the procedures performed by that surgeon. As the team works together over time, the members will become more efficient and more comfortable with one another.

When a case is scheduled, the surgical team comes together in the operating-room area to mark the site of the surgery and briefly review the surgical plan. Led by the surgeon, the entire team, including the patient, discuss the procedure and goals, along with any potential complications. Any questions from a team member are answered. The team can then approach the surgery with a goal-oriented approach and can complete it successfully, without errors. Once the surgery has been completed, the team can briefly discuss any problems that occurred with the surgery and with team process and how to avoid the same problems in the future. A similar plan can be crafted for teams in other areas of the hospital.

Workplace communication skills

To prevent medical errors and facilitate efficient functioning within a health-care team, communication skills are paramount, as are listening skills. These topics are reviewed in depth in chapter 11, "Professionalism." Recall that a message that is brief, fact-based, and direct has the greatest chance of being accurately registered by the listener and is, therefore, optimal in a professional situation. This kind of message is free of hidden content that could arouse the listener's emotions and, thus, distort the message by subjective interpretation. In addition to being objective, reality-based, and focused, good workplace and team communication must be complete. Communication is considered incomplete when information is withheld for any reason. This type of communication breakdown tends to occur in cases of disagreement, confusion, or fear. The speaker withholds content in anticipation of a negative reaction on the part of the listener (or other team members). For example, when the speaker is of lower status or feels less powerful than the listener, content is withheld to avoid retribution or being fired. In an effectively functioning team, all members must feel free to, and be safe to, speak so that all communication can be authentic and complete.

Marsha W. Snyder, MD., MAPP.

Emphasizing professionalism

Several common mistakes are made in health-care organizations that can undermine professionalism and the well-being of patients. The most common mistake is the disempowering of frontline caregivers to solve their own problems. This situation tends to occur when a decision regarding clinical patient care is made at the administrative level and is then presented to frontline staff as something that they must or must not do concerning the care of the patients. Policies and decisions such as these, made in the absence of clinical staff, can easily conflict with professional ethics and knowledge and can undermine the professionalism of the clinical staff. An example of this type of occurrence in the outpatient setting is when a practice is losing revenue and an administrative decision is made to schedule a clinician to see more patients in an hour than is reasonable and safe based upon the work that is required for each patient and the time that is needed to safely complete it. This scenario creates moral conflict, anxiety, and resentment in the clinician, which impairs professional behavior and increases the likelihood of errors. However, if the administrator met with the frontline staff, observed their work, and presented the financial challenge, it is likely that the clinical staff could then brainstorm many creative cost-saving strategies that would resolve the problem of lost revenue without undermining the quality and safety of patient care.

Other factors that undermine professional behavior include a lack of respect for the clinicians' skills and their unique contribution to the organization and not allowing (or trusting) the frontline multidisciplinary team to self-regulate and problem solve on its own. Keep in mind that the unit administrator is an integral part of that frontline team, and the interests of the administrative sector of the organization are, therefore, well-represented at each and every team meeting.

Even in the case of a fully supportive organization and an empowered team, there are factors that can undermine professional behavior within the team. Avoiding disruptive behavior through self-regulation was addressed in chapter 11, "Professionalism." Other factors that undermine professionalism include physical or emotional illness, burnout, substance abuse, severe personal problems, and other stressors (e.g., divorce, death, birth of a child). Many health-care organizations have a professional health committee set up specifically for the medical staff to confidentially advise, mentor, and support their colleagues who are ill or under unusual stress. Many states offer a similar program through their medical societies. These complex personal issues of physician ill-being must be addressed immediately, confidentially, and respectfully when they arise.

One of the principal goals of practicing positive health is to prevent such undermining factors to the health and well-being of every physician and to employ the practices of resilient thinking to cope with stressful situations when those events do occur.

Group process and problem solving

There is no doubt that an effectively functioning health-care team, in all health-care settings, can decrease medical errors, improve communication among health-care providers, empower patients to participate in their own care, facilitate early problem solving, and decrease the cost of care. The key to a successful team, however, lies in its process.

Physicists tell us that nature is composed of an infinite series of rhythmic fields. Similarly, team process is a rhythmic field with its own set of harmonic qualities, both consonant and dissonant (Heermann, 1997). The Dutch scientist Christian Huygens in 1665 conducted experiments with pendulum clocks mounted side by side and discovered that, over time, the pendulums would begin to swing together in precise time. Later scientists referred to this mutual phase locking of two oscillators as *entrainment*. It is easy to observe entrainment when watching a small chamber music group play together. Members of a chamber group play without a conductor. The musicians begin to move as one as they sense and feel the music that they are creating together. Margaret Wheatley later applied this concept to the work of organizations and teams (1992). Wheatley noted that, through this self-organizing process, systems regenerate themselves and move to higher levels of harmony and effectiveness. Through these concepts, we can understand that, in spite of the stress and differences within a team, its ability to problem solve actually brings the members closer and makes them more effective as a unit. They begin to *move together* and function ever more effectively as a unit.

Allan Drexler and associates' work on team process led to their proposal of a seven-stage model, in which each stage represents a set of concerns that team members face as they work together (Drexler, Sibbet, & Forrester, 1988). These interdependent stages are: (1) orientation, (2) trust building, (3) goal/role clarification, (4) commitment, (5) implementation, (6) high performance, and (7) renewal. If the team gets stuck in any one of these stages, resolution must occur before the team is able to move ahead to the next stage. Matthew Fox's work added to this concept by emphasizing the unifying value of recognizing and celebrating the experiences of unbounded possibility that can arise from a successful group dynamic (1994). Fox also notes the cleansing force found in the recognition of the darker, more difficult aspects of the group experience and how this recognition can be transformed into an energizing dynamic that gives life and power to the team.

All of these contributions to the understanding of effective group process help us to understand that the ability of human beings to work in teams is natural and that, in a healthy team, the whole is greater than the sum of its parts. It further points out that when a group of health-care workers unite behind a common goal, the tensions that inevitably arise within the group can actually facilitate a stronger and more cohesive unit—versus a negative force that leads to communication breakdown and errors. We can further conclude that there is a process or *flow* that can help us to create a model for effective and empowered health-care teams that are professional and can communicate openly with both patients and one another.

At the team's core, the goal that unifies focus and purpose is outstanding service to their "*customers.*" In this case, *service* reflects Robert Greenleaf's notion of *servant leadership* (1977), wherein the ultimate concern of the effort is contributing to those being served by the team, as well as other team members, and the well-being of the self. The idea of serving oneself and other team members—in addition to patients—is a marked departure from the current state of health care, in which there is a preponderance of burned-out professionals within a system that creates divisiveness among them. This *spirit of service* is manifested in the sense of wonder that is experienced by the team as it discovers its own power to provide amazing service—both to one another and self, as well as to those they serve. The more nurtured and empowered that the team feels in taking care of its own needs, the more energy, enthusiasm, and creativity they generate in meeting the needs of those they serve.

To achieve high performance, the team must be able to function as a harmonious unit. There are often challenges to this harmony, such as differences of opinion or a breakdown in trust. The team must be empowered to deal with these difficulties and be able to resolve them. Both the harmonious function and the ability to resolve negative issues help the team—and each individual member—to grow and blossom. Hence, the dynamic of team growth can be seen as a continual ebb and flow, or rhythm, that is experienced by the team as it embraces and builds on its consonances while working through its dissonances. The team enhances its own performance and learns to solve its own problems proactively, which in turn, strengthens the team's evolving sense of purpose, unity, and worth. Imagine the amount of administrative time and dollars this approach could potentially save the health-care industry!

Figure 15-2 shows a model of the processes that the team must go through to reach peak performance and function, thereby enhancing communication and decreasing medical errors. It is important to note that these processes are neither linear nor sequential in occurrence; this is the reason why the figure is depicted as a spiral that reflects back on itself. The team is constantly using each of these processes to strengthen itself and to provide outstanding, cost-effective, error-free service to patients. This model also emphasizes how service, as described above, is the centerpiece and the glue that unites the team and all of its processes. (Note the similarities with the noble purpose spiral of chapter 8.)

Figure 15-2. The Spirited Multidisciplinary Team spiral

The core integrating phase of Service
Quality of spirit: The team experiences contribution and service to customers and to the team.

Letting Go phase
Quality of spirit: A sense of freedom and completion arises from being forthright and sharing with full integrity.

Celebrating phase
Quality of spirit: There is a presence of awe, wonder, and an appreciation for the contribution of the team and team members.

Claiming phase
Quality of spirit: The team experiences solidarity, single-minded purpose, and assurance about what needs to be accomplished.

Visioning phase
Quality of spirit: An extraordinary sense of possibility for what can be created is alive and present for the team.

Initiating phase
Quality of spirit: A profound sense of relationship exists, wherein team members feel belonging and trust in their work together.

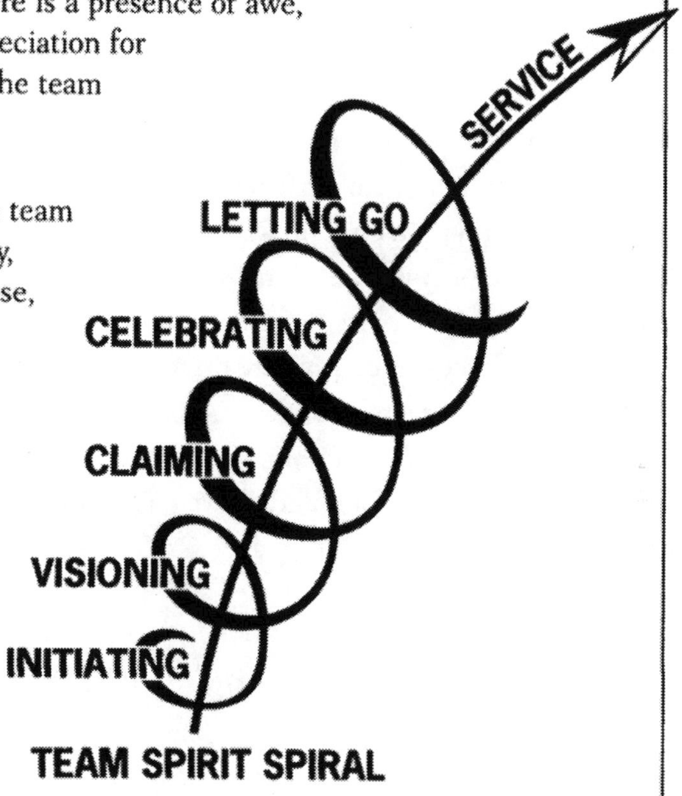

Note: The qualities of spirit represented in the Spiral interact in complex ways, as they blend and fuse throughout the life of the team. For example, the Letting Go quality of spirit is ideally occurring in every phase of the team's work together.

SERVICE

LETTING GO

CELEBRATING

CLAIMING

VISIONING

INITIATING

TEAM SPIRIT SPIRAL

Figure 1-1. The Team Spirit Spiral

Team process and phases of the spiral

In this section, the finer points of the group process-in-team spiral will be explained and demonstrated. If you are already part of an intact team, it is best to carry out the exercises discussed here with your team, but if that is not possible or if you are an independent learner, it is best to join with one team of other learners (three or four individuals) for all of the activities in the remainder of this chapter. The primary reason for this advice is that team process is not concrete and is, therefore, difficult to describe clearly without experiential context and demonstration. For those who have no access to others to complete the exercises, my suggestion would be to read and understand the exercises and to try and relate them to any prior experiences that you have had working with intact teams.

As mentioned many times throughout this chapter, it is when health-care teams are constant and consistent in membership that they learn best to work effectively together. However, realizing that this is impractical in some situations, it is also important to note that the degree of investment in the process, particularly early in the life of the team, will determine its success. In the sections that follow, you will note a reference to *process meetings*. Process meetings are brief meetings that the team must have to deal solely with the issues of team process, such as getting to know one another and trust building. These meetings need to be separate from the clinical work of the team. They should be open, nonthreatening, and viewed as a safe place to work together on team-building issues.

Phase 1: Trust building (initiating)

When people initially come together to work as a team, a certain level of awkwardness and uncertainty is natural. To build a sense of trust and belonging, team members must devote time to getting to know one another. This process can be accomplished at an initial meeting in which each team member is given the opportunity to introduce himself or herself to the group. The introduction should include discipline and training, current work role or function, personal strengths, hopes for the team, and the unique contribution that the individual hopes to make to the team. Once each member is given time for his or her introduction, time should be allowed for questions and open discussion. This process of creating a sense of belonging and trust is continuously improved and enhanced throughout the life of the team through mutual goal creation, working together, and working on consonances and dissonances within the team. Each time a new member joins the team, he or she should be given the opportunity to experience this kind of welcome and introductory process.

With effective trust building, each member of the team has a sense of belonging and clarity of direction that empowers the team to define and accomplish its work effectively. A sign of mistrust, fear, or disorientation among team members signals a need for the team to undertake work in the trust-building process.

Key processes for fostering belonging and trust include the following:

1) Create a context for relationship, seeking out team members and exploring commonalities.
2) Determine ways that you can support one another and the work of the team.
3) Agree on what you will do to provide support.
4) Welcome new team members and others warmly and openly, which creates a relationship.

Trust-building exercise

Learning Goal: To provide a trust-building experience by promoting communication and a relationship among team members through visual expression and telling their stories both as individuals and members of a team.

Learning Activity: A mandala is a visual representation of prized values, beliefs, and viewpoints held by an individual or group that captures their essence or spirit. *Mandala* is the Sanskrit word for *circle*. These art forms are particularly common in the East, especially in India.

1) Take a large piece of blank paper, preferably the size of flip-chart paper. Have at least two or three colored markers ready to use.
2) Draw a large circle on your paper, similar to what is pictured in figure 15-3, and divide the circle into four quadrants as shown in the figure.
3) Beginning with the upper-right quadrant and moving clockwise, you are to pictorially represent in each quadrant the following four things:
    a. Your source of personal pride (work or personal life)
    b. A gift or a personal strength that you bring to the team
    c. A source of frustration with the team (or another team if you are alone)
    d. Your intention for the team to help it become a spirited, high-performance team

Figure 15-3. Personal mandala

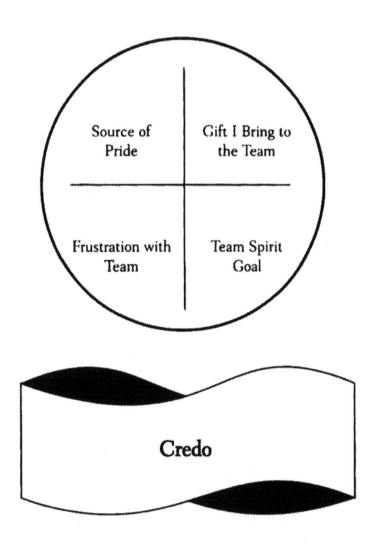

Photocopied from *Building Team Spirit* by Barry Heermann.
Published by McGraw-Hill. ISBN 0-07-028472-5. To order, call 1-800-2MCGRAW.

4) As shown in figure 15-3, draw a ribbon at the bottom of your circle, in which you write a personal credo—an essential guiding principle or perspective that you rely on as a guide to everyday life.

5) Use only images, icons, or pictures when completing step 3 in each of the four quadrants. Do not use words. The credo must be only words—no images or icons.

6) Take twenty minutes to complete steps 1 to 5 above. Put your name on your finished work and, using masking tape or tacks, secure it to a wall alongside your team members' mandalas.

7) When all team members are finished, arrange your chairs in a circle around the posted mandalas. One by one, each team member should stand and explain to the others the significance of each of his or her drawings and creed. Team members should be allowed to ask questions before moving on. A time slot of three to five minutes per individual presentation is usually sufficient to complete the exercise.

Discussion questions

- What did you learn about your teammates? How is this knowledge important to your ability to effectively work together in a team?

- Did you learn anything about yourself? What new piece of self-knowledge surprised you the most?

- How did it feel to share your goals for the team as opposed to your frustrations with the team? Does this revelation give you any important insights?

- How did it feel to share the gift that you feel you bring to the team? How was listening to your teammates' gifts helpful to you?

Team exercise

Before continuing with this chapter, you and your team should complete the following exercise. The mandala exercise can take as long as an hour to complete. When your frontline multidisciplinary team is struggling with a trust-building issue, you generally do not have the luxury of an hour to complete such an exercise. Therefore, you should devise a trust-building mechanism that can be used by your team or any clinical team and be completed within fifteen to twenty minutes.

Phase 2: Visioning

Phase 2, which is focused on visioning possibilities and goal creation, is actually quite interdependent with phase 1, because each greatly enhances the success of the other. Often they occur simultaneously.

Visioning engages the team in considering the very essence of its work. Through visioning, the team defines its purpose, its core values and beliefs, and its own highest goals for serving patients, other customers, and one another. With good visioning, the team is filled with a sense of wonder and enthusiasm and a clear view of the heights that they hope to achieve together. Because the team includes doctors, nurses, administrators, social workers, pharmacists, case managers, and allied therapists, the vision can be creative and broad and designed to make the best use of the limited resources that are available to the team. This approach helps to achieve the goal of cost-effectiveness for the organization and can help to increase efficiency and decrease length-of-stay in the inpatient setting. By maintaining a focus on the team's vision of excellence in patient care, behavior of team members remains cooperative, professional, harmonious, and highly motivated.

Dissonances that can occur due to inadequate visioning include a feeling of emptiness or aridness in team members or a vision and values that lack clarity. Should these feelings arise, it is a signal that the team is in need of additional process work related to their common vision and values.

Key processes for excellent visioning include:

1) Discovering and cocreating what the team stands for.
2) Articulating the values and purposes that are of overriding importance to individual team members, to the team as a whole, and in the service of patients.
3) Establishing in visual and verbal forms what the team stands for.
4) Creating a mental image of exactly how the team will contribute to patients through excellent, error-free, and compassionate care, teaching positive health, and distinguishing current reality from the intended results.
5) Ensuring that each and every team member has participated in and fully accepts the goals and values of the team.

Visioning exercise

Learning Goals:

1) To assist a team in identifying achievements, values, and areas of improvement in their work together.

2) To support the team in envisioning the future and claiming their role in creating that positive future.

Learning Activity: This activity works best if you are comfortably seated in a circle, with access to a flip chart for recording the results of the activity. If you are performing this exercise with an intact team, simply follow the steps as they are stated. If you are working with a team that was formed solely for the purpose of these exercises, alternatives will be given in parentheses.

1) Begin by brainstorming about the work of the team during the past five years or the life span of the team if it is less than five years old. This exercise should include having team members tell stories of the team's past achievements, values, successes, errors, frustrations, and high points. You should reflect on how these events contributed to or detracted from the team's sense of meaning and purpose. Record the responses on the flip chart and label it *Team Heights and Depths*. (If you are not an intact team, each individual should relate stories from his or her own past experiences with intact teams.) (20 minutes)

2) Once that discussion is complete, each team member should relax, close his or her eyes, and focus on the work of the team as he or she sees it five years into the future. Take a flight of fancy, imagining that it is five years from now and that, in your fanciful flight, you are able to create the ideal team in the ideal work setting. It is the same setting in which you currently work, but you have, magically, been able to change and fashion it into the ideal place to work and the ideal team with whom to work. Give yourself several minutes to relax and focus on the details of your vision. Once your vision is clear, open your eyes.

3) Have a discussion with your teammates regarding each person's ideal vision. What does the work setting look like? What are the services that the team is providing? How is the team different? In what ways is it the same? What are key changes that need to be made? Record all of these responses on a flip chart labeled *Flight of Fancy*. (20 minutes)

4) As a team, identify the most common and most outstanding patterns of change and progress that emerged from step 3. Record these on a flip chart labeled *Shared Positive Vision*.

5) Combine the items in step 4 and formulate the team vision for the future in a single sentence. Write this sentence at the top of a flip-chart page. (15 minutes)

6) Finally, brainstorm action steps for realizing this shared vision. Record these action steps under the vision statement.

Discussion questions

- Based on your experience with the above exercise, how can individuals who come from different disciplines and backgrounds with various points of view come together harmoniously behind a shared vision?
- In your magical flight of fancy, how did it feel to be at work? How does that feeling compare with how you currently feel at your workplace? Are there issues of focus beyond those of the team that were prominent in your ideal fantasy? Discuss those issues and how a trusted multidisciplinary team might assist you in formulating and achieving realistic goals for change.
- How does a shared vision and values unite and equalize a team that might otherwise be regarded as having unequal employee status within an organization?
- When you find a group of individuals who share your vision of excellence and compassion in patient care and your desire for the creation of positive health and a thriving life, how does it impact your feelings about coming to work? How does it impact your desire to care for yourself and your team, as well as your patients? When you brainstormed action steps for achieving your shared vision, did you include steps concerning caring for yourself and your teammates? If not, what steps would you now add?

Team exercise

The above visioning exercise takes at least one and a half hours to fully process and complete. In the work setting, the team often does not have the luxury of that amount of time to work on visioning. Together with your team members, develop a visioning exercise that can be completed in fifteen to twenty minutes and is appropriate for your work setting. Once you have formulated the exercise, discuss it together with your teammates. If successful, this exercise should give you a result similar to the full-length exercise in terms of goals alignment, spirit of service, and enthusiasm, but with, perhaps, a more limited focus.

Phase 3: Implementation (claiming)

With a shared vision and values, the team can brainstorm what is needed to implement the vision and the important role of each team member in successful achievement of that vision. This brainstorming includes what is needed from the parent organization, along with the skills, strengths, and resources of each team member. In the classic frontline multidisciplinary team, implementation most often occurs in the context of walking daily rounds in an inpatient setting or planning rounds in an outpatient setting.

In terms of performance improvement (quality and cost) within an organization, particularly a vertical health-care organization, most of the planning and strategizing occur at the vice president and director/administrator levels. As a result, there is no clear understanding or acceptance of the performance-improvement strategies at the staff level. From the perspective of the frontline, it appears as if they are expected to improve performance with fewer staff and by using the same inefficient processes or, worse, new strategies formulated by administrators who are remote from direct patient care and the knowledge of their challenges. Quality, service, and employee satisfaction consequently suffer.

One of the greatest stressors for any human being is the perception of complete loss of control. This feeling, unfortunately, is what results from a vertical model of quality and cost improvement. The frontline staff develops a "management versus us" mentality. "They do not know what they are doing, and they do not care about us," is what the staff whispers to one another as stress builds and divisiveness grows. Furthermore, the staff does not cooperate with the proposed changes simply as a way to retain some degree of control in a passive-aggressive fashion.

With empowerment of the frontline multidisciplinary team, the organization's goals, which are incorporated into the team's own vision, become clear. Then, through implementation, the team can creatively brainstorm how to accomplish their goals in an educated and professional way that is best suited to the needs of the patient, the clinical situation, and their skills. Thus, they share and support the goals of the organization and have input into how these goals can be accomplished and implemented. The result is total organization-wide acceptance of high-quality, safe, compassionate, cost-effective service to patients and all customers. Implementation strategies obviously will differ from department to department and team to team as each determines the best fit for their clinical situation and resources, but the organizational goal of outstanding care ultimately is realized in a way that delights both staff and patients.

Dissonant feelings regarding implementation include a lack of agreement on the roles of each member or a perceived lack of needed skills, attitudes, and resources. Should these feelings arise, it is a clue that the team is in need of additional process work on implementation.

Key processes for implementation include the following:

1) Maintaining a firm base in the team's shared vision, values, and purpose.
2) Developing a plan that will allow the team to accomplish its shared goals.
3) Agreement on the roles and responsibilities of each team member.

4) Fostering team commitment to the roles and responsibilities that support the team's vision, values, and goals.

5) Determining ways in which the team members can educate and support one another.

6) Establishing a follow-up plan to reinforce successful processes and improve those processes that do not lead to success.

Implementation exercise

This learning activity focuses on a key aspect of implementation: spirited role clarification. In a clinical team in which the physician has clinical leadership but each member's role is equally important and valued, this particular activity can be extremely instructive and helpful.

Learning Goals:

1) To clarify the critical roles of each team member as perceived by the team.

2) To allow all team members to reflect and comment on the critical roles of their colleagues.

Learning Activity:

1) Each team member will need a piece of flip-chart paper and black, green, red, and blue markers. Work individually and silently in this first part of the activity. Put your name at the top of your paper in black. Then, below your name, make a list of all of your roles and responsibilities within the team, including responsibilities that you might carry out individually when other team members are not present. Please be as inclusive as possible. (If you are not working with an intact team, reference a role that you actively played in a prior health-care team experience.)

2) Once you have completed your list, underline with green marker those roles that provide you with the greatest passion and spirit. Underline with red marker those roles that you would be happy to get rid of. Underline with blue marker those roles in which you would appreciate assistance or clarification from other team members to help you fulfill the task. Once you have completed this exercise, use masking tape and post your list on the wall in front of the team and return to your seat.

3) Once all lists are complete and displayed, each team member should silently circulate, read, and absorb the content on each member's list. As you do this, make notes directly on your colleagues' displays, such as constructive comments,

questions that come to mind, helpful ideas or suggestions. The idea is to take your time and consider what your teammate has expressed in an appreciative and helpful manner. It is important that respectful silence is maintained until all members of the team have completed this step.

4) Finally, each team member should verbally discuss his or her unique role, with the rest of the team listening, referring to his or her display and reflecting on comments and suggestions that were added by other team members. It is important to ask for clarification of any questions that remain regarding fulfillment of role (areas underlined in blue) or any creative suggestions for areas underlined in red, if not already given.

5) Once each team member has had the opportunity to discuss his or her role with the rest of the team, the team should have a greater awareness of its depth and breadth of strengths and how each team member, who is now encouraged to use these strengths in a coordinated fashion, creates the miracle of outstanding, giving, and committed service.

Discussion questions

*   How can lack of clarity of team members' roles undermine the spirit of an intact team?
*   Clinical team A is making its morning inpatient rounds. Once assembled, they walk into the room of Mrs. Jones, a fifty-eight-year-old female who has newly diagnosed systemic lupus erythematosis (SLE) and was admitted in acute renal failure. Dr. Smith greets Mrs. Jones, looks at her laboratory report, and says, "Your renal failure has been resolved, Mrs. Jones. This is good news! I am discharging you today." Was this sequence of behavior optimal? How would you have felt if you were the social worker on the team who had to arrange the discharge? How would you have felt if you were Mrs. Jones? Recreate the scene in a way that includes and considers all team members' knowledge and input, including the patient herself.

Team exercise

As a team, brainstorm a script for an ideal morning of rounds. The script should focus on your team in your routine clinical setting. It must involve the active participation of every team member and include the team's interaction with at least two or three different patients. Work on the script until every team member can accept the finished product. Notice the vital role that each person contributes and the areas around which the team has great enthusiasm and spirit of service.

Phase 4: Celebrating

In a work situation, particularly in the health-care setting, much time and attention are devoted to problems and perceived inadequate performance on the part of individuals, teams, and departments. This sole focus on negative behavior creates a sense of discouragement and pessimism that pervades the team and the organization.

When the Philadelphia Phillies won baseball's World Series in 2008 for the first time in many years, what did they do first? They all ran out to the pitcher's mound, hugged and jumped on top of one another, and high-fived one another in victory. They then ran directly into their clubhouse, where they opened bottles of champagne and celebrated their triumph and each another. Most outstanding professional athletic teams behave in the same way.

The celebration of victories and achievement of goals ignites and nurtures enthusiasm and spirit. Each team member feels appreciated and acknowledged. This phase is life-giving and illuminating to the ongoing work of the team. Celebrating adds to the sense of solidarity and spirit within the team. It generates optimism and a desire to take on new challenges and new opportunities for service to patients and to the organization. Even the smallest victories should be acknowledged in celebration with the team. Each victory is another step toward outstanding, safe, compassionate care of patients and the creation of a thriving population. Celebrating increases self-respect and mutual respect within the team. Celebrating is joyful and fun. It gives the team the opportunity to positively practice gratitude as a group for its bountiful gifts and talents that allow them to bring joy and healing to others.

Key processes for celebrating include:

1) Recognizing the gifts and accomplishments of each team member and the team as a whole.
2) Acknowledging the results produced by the efforts of the team or team members.
3) Expressing mutual appreciation within the team.
4) Affirming all team members for their skills and contributions to the team and to a job well done.

Celebrating exercise

This exercise is carried out with the team subdivided into two smaller groups. It will not matter if the two groups do not have an equal number of members. However, the division should be random. This exercise is also done in two phases, a planning phase and an execution phase. The two phases may be done one right after the other, as long as adequate preparation time is allowed.

Learning Goals:

1) To heighten team spirit through a conscious reflection on the team's positive work.
2) To learn how to regularly acknowledge and celebrate positive work through celebration and gratitude.

Learning Activity:

1) The team has been subdivided into two celebration teams to commemorate the entire team's work together. The celebration should acknowledge and ritualize the spirit of the team in its work together as a unit, acknowledging milestones, accomplishments, highlights, strengths, and any other positives for which gratitude and appreciation is felt.
2) Each sub-team must plan its celebration independent of the other. The celebration must take no more than twenty minutes, be held in the training room, take no more than five minutes to set up and five more to clean up, and not involve any food, beverages, or dangerous materials such as lighted candles. The cost of the materials for the celebration must not exceed $20. Special audiovisual materials may be used if the team has them available and ready to go.
3) Each celebration team should take thirty minutes to meet and plan their celebration. If the planning half of this exercise and the execution half of this exercise are separated by a meal break or an overnight break, the sub-teams may decide to reconvene at a later time to fine-tune their celebrations. Given that a celebration is happy and joyous, this event should be a fun, creative exercise.
4) Once the planning phase is complete and the room is returned to its original setup, the first sub-team is given five minutes to set up for their celebration, thirty minutes in which to carry it out, and then five minutes for cleanup. The second sub-team follows the same procedure.

Discussion questions

- What is the importance of celebration for the renewal of the spirit of the team?
- In what other significant ways is celebration a vital part of the team's process? What other team functions and relationships are strengthened through celebration?
- What did you learn through your participation in the preparation of a celebration? How is this experience related to the character strength of gratitude or the "three good things" positive intervention?

- Because we, as physicians, are always too busy going from one crisis to another, we tend to—disastrously—ignore the positive as an unnecessary luxury. How will you, as the clinical team leader, stay focused and keep your team focused on celebrating?

Team exercise

There are many different ways in which we can celebrate our work together as a team and show our gratitude and respect to others, as well as to ourselves. Not all of these exercises take hours or days. Some take only a minute. As a team, develop two or three regular rituals that take ten minutes or less in which you can celebrate your accomplishments and express your respect and gratitude toward your team, yourselves, and each other. Write them down and practice them, using each one for a week after daily rounds.

Phase 5: Resolving dissonances (letting go)

Inevitably, when a group of people come together, particularly in high-stress conditions and life-and-death situations, dissonances can develop. Even in the best of circumstances and relationships, interpersonal tensions and misunderstandings can and do develop.

Similarly, breakdown occurs even in the best of teams. Team members can experience disappointment, for example, when they are unable to provide a patient with the outstanding service for which they strive. They can then become frustrated with their own performance or that of others. Frustrations with the organization can also occur. Conflict that results from committed team members having honest differences of opinion as to how best to serve a patient also happens in the best of teams. Therefore, even in successful teams, there is a dark side that must be addressed.

In the vertical health-care organization, these issues tend to be addressed through the chain of command of one's own discipline. This scenario often sets up a situation in which disciplines blame one another for causing the problem, which results in even further breakdown in communication and the ability to work together. As the unsolved problem continues, frustration and a feeling of loss of control grow, thereby increasing the likelihood of acting out or disruptive behavior.

However, when empowered health-care teams encounter this dark side, it actually presents an opportunity for increased cohesiveness within the team. How? By working in an intact team in which there is trust and consistency, team members are free to embrace these dissonances, rather than withhold feelings or repress differences. How does this happen? The team sets aside time on a weekly basis to work on issues related to team process. During these meetings, no clinical issues or business are discussed. Members are encouraged to express any problems, conflicts, or frustrations related to the team and its function. Each issue is discussed by the team until the problem is resolved, an understanding is reached, and each team member feels complete in his or her communication—with nothing held back. In addressing difficult issues and coming to creative solutions as a team, each team member learns more about the others on the team and cohesion grows. The problem is resolved directly as a team without any disruptive behavior or acting out, because no one feels helpless and everyone is empowered to solve the problem together. Because everyone on the team remains focused on the same vision and goals, this scenario provides a basis for a professional discussion with a win-win outcome.

As you can see, this phase of resolving dissonances is a key step in the evolving trust and communication within the team. The more each team member is able to comfortably reveal uncertainties or disagreements to the rest of the team, with a positive reception and resolution, the more open and authentic the communication becomes. This, in turn, results in decreased medical errors and increased efficiency of care. Employee satisfaction increases, patient satisfaction increases, and staff retention ceases to be a problem.

Key processes for resolving dissonances include:

1) Describing the high purpose of a team member's feedback and its relevance to team goals prior to giving it.
2) Feedback begins with providing observations (facts, issues, situations, and behaviors) and then following with one's relevant reactions.
3) After this initial statement, responses are invited by team members.
4) Stating your understanding of what you are hearing clarifies that you have received the intended message.

Resolving-dissonance exercise

It is natural for team members to experience dissonances with the team or with organizational colleagues. When these problems are effectively processed, they are easily solvable. How is it done? This exercise will guide you naturally and wisely through this process.

Learning Goal: To gain insight on how to handle a dissonant work relationship.

Learning Activity:

1) Begin by working individually. Each team member should take a piece of paper and a pen. Identify and record at the top of the paper someone with whom you currently feel some level of dissonance in some domain of your work relationship:

287

a colleague, a team member, an administrator, or a patient. Spend a few minutes reflecting on the important relevant facts and issues surrounding the dissonant relationship and write them down on the paper below the person's name.

2) Next, turn the piece of paper over. Put the pen down, relax your body and mind, and close your eyes. Think of a person, living or dead, real or fictional, for whom you have always had great respect and admiration. This individual is full of love and grace, always having the insight to understand difficult human situations and the wisdom to know the best way forward so that everyone benefits. You can always look up to this wisdom figure and trust him or her. Open your eyes and write his or her name at the top of the opposite side of the paper, along with a brief statement as to why you chose this wisdom figure.

3) Take a second piece of paper and fold it in half lengthwise, creating two long columns. At the top of the left-hand column, write "Me." At the top of the right-hand column, write the name of your wisdom figure.

4) Enter into a written, imaginary dialogue with your wisdom figure about this dissonant relationship, with each of you taking a turn to speak and reply to one another. Feel free to ask your wisdom figure for help or advice and then, in turn, provide the responses that you intuit your wisdom figure would give. Continue the dialogue until you feel a sense of resolution or completeness regarding your dissonance. (20–30 minutes)

5) When all team members have completed their dialogues, reconvene in a group and share what you learned from the exercise.

Discussion questions

- Why is it so difficult to open up to others on the team when we have dissonant feelings versus positive feelings to share?
- What advice did you get from your wisdom figure about sharing dissonant feelings that differs from how you share positive feelings with your team?
- Reflecting back on chapter 7 about resilient thinking, what thinking trap might be creating the distortion of reality that makes resolving dissonances more fearsome?
- Why is it crucial that the team devote some time, apart from clinical time, to a weekly process meeting, particularly when the team is young?

Team exercise

Because resolving dissonances is so crucial to the life, growth, and success of the team, and yet rather awkward at first, develop an exercise as a team that all team members can participate in and that exercises your resolving-dissonances team muscle. The exercise must be able to be completed in ten minutes or less. Practice it weekly each time that you gather for a process meeting.

Spirit of service

The outcome of a spirited multidisciplinary health-care team that practices the five phases explained above is outstanding service to self, patients, and fellow human beings. The magic happens when the combined strengths and talents of all team members are uniquely devoted to the deep meaning and purpose of healing. Such service is passionate and heartfelt, and it creates thriving, fortification, and flourishing in both the recipients and caregivers.

In the words of Mother Theresa, "There is a joy in transcending self to serve others." May we all serve one another in joy!

Author Note: More information about spirited multidisciplinary teams and workshops specifically devoted to spirited health-care teams can be found at www.creatingpositivehealth. com, under meaning and purpose.

References

Affleck, G., & Tennen, H. (1996). Construing benefits from adversity: Adaptational significance and dispositional underpinnings. *Journal of Personality, 64*(4), 899-922.

Ai, A. L., Cascio, T., Santangelo, L. K., & Evans-Campbell, T. (2005). Hope, meaning, and growth following the September 11, 2001, terrorist attacks. *Journal of Interpersonal Violence, 20*(5), 523-548.

Allport, G. W., & Ross, J. M. (1967). Personal religious orientation and prejudice. *Journal of Personality and Social Psychology, 5*, 432-443.

American Medical Association. (2001). *AMA principles of medical ethics.* Retrieved from http://www.ama-assn.org/ama/pub/physician-resources/medical-ethics/code-medical-ethics/principles-medical-ethics.page

Archer, S. (2005). *The walking deck.* San Francisco: Chronicle Books.

Aristotle. (2000). *Nicomachean ethics.* (R. Crisp, Trans.) Cambridge, UK: Cambridge University Press.

Armstrong, K. (2010). *Twelve steps to a compassionate life.* New York: Knopf.

Atchley, R. (2004). *Social forces and aging: An introduction to social gerontology.* New York: Wadsworth Publishing.

Baer, R. (2003). Mindfulness training as a clinical intervention: A conceptual and empirical review. *Clinical Psychology: Science and Practice, 10*, 125-143.

Baer, R. A. (2006). *Mindfulness-based treatment approaches: Clinician's guide to evidence base and applications.* Boston, MA: Academic Press.

Baile, W. F., Buckman, R., Lenzi, R., Glober, G., Beale, E. A., & Kudelka, A. P. (2000). SPIKES-A six-step protocol for delivering bad news: Application to the patient with cancer. *Oncologist, 5*(4), 302-311.

Baldwin, D. C., Daugherty, S. R., & Eckenfels, E. J. (1991). Student perceptions of mistreatment and harassment during medical school. A survey of ten United States schools. *Western Journal of Medicine, 155*(2), 140-145.

Baldwin, D. C., Daugherty, S. R., Eckenfels, E. J., & Leksas, I. (1988). The experience of mistreatment and abuse among medical students. *Proceeding of Annual Conference on Research in Medical Education*, (pp. 80-84).

Bandura, A. (2001). Social cognitive theory: An agentic perspective. *Annual Review of Psychology, 52*, 1-26.

Barber, B. (1976). Compassion in medicine: Toward new definitions and new institutions. *New England Journal of Medicine, 295*(17), 939-943.

Barnet, K., Mercer, S. W., Norbury, M., Watt, G., Wyke, S., & Guthrie, B. (2012). Epidemiology of multimorbidity and implications for health care, research, and medical education: A cross-sectional study. *Lancet, 380*, 37-43.

Batson, C. D. (2014). *The altruism question: Toward a social-psychological answer.* Hillside, NJ: Psychology Press.

Batson, C. D., Ahmad, N., & Lishner, D. A. (2009). Empathy and altruism. In C. R. Snyder, & S. J. Lopez (Eds.), *Handbook of Positive Psychology* (2nd ed., pp. 417-426). New York: Oxford University Press.

Beach, M. C., Roter, D., Korthuis, P. T., Epstein, R. M., Sharp, V., Ratanawongsa, N., . . . Saha, S. (2013). A multicenter study of physician mindfulness and health care quality. *Annals of Family Medicine, 11*(5), 421-428.

Benight, C. C., & Bandura, A. (2004). Social cognitive theory of posttraumatic recovery: the role of perceived self-efficacy. *Behaviour Research and Therapy, 42*(10), 1129-1148.

Bishop, S. R., Lau, M., Shapiro, S. L., Carlson, L., Anderson, N. D., Carmody, J., . . . Devins, G. (2004). Mindfulness: A proposed operational definition. *Clinical Psychology: Science and Practice, 11*, 230-241.

Biswas-Diener, R. (2006). From the equator to the North Pole: A study of character strengths. *Journal of Happiness Studies, 7*, 293-310.

Biswas-Diener, R., Kashdan, T. B., & Minhas, G. A. (2011). A dynamic approach to psychological strength development and intervention. *Journal of Positive Psychology, 6*(2), 106-118.

Black, D. S. (2010). Mindfulness research guide: A new paradigm for managing empirical health. *Mindfulness, 1*(3), 174--176.

Blair, S. N. (2009). Warm up: Physical inactivity: The biggest public health problem of the 21st century. *British Journal of Sports Medicine, 43*, 1-2.

Bonanno, G. A. (2004). Loss, trauma, and human resilience: Have we underestimated the human capacity to thrive after extremely aversive events? *American Psychologist, 59*(1), 20-28.

Bonanno, G. A. (2005). Resilience in the face of potential trauma. *Current Directions of Psychological Science, 14*(3), 135-138.

Bond, A. R., Mason, H. F., Lemaster, C. M., Shaw, S. E., Mulllin, C. S., Holick, E. A., & Saper, R. B. (2013). Embodied health: The effects of a mind-body course for medical students. *Medical Education Online, 18*, 1-8.

Borghans, L., Duckworth, A. L., Heckman, J. J., & ter Weel, B. (2008). The economics and psychology of personality traits. *Journal of Human Resources, 43*(4), 972-1059.

Bravata, D. M., Smith-Spangler, C., Sundaram, V., Gienger, A. L., Lin, N., Lewis, R., . . . Sirard, J. R. (2007). Using pedometers to increase physical activity and improve health: A systematic review. *JAMA, 298*(18), 2296-2304.

Breslau, N., Chilcoat, H. D., Kessler, R. C., & Davis, G. C. (1999). Previous exposure to trauma and PTSD effects of subsequent trauma: Results from the Detroit Area Survey of Trauma. *American Journal of Psychiatry, 156*(6), 902-907.

Brown, K. W., & Ryan, R. M. (2004). Fostering healthy self-regulation from within and without: A self-determination theory perspective. In A. P. Linley, & S. Joseph (Eds.), *Positive psychology in practice* (pp. 105-124). Hoboken, NJ: John Wiley & Sons.

Brown, K. W., Ryan, R. M., & Creswell, J. D. (2007). Mindfulness: Theoretical foundations and evidence for its salutary effects. *Psychological Inquiry, 18*, 211-237.

Brunwasser, S. M., Gillham, J. E., & Kim, E. S. (2009). A meta-analytic review of the Penn Resiliency Program's effect on depressive symptoms. *Journal of Consulting and Clinical Psycholog, 77*(6), 1042-1054.

Bryant, F. (2003). Savoring Beliefs Inventory (SBI): A scale for measuring beliefs about savouring. *Journal of Mental Health, 12*(2), 175-196.

Bryant, F., & Veroff, J. (2007). *Savoring: A new model of positive experience.* Mahwah, NJ: Lawrence Erlbaum.

Butler, L. D., Blasey, C. M., Garlan, R. W., McCaslin, S. E., Azarov, J., Chen, X.-H., . . . Spiegler, D. (2005). Posttraumatic growth following the terrorist attacks of September 11, 2001: Cognitive, coping, and trauma symptom predictors in an Internet convenience sample. *Traumatology, 11*(4), 247-267.

Calado, R. T., & Young, N. S. (2009). Telomere diseases. *New England Journal of Medicine, 361*(24), 2353-2365.

Cann, A., Calhoun, L. G., Tedeschi, R. G., Taku, K., Vishnevsky, T., Triplett, K. N., & Danhauer, S. C. (2010). A short form of the Posttraumatic Growth Inventory. *Anxiety, Stress, and Coping, 23*(2), 127-137.

Carlson, E. N. (2013). Overcoming the barriers to self-knowledge: Mindfulness as a path to seeing yourself as you really are. *Perspectives on Psychological Science, 8*, 173-186.

Carver, C. S., Pozo, C., Harris, S. D., Scheier, M. F., Robinson, D. S., Ketcham, A. S., . . . Clark, K. C. (1993). How coping mediates the effect of optimism on distress: A study of women with early stage breast cancer. *Journal of Personality and Social Psychology, 65*(2), 375-390.

Cassell, E. J. (2009). Compassion. In C. R. Snyder, & S. J. Lopez (Eds.), *Oxford handbook of positive psychology* (2nd ed., pp. 393-404). New York: Oxford University Press.

Chiesa, A., & Serretti, A. (2014). Are mindfulness-based interventions effective for substance use disorders? A systematic review of the evidence. *Substance Use and Misuse, 49*(5), 492-512.

Christakis, N. A. (2003). On the sociological anxiety of physicians. In C. M. Messikomer, J. P. Swazey, & A. Glicksman (Eds.), *Society and medicine: Essays in honor of Renee C. Fox* (pp. 135-143). New Brunswick, NJ: Transaction Publishers.

Clark, N. (1996). The power of protein. *The Physician and Sportsmedicine, 24*(4), 22-27.

Cohen, S. (2004). Social relationships and health. *American Psychologist, 59*(8), 676-684.

Cohen, S., & Hoberman, H. (1983). Positive events and social supports as buffers of life change stress. *Journal of Applied Social Psychology, 13*(2), 99-125.

Cohen, S., & Janicki-Deverts, D. (2009). Can we improve our physical health by altering our social networks? *Perspectives on Psychological Science*, 375-378.

Cohen, S., Alper, C. M., Doyle, W. J., Treanor, J. J., & Turner, R. B. (2006). Positive emotional style predicts resistance to illness after experimental exposure to Rhinovirus or Influenza A virus. *Psychosomatic Medicine, 68*, 809-815.

Cooper, K. H. (1968). *Aerobics*. Lanham, MD: Evans and Company.

Csikszentmihalyi, M. (1990). *Flow: The psychology of optimal experience*. New York: Harper & Row.

Csikszentmihalyi, M. (1997). *Finding flow: The psychology of engagement with everyday life*. New York: Basic Books.

Csikszentmihalyi, M., & LeFevre, J. (1989). Optimal experience in work and leisure. *Journal of Personality and Social Psychology, 56*(5), 815-822.

Damon, W., Menon, J. L., & Bronk, K. C. (2003). The development of purpose during adolescence. *Applied Developmental Science, 7*(3), 119-128.

Davis, T. C., Dolan, N. C., Ferreira, M. R., Tomori, C., Green, K. W., Sipler, A. M., & Bennett, C. L. (2001). The role of inadequate health literacy skills in colorectal cancer screening. *Cancer Investigation, 19*(2), 193-200.

De Vibe, M., Solhaug, I., Tyssen, R., Friborg, O., Rosenvinge, J. H., Sørlie, T., & Bjørndal, A. (2013). Mindfulness training for stress management: A randomised controlled study of medical and psychology students. *BMC Medical Education, 13*, 107.

Deci, E. L., & Ryan, R. M. (2000). The "what" and "why" of goal pursuits: Human needs and the self-determination of behavior. *Psychological Inquiry, 11*, 227-268.

Dimatteo, M. R., Sherbourne, C. D., Hays, R. D., Ordway, L., Kravitz, R. L., McGlynn, E. A., . . . Rogers, W. H. (1993). Physicians' characteristics influence patients' adherence to medical treatment: results from the Medical Outcomes Study. *Health Psychology, 12*(2), 93-102.

Dobkin, P. L., & Hutchinson, T. A. (2013). Teaching mindfulness in medical school: Where are we now and where are we going? *Medical Education, 47*(8), 768-779.

Drexler, A., Sibbet, D., & Forrester, R. (1988). Team performance model. In J. B. Reddy, & K. Jamison (Eds.), *Team building: Blueprints for productivity and satisfaction.* Alexandria, VA: NTL Institute for the Applied Behavioral Sciences.

Duckworth, A. L., Peterson, C., Matthew, M. D., & Kelly, D. R. (2007). Grit: Perseverance and passion for long-term goals. *Journal of Personality and Social Psychology, 92*(6), 1087-1101.

Dunn, P. M., Arnetz, B. B., Christensen, J. F., & Homer, L. (2007). Meeting the imperative to improve physician well-being: Assessment of an innovative program. *Journal of General Internal Medicine, 22*(11), 1544-1552.

Dutton, J. E. (2003). *Energize your workplace: How to create and sustain high-quality connections at work.* San Francisco, CA: Jossey-Bass.

Dyrbye, L. N., & Shanafelt, T. D. (2011). Commentary: Medical student distress: A call to action. *Academic Medicine, 86*(7), 801-803.

Dyrbye, L. N., Shanafelt, T. D., Thomas, M. R., & Durning, S. J. (2009). Brief observation: A national study of burnout among internal medicine clerkship directors. *American Journal of Medicine, 122*(3), 310-312.

Dyrbye, L. N., Thomas, M. R., & Shanafelt, T. D. (2006). Systematic review of depression, anxiety, and other indicators of psychological distress among U.S. and Canadian medical students. *Academic Medicine, 81*(4), 354-373.

Eisenberg, N., & Miller, P. A. (1987). The relation of empathy to prosocial and related behaviors. *Psychological Bulletin, 101*(1), 91-119.

Elkind, D. (2007). *The power of play.* Philadelphia, PA: Da Capo Books.

Emmons, R. A., & McCullough, M. E. (2003). Counting blessings versus burdens: An experimental investigation of gratitude and subjective well-being in daily life. *Journal of Personality and Social Psychology, 84*(2), 377-389.

Emmons, R. A., & Mishra, A. (2011). Why gratitude enhances wellbeing: What we know, what we need to know. In K. M. Sheldon, T. B. Kashdan, & M. F. Steger (Eds.), *Designing positive psychology: Taking stock and moving forward* (pp. 248-262). New York: Oxford University Press.

Escott-Stump, S. (2008). *Nutrition and diagnosis-related care.* Baltimore, MD: Lippincott Williams & Wilkins.

Evans, W. (1993). Exercise and protein metabolism. In A. P. Simopoulos, & K. N. Pavlou (Eds.), *Nutrition and fitness for athletes.* Washington, DC: Basel, Karger Ag.

Feder, A., Nestler, E. J., & Charney, D. S. (2009). Psychobiology and molecular genetics of resilience. *Nature Reviews. Neuroscience, 6*, 446-457.

Fenton, M. (2008). *The complete guide to walking.* Guilford, CT: Globe Pequot.

Feudtner, C. (2005). Hope and the prospects of healing at the end of life. *Journal of Alternative and Complementary Medicine, 11*(Suppl 1), S23-S30.

Feudtner, C., Christakis, D. A., & Christakis, N. A. (1994). Do clinical clerks suffer ethical erosion? Students' perceptions of their ethical environment and personal development. *Academic Medicine, 69*(8), 670-679.

Foa, E. B., Keane, T. M., Friedman, M. J., & Cohen, J. A. (2008). *Effective Treatments for PTSD: Practice guidelines from the International Society for Traumatic Stress Studies* (2nd ed.). New York: Guilford Press.

Fortney, L., Luchterhand, C., Zakletskaia, L., Zgierska, A., & Rakel, D. (2013). Abbreviated mindfulness intervention for job satisfaction, quality of life, and compassion in primary care clinicians: A pilot study. *Annals of Family Medicine, 11*(5), 412-420.

Fox, M. (1994). *The reinvention of work: A new vision of livelihood for our time.* San Francisco, CA: Harper.

Frank, E., Carrera, J. S., Elon, L., & Hertzberg, V. S. (2007). Predictors of US medical students' prevention counseling practices. *Preventive Medicine, 44*(1), 76-81.

Frank, E., Carrera, J. S., Stratton, T., Bickel, J., & Nora, L. M. (2006). Experiences of belittlement and harassment and their correlates among medical students in the United States: longitudinal survey. *British Medical Journal, 333*(7570), 682.

Frank, E., Segura, C., Shen, H., & Oberg, E. (2010). Predictors of Canadian physicians' prevention counseling practices. *Canadian Journal of Public Health, 101*(5), 390-395.

Frankl, V. E. (1946; 1985). *Man's search for meaning: An introduction to Logotherapy.* Boston: Beacon Press.

Fredrickson, B. L. (2001). The role of positive emotions in positive psychology: The broaden-and-build theory of positive emotions. *American Psychologist, 56*(3), 218-226.

Fredrickson, B. L. (2003). The value of positive emotions. *American Scientist, 91*, 330-335.

Fredrickson, B. L. (2004). The broaden-and-build theory of positive emotions. *Philosophical Transactions of The Royal Society Biological Sciences, 359*(1449), 1367-1378.

Fredrickson, B. L. (2009). *Positivity.* New York: Crown.

Fredrickson, B. L. (2013). *Love 2.0: How our supreme emotion affects everything we feel, think, do, and become.* London: Hudson St. Press.

Fredrickson, B. L. (2013). Updated thinking on positivity ratios. *American Psychologist, 68*(9), 814-822.

Fredrickson, B. L., & Branigan, C. (2005). Positive emotions broaden the scope of attention and thought-action repertoires. *Cognition and Emotion, 19*(3), 313-332.

Fredrickson, B. L., & Cohn, M. A. (2008). Positive emotions. In M. Lewis, J. M. Haviland-Jones, & L. F. Barrett (Eds.), *Handbook of emotions* (3rd ed., pp. 777-796). New York: Guilford Press.

Fredrickson, B. L., & Joiner, T. (2002). Positive emotions trigger upward spirals toward emotional well-being. *Psychological Science, 13*(2), 172-175.

Fredrickson, B. L., Cohn, M. A., Coffey, K. A., Pek, J., & Finkel, S. M. (2008). Open hearts build lives: Positive emotions, induced through loving-kindness meditation, build consequential personal resources. *Journal of Personality and Social Psychology, 95*(5), 1045-1062.

Fredrickson, B. L., Mancuso, R. A., Branigan, C., & Tugade, M. M. (2000). The undoing effect of positive emotions. *Motivation and Emotion, 24*(4), 237-258.

Fried, R. (1990). Integrating music in breathing, training and relaxation: 1. Background, Rationale and relevant elements. *Journal of Applied Psychology, 15*(2), 161-169.

Gable, S. L., & Gosnell, C. L. (2011). The positive side of close relationships. In K. M. Sheldon, T. B. Kashdan, & M. F. Steger (Eds.), *Designing positive psychology, Taking stock and moving forward* (pp. 265-279). New York: Oxford University Press.

Gable, S. L., Gonzaga, G. C., & Strachman, A. (2006). Will you be there for me when things go right? Supportive responses to positive event disclosures. *Journal of Personality and Social Psychology, 91*(5), 904-917.

Gable, S. L., Reis, H. T., Impett, E. A., & Asher, E. R. (2004). What do you do when things go right? The intrapersonal and interpersonal benefits of sharing positive events. *Journal of Personality and Social Psychology, 87*(2), 228-245.

Gander, F., Proyer, R. T., Ruch, W., & Wyss, T. (2012). Strength-based positive interventions: Further evidence for their potential in enhancing well-being. *Journal of Happiness Studies.*

Gavin, J. (2004). Pairing personality with activity: New tools for inspiring active lifestyles. *The Physician and Sportsmedicine, 32*(12), 17-34.

Gavin,, J., Seguin, S., & McBrearty, M. (2006). The psychology of exercise. *IDEA Fitness Journal.* Retrieved from http://www.ideafit.com/fitness-library/psychology-exercise-1

Gaylord, S. A., Palsson, O. S., Garland, E. L., Faurot, K. R., Coble, R. S., Mann, J. D., . . . Whitehead, W. E. (2011). Mindfulness training reduces the severity of irritable bowel syndrome in women: Results of a randomized controlled trial. *American Journal of Gastroenterology, 106*(9), 1678-1688.

Gilbert, B., & Jamison, S. (1993). *Winning ugly: Mental warfare in tennis-- lessons from a master.* New York: Citadel Press.

Gillham, J., Brunwasser, S. M., & Freres, D. (2008). Preventing depression in early adolescence: The Penn Resiliency Program. In J. R. Abela, & B. L. Hankin (Eds.), *Handbook of depression in children and adolescents* (pp. 309-332). New York: Guilford Press.

Gillick, M. R. (2013). The critical role of caregivers in achieving patient-centered care. *JAMA, 310*(6), 574-576.

Goleman, D. (2011). *The brain and emotional intelligence.* Northhampton, MA: More Than Sound.

Gottman, J. M., & Silver, N. (1999). *The seven principles for making marriage work.* New York: Three Rivers Press.

Greenleaf, R. K. (1977). *Servant leadership: A journey into the nature of legitimate power and greatness.* New York: Paulist Press.

Gregg, J. A., Callaghan, G. M., Hayes, S. C., & Glenn-Lawson, J. L. (2007). Improving diabetes self-management through acceptance, mindfulness, and values: A randomized controlled trial. *Journal of Consulting and Clinical Psychology, 75*(2), 336-343.

Greider, K. (2011). The real fountain of youth: Exercise. *AARP Health Newsletter,* 1.

Grob, G. M. (1991). Origins of DSM-I: A study in appearance and reality. *American Journal of Psychiatry, 148*(4), 421-431.

Grol, R., & Grimshaw, J. (2003). From best evidence to best practice: Effective implementation of change in patients' care. *Lancet, 362*(9391), 1225-1230.

Grossman, P., Niemann, L., Schmidt, S., & Walach, H. (2004). Mindfulness-based stress reduction and health benefits: A meta-analysis. *Journal of Psychosomatic Research, 57*(1), 35-43.

Grossman, P., Tiefenthaler-Gilmer, U., Raysz, A., & Kesper, U. (2007). Mindfulness training as an intervention for fibromyalgia: Evidence of postintervention and 3-year follow-up benefits in well-being. *Psychotherapy and Psychosomatics, 76*(4), 226-233.

Halbesleben, R., & Rathert, C. (2008). Linking physician burnout and patient outcomes: Exploring the dyadic relationship between physicians and patients. *Health Care Management Review, 33*(1), 29-39.

Harvey, J. H., & Pauwels, B. G. (2009). Relationship connections: A redux on the role of minding and the quality of feeling special in the enhancement of closeness. In C. R. Snyder, & S. J. Lopez (Eds.), *Handbook of positive psychology* (2nd ed., pp. 385-390). New York: Oxford University Press.

Hassed, C., De Lisle, S., Sullivan, G., & Pier, C. (2009). Enhancing the health of medical students: Outcomes of an integrated mindfulness and lifestyle program. *Advances in Health Sciences Education: Theory and Practice, 14*(3), 387-98.

Haubenstricker, J., & Seefeldt, V. (1986). In V. Seeveldt (Ed.), *Physical activity and well-being.* Reston, VA: AAHPERD.

Haviland, M. G., Yamagata, H., Werner, L. S., Zhang, K., Dial, T. H., & Sonne, J. L. (2012). Student mistreatment in medical school and planning a career in academic medicine. *Teaching and Learning in Medicine, 24*(1), 100.

Heermann, B. (1997). *Building team spirit: Activities for inspiring and energizing teams.* New York: McGraw-Hill Company.

Heermann, B. (2004). *Noble purpose: Igniting extraordinary passion for life and work.* Fairfax, VA: QSU Publishing.

Hefferon, K., Grealy, M., & Mutrie, N. (2009). Post-traumatic growth and life threatening physical illness: A systematic review of the qualitative literature. *British Journal of Health Psychology, 14*(Pt 2), 343-378.

Helgeson, V. S., Reynolds, K. A., & Tomich, P. L. (2006). A meta-analytic review of benefit finding and growth. *Journal of Consulting and Clinical Psychology, 74*(5), 797-816.

Henning, M. A., Hawken, S. J., & Hill, A. G. (2009). The quality of life of New Zealand doctors and medical students: What can be done to avoid burnout? *New Zealand Medical Journal, 122*(1307), 102-110.

Heymann, D. L. (2008). *Control of communicable diseases manual.* American Public Health Association.

Hojat, M., Gonnella, J. S., Nasca, T. J., Mangione, S., Vergare, M., & Magee, M. (2002). Physician empathy: Definition, components, measurement, and relationship to gender and specialty. *American Journal of Psychiatry, 159*(9), 1563-1569.

Holmes, T. H., & Rahe, R. H. (1967). The Social Readjustment Rating Scale. *Journal of Psychosomatic Medicine, 11*(2), 213-218.

Hope, J. (2001). *The meditation year.* New York: Storey Books.

Hu, Y. Y., Fix, M. L., Hevelone, N. D., Lipsitz, S. R., Greenberg, C. C., Weissman, J. S., & Shapiro, J. (2012). Physicians' needs in coping with emotional stressors: The case for peer support. *Archives of Surgery, 147*(3), 212-217.

Huenther, G. (2010). Das Glück und die Neurowissenschaften. *Berliner Symposium der Positiven Psychologie.* Berlin, Germany.

Jonas, S., & Phillips, E. M. (2009). *ACSM's Exercise is Medicine(TM): A clinician's guide to exercise prescription.* Philadelphia, PA: Lippincott, Williams, & Wilkins.

Joy, E., Blair, S. N., McBride, P., & Sallis, R. (2013). Physical activity counseling in sports medicine: A call to action. *British Journal of Sports Medicine, 47*(1), 49-53.

Kabat-Zinn, J. (1990). *Full catastrophe living: Using the wisdom of your body and mind to face stress, pain, and illness.* New York: Dell.

Kabat-Zinn, J., Lipworth, L., Burney, R., & Sellers, W. (1986). Four year follow-up of a meditation-based program for the self-regulation of chronic pain: Treatment outcomes and compliance. *Clinical Journal of Pain, 2*(3), 159-173.

Kabat-Zinn, J., Wheeler, E., Light, T., Skillings, A., Scharf, M. J., Cropley, T. G., . . . Bernhard, J. D. (1998). Influence of a mindfulness meditation-based stress reduction intervention on rates of skin clearing in patients with moderate to severe psoriasis undergoing phototherapy (UVB) and photochemotherapy (PUVA). *Psychosomatic Medicine, 60*(5), 625-632.

Kashdan, T. B. (2009). *Curious? Discover the missing ingredient to a fulfilling life.* New York: William Morrow.

Kashdan, T. B., & Rottenberg, J. (2010). Psychological flexibility as a fundamental aspect of health. *Clinical Psychology Review, 30*(7), 865-878.

Keltner, D., & Haidt, J. (2003). Approaching awe, a moral, spiritual, and aesthetic emotion. *Cognition and Emotion, 17*(2), 297-314.

Killingsworth, M. A., & Gilbert, D. T. (2010). A wandering mind is an unhappy mind. *Science, 330*(6006), 932.

Kim, E. S., Park, N., & Peterson, C. (2011). Dispositional optimism protects older adults from stroke: The Health and Retirement Study. *Stroke, 42*(10), 2855-2859.

King, J. (2003). Nutritional genomics: Interview by Deborah Shattuck. *Journal of the American Dietetic Association, 103*(1), 16, 18.

Krasner, M. S., Epstein, R. M., Beckman, H., Suchman, A. L., Chapman, B., Mooney, C. J., & Quill, T. E. (2009). Association of an educational program in mindful communication with burnout, empathy, and attitudes among primary care physicians. *JAMA, 302*(12), 1284-1293.

Krasner, M. S., Epstein, R. M., Beckman, H., Suchman, A. L., Chapman, B., Mooney, C. J., & Quill, T. E. (2009). ssociation of an educational program in mindful communication with burnout, empathy, and attitudes among primary care physicians. *JAMA, 302*(12), 1284-93.

Kubzansky, L. D., & Thurston, R. C. (2007). Emotional vitality and incident coronary heart disease: Benefits of healthy psychological functioning. *Archives of General Psychiatry, 64*(2), 1393-1401.

Kushner, R. F., Kessler, S., & McGaghie, W. C. (2011). Using behavior change plans to improve medical student self-care. *Academic Medicine, 86*(7), 901-906.

Langer, E. (2009). *Counterclockwise: Mindful health and the power of possibility.* New York: Ballantine Books.

Larner, B., & Blow, A. (2011). A model of meaning-making coping and growth in combat veterans. *Review of General Psychology, 15*(3), 187-197.

Leidy, H. J., Hoertel, H. A., Douglas, S. M., & Shafer, R. S. (2013). Daily addition of a protein-rich breakfast for long-term improvements in energy intake regulation and body weight management in overweight & obese 'breakfast skipping' young people. *The FASEB Journal, 27,* 249.7.

Lemaire, J. B., & Wallace, J. E. (2010). Not all coping strategies are created equal: A mixed methods study exploring physicians' self reported coping strategies. *BMC Health Services Research, 10,* 208.

Lemon, P. W. (1995). Do athletes need more dietary protein and amino acids? *International Journal of Sports Nutrition, 5 Suppl,* S39-S61.

Leontopoulou, S., & Triliva, S. (2012). Explorations of subjective wellbeing and character strengths among a Greek university student sample. *International Journal of Wellbeing, 2*(3), 251-270.

Lerman, R., Jarski, R., Rea, H., Gellish, R., & Vicini, F. (2012). Improving symptoms and quality of life of female cancer survivors: A randomized controlled study. *Annals of Surgical Oncology, 19*(2), 373-378.

Lesser, C. S., Lucey, C. R., Egener, B., Braddock, C. H., Linas, S. L., & Levinson, W. (2010). behavioral and systems view of professionalism. *JAMA, 304*(24), 2732-2737.

Levine, S. Z., Laufer, A., Stein, E., Hamama-Raz, Y., & Solomon, Z. (2009). Examining the relationship between resilience and posttraumatic growth. *Journal of Traumatic Stress, 22*(4), 282-286.

Lindstrøm, B. (2001). The meaning of resilience. *International Journal of Adolescent Medicine and Health, 13*(1), 7-12.

Lineham, M. M. (1993). *Cognitive-behavioral treatment of borderline personality disorder.* New York: Guilford Press.

Linley, P. A. (2008). *Average to A+, Realising strengths in yourself and others.* Coventry, UK: CAPP Press.

Linn, L. S., Brook, R. H., Clark, V. A., Davies, A. R., Fink, A., & Kosecoff, J. (1985). Physician and patient satisfaction as factors related to the organization of internal medicine group practices. *Medical Care, 10,* 1171-1178.

Losada, M., & Heaphy, E. (2004). The role of positivity and connectivity in the performance of business teams: A non-linear dynamics model. *American Behavioral Science, 47,* 740-765.

LoSavio, S. T., Cohen, L. H., Laurenceau, J. P., Dasch, K. B., Parrish, B. P., & Park, C. L. (2011). Reports of stress-related growth from daily negative events. *Journal of Social and Clinical Psychology, 30*(7), 760-785.

Ludwig, D. S., & Kabat-Zinn, J. (2008). Mindfulness in medicine. *JAMA, 300*(11), 1350-1352.

Lyubomirsky, S., King, L., & Diener, E. (2005). The benefits of frequent positive affect: Does happiness lead to success? *Psychological Bulletin, 131*(6), 803-855.

Lyubomirsky, S., Sheldon, K. M., & Schkade, D. (2005). Pursuing happiness: The architecture of sustainable change. *Review of General Psychology, 9,* 111-131.

Ma, M., Kibler, J. L., Dollar, K. M., Sly, K., Samuels, D., Benford, M. W., . . . Wiley, F. (2008). The relationship of character strengths to sexual behaviors and related risks among African American adolescents. *International Journal of Behavioral Medicine, 15*(4), 319-327.

Mahan, L. K., & Escott-Stump, S. (2000). *Krause's food, nutrition, & diet therapy.* Philadelphia, PA: W. B. Saunders Company.

Mancini, A. D., & Bonanno, G. A. (2006). Resilience in the face of potential trauma: Clinical practices and illustrations. *Journal of Clinical Psychology, 62*(8), 971-985.

Marroqui, L., Batista, T. M., Gonzalez, A., Vieira, E., Colleta, S. J., Taboga, S. R., . . . Quesada, I. (2012). Functional and structural adaptations in the pancreatic α-cell and changes in glucagon signaling during protein malnutrition. *Endocrinology, 153*(4), 1663-1672.

Martin Asuero, A., Rodriguez Blanco, T., Pujol-Ribera, E., Berenquera, A., & Moix Queraltó, J. (2013). [Effectiveness of a mindfulness program in primary care professionals]. *Gaceta Sanitaria, 27*(6), 521-528.

Martin, A. B., Lassman, D., Washington, B., & Catlin, A. (2012). Growth in US health spending remained slow in 2010; Health share of gross domestic product was unchanged from 2009. *Health Affairs, 31*(1), 208-219.

Marvel, M. K., Epstein, R. M., Flowers, K., & Beckman, H. B. (1999). Soliciting the patient's agenda: Have we improved? *JAMA, 281*(3), 283-287.

Maslach, C. (1982). *Burnout: The cost of caring.* Englewood Cliffs, NJ: Prentice-Hall.

Masten, A. S. (2001). Ordinary magic: Resilience processes in development. *American Psychologist, 56*(3), 227-238.

Masten, A. S., Cutuli, J. J., Herbers, J. E., & Reed, M. J. (2009). Resilience in development. In C. R. Snyder, & S. J. Lopez (Eds.), *Handbook of positive psychology* (2nd ed.). New York: Oxford University Press.

Mattke, A., Schmitz, J. J., & Zink, T. (2009). Call it what it is: Sexual harassment. *Academic Medicine, 84*(2), 191.

Mayer, J. D., Salovey, P., & Caruso, D. R. (2002). *Mayer-Salovey-Caruso emotional intelligence test (MSCEIT) item booklet.* Toronto, ON: MHS Publishers.

McArdle, W. D., Katch, F. I., & Katch, V. L. (1999). *Sports & exercise nutrition.* New York: Lippincott Williams & Wilkins.

McCracken, L. M., Gauntlett-Gilbert, J., & Vowles, K. E. (2007). The role of mindfulness in a contextual cognitive-behavioral analysis of chronic pain-related suffering and disability. *Pain, 131*(1-2), 63-69.

McCray, L. W., Cronholm, P. F., Bogner, H. R., Gallo, J. J., & Neill, R. A. (2008). Resident physician burnout: Is there hope? *Family Medicine, 40*(9), 626-632.

McFarlane, A. C., & Yehuda, R. (1996, 2007). Resilience, vulnerability and the course of posttraumatic reactions. In B. A. Kolk, A. C. McFarlane, & L. Weisaeth (Eds.), *Traumatic Stress: The effects of overwhelming experience on mind, body, and society* (pp. 155-181). New York: Guilford Press.

McGill, J. S. (1980). *The joy of effort: A biography of R. Tait McKenzie.* Columbia: Clay Publishing Company.

McGonigal, K. (2007). Facilitating fellowship. *IDEA Fitness Journal, 4*(6), 72-79.

McGrath, R. E. (2014). Character strengths in 75 nations: An update. *Journal of Positive Psychology.*

McKenzie, R. T. (1909). *Exercise in education and medicine.* Philadelphia, PA: W. B. Saunders Company.

Mitchell, J., Stanimirovic, R., Klein, B., & Vella-Brodrick, D. (2009). A randomised controlled trial of a self-guided Internet intervention promoting well-being. *Computers in Human Behavior, 25*(3), 749-760.

Mongrain, M., & Anselmo-Matthews, T. (2012). Do positive psychology exercises work? A replication of Seligman et al. (2005). *Journal of Clinical Psychology, 68*(4), 382-389.

Morris, J. N., Heady, J. A., Raffle, P. A., Roberts, B. A., & Parks, J. (1953). Coronary heart disease and physical activity of work. *The Lancet, 262*(6796), 1111-1120.

Moskowitz, J. T., Folkman, S., & Acree, M. (2003). Do positive psychological states shed light on recovery from bereavement? Findings from a 3-year longitudinal study. *Death Studies, 27*(6), 471-500.

Nielsen-Bohlman, L., Panzer, A. M., & Kindig, D. A. (2004). *Health literacy: A prescription to end confusion.* Washington, DC: National Academies Press.

Niemiec, R. M. (2012a). Mindful living: Character strengths interventions as pathways for the five mindfulness trainings. *International Journal of Wellbeing, 2*(1), 22-33.

Niemiec, R. M. (2012b). VIA character strengths–research and practice: The first 10 years. In H. H. Knoop, & A. Delle Fave (Eds.), *Well-being and cultures: Perspectives from positive psychology* (Vol. 3, pp. 11-31). New York: Springer.

Niemiec, R. M. (2014). *Mindfulness and character strengths: A practical guide to flourishing.* Boston, MA: Hogrefe.

Niemiec, R. M., Rashid, T., & Spinella, M. (2012). Strong mindfulness: Integrating mindfulness and character strengths. *Journal of Mental Health, 34*(3), 240-253.

Norlander, T., Schedvin, H., & Archer, T. (2005). Thriving as a function of affective personality: Relation to personality factors, coping strategies and stress. *Anxiety, Stress, and Coping, 18*(2), 105-116.

Nyklicek, I., Vingerhoets, A., & Zeelenberg, M. (2010). *Emotional regulation and well-being.* New York: Springer.

Paffenbarger, R. S., Gima, A. S., Laughlin, E., & Black, R. A. (1971). Characteristics of longshoremen related fatal coronary heart disease and stroke. *American Journal of Public Health, 61*(7), 1362-1370.

Palmer, M. A., Capra, S., & Baines, S. (2006). Smaller, more frequent meals are associated with greater reduction in total cholesterol and triglycerides in obese adults after three months on isocaloric weight loss regimens. *Journal of the American Dietitic Association*, 106-108.

Pargament, K. I. (2002). The bitter and the sweet: An evaluation of the costs and benefits of religiousness. *Psychological Inquiry, 13*(3), 168-181.

Pargament, K. I., & Mahoney, A. (2009). Spirituality: The search for the sacred. In C. R. Snyder, & S. J. Lopez (Eds.), *Oxford handbook of positive psychology* (pp. 611-620). New York: Oxford University Press.

Park, C. L., & Ai, A. L. (2006). Meaning making and growth: New directions for research on survivors of trauma. *Journal of Personality, 11*(5), 389-407.

Park, C. L., Cohen, L. H., & Murch, R. L. (1996). Assessment and prediction of stress-related growth. *Journal of Personality, 64*(1), 71-105.

Park, N., Peterson, C., & Seligman, M. E. (2004). Strengths of character and well-being. *Journal of Social and Clinical Psychology, 23*(5), 603-619.

Pennington, J. A. (Ed.). (1998). *Bowes & Church's food values of portions commonly used.* Philadelphia, PA: Lippincott Williams & Wilkins.

Peterson, C. (2000). The future of optimism. *American Psychologist, 55*(1), 44-55.

Peterson, C. (2006). *A primer in positive psychology.* New York: Oxford University Press.

Peterson, C. (2013). *Pursuing the good life: 100 reflections in positive psychology.* New York: Oxford University Press.

Peterson, C., & Seligman, M. E. (2002). *Character strengths before and after September 11.* Retrieved from http://www.psychologicalscience.org/pdf/14_4Peterson.cfm

Peterson, C., & Seligman, M. E. (2004). *Character strengths and virtues: A handbook and classification.* New York: Oxford University Press.

Peterson, C., Park, N., & Seligman, M. E. (2006). Greater strengths of character and recovery from illness. *Journal of Positive Psychology, 1*(1), 17-26.

Peterson, C., Park,, N., & Kim, E. S. (2012). Can optimism decrease the risk of illness and disease among the elderly? *Aging Health, 8*(1), 5-8.

Peterson, C., Seligman, M. E., Yurko, K. H., Martin, L., & Friedman, H. S. (1998). Catastrophizing and untimely death. *Psychological Science, 9*(2), 127-130.

Peterson, T. D., & Peterson, E. W. (2009). Stemming the tide of law student depression: What law schools need to learn from the science of positive psychology. *Yale Journal of Health Policy & Ethics, 9*(2), 357-434.

Pezzolesi, C., Ghaleb, M., Kostrzewski, A., & Dhillon, S. (2013). Is Mindful Reflective Practice the way forward to reduce medication errors? *International Journal of Pharmacy Practice, 21*(6), 413-416.

Pololi, L. H., Krupat, E., Civian, J., Ash, A. S., & Brennan, R. T. (2012). Why are a quarter of faculty considering leaving academic medicine? A study of their perceptions of institutional culture and intentions to leave at 26 representative U.S. medical schools. *Academic Medicine, 87*(7), 859-869.

Powell, D. R. (1999). Characteristics of successful wellness programs. *Employee Benefits Journal, 24*(3), 15-21.

Pradhan, E. K., Baumgarten, M., Langenberg, P., Handwerger, B., Gilpin, A. K., Magyari, T., . . . Berman, B. M. (2007). Effect of Mindfulness-Based Stress Reduction in rheumatoid arthritis patients. *Arthritis and Rheumatism, 57*(7), 1134-1142.

Prati, G., & Pietrantoni, L. (2009). Optimism, social support, and coping strategies as factors contributing to posttraumatic growth: A meta-analysis. *Journal of Loss and Trauma, 14*(5), 364-388.

President's Council on Fitness, Sports and Nutrition. (2011). Healthy people 2020: Physical activity objectives for the future. *Physical Activity and Fitness Digest, 12*(2). Retrieved from http://www.fitness.gov/pdfs/research-digest-june-2011.pdf

Prochaska, J. O., Norcross, J. C., & DiClemente, C. C. (1994). *Changing for good.* New York: HarperCollins.

Proctor, C., Maltby, J., & Linley, P. A. (2009). Strengths use as a predictor of well-being and health-related quality of life. *Journal of Happiness Studies, 10*, 583-630.

Proyer, R. T., Gander, F., Wellenzohn, S., & Ruch, W. (2013). What good are character strengths beyond the subjective well-being? The contribution of the good character on self-reported health-oriented behavior, physical fitness, and the subjective health status. *Journal of Positive Psychology, 8*(3), 222-232.

Proyer, R. T., Ruch, W., & Buschor, C. (2013). Testing strengths-based interventions: A preliminary study on the effectiveness of a program targeting curiosity, gratitude, hope, humor, and zest for enhancing life satisfaction. *Journal of Happiness Studies, 14*(1), 275-292.

Rakel, D. P., & Hedgecock, J. (2008). Healing the healer: A tool to encourage student reflection towards health. *Medical Teacher, 30*(6), 633-635.

Ratey, J. (2008). *Spark: The revolutionary new science of exercise and the brain.* New York: Little, Brown and Company.

Reivich, K. J., & Shatté, A. J. (2002). *The resilience factor: 7 keys to finding your inner strengths and overcoming life's hurdles.* New York: Broadway.

Reivich, K. J., Gillham, J. E., Chaplin, T. M., & Seligman, M. E. (2005). From helplessness to optimism: The role of resilience in treating and preventing depression in youth. In S. Goldstein, & R. B. Brooks (Eds.), *Handbook of resilience in children* (pp. 223-237). New York: Kluwer Academic/Plenum Publishers.

Reivich, K. J., Seligman, M. E., & McBride, S. (2011). Master resilience training in the U.S. Army. *American Psychologist, 66*(1), 25-34.

Reynolds, G. (2007). Lobes of steel. *The New York Times.* Retrieved from ttp://www.nytimes.com/2007/08/19/sports/playmagazine/0819play-brain.html

Ricard, M. (2011). The Dalai Lama: Happiness from within. *International Journal of Wellbeing, 1*(2), 274-290.

Roberts, C., Kane, R., Thomson, H., Bishop, B., & Hart, B. (2003). The prevention of depressive symptoms in rural school children: A randomized controlled trial. *Journal of Consulting and Clinical Psychology, 71*(3), 622-628.

Robitschek, C., Ashton, M. W., Spering, C. C., Geiger, N., Byers, D., Schotts, G. C., & Thoen, M. A. (2012). Development and psychometric evaluation of the Personal Growth Initiative Scale-II. *Journal of Counseling Psychology, 59*(2), 274-287.

Roepke, A. M. (2013). Gains without pains? Growth after positive events. *Journal of Positive Psychology, 8*(4), 280-291.

Rogers, B., Christopher, M., Sunbay-Bilgen, Z., Pielage, M., Fung, H., Dahl, L., . . . Beale, N. (2013). Mindfulness in participatory medicine: Context and relevance. *Journal of Participatory Medicine, 5*, e7.

Rosenberg, D. A., & Silver, H. K. (1984). Medical student abuse. An unnecessary and preventable cause of stress. *JAMA, 251*(6), 739-742.

Rosenbloom, C. A. (Ed.). (2000). *Sports nutrition: A guide for the professional working with active people.* Chicago, IL.

Rosenthal, J. M., & Okie, S. (2005). White coat, mood indigo—Depression in medical school. *New England Journal of Medicine, 353*(11), 1085-1088.

Rozanski, A., & Kubzansky, L. D. (2005). Psychologic functioning and physical health: A paradigm of flexibility. *Psychosomatic Medicine, 67*(Suppl. 1), 547-553.

Rozin, P., & Royzman, E. B. (2001). Negativity bias, negativity dominance and contagion. *Personality and Social Psychology Review, 5*(4), 296-320.

Rust, T., Diessner, R., & Reade, L. (2009). Strengths only or strengths and relative weaknesses? A preliminary study. *Journal of Psychology, 143*(5), 465-476.

Ryan, K. D., Gottman, J. M., Murray, J. D., Carrere, S., & Swanson, C. (2000). Theoretical and mathematical modeling of marriage. In M. D. Lewis, & I. Granic (Eds.), *Emotion, development, and self-organization: Dynamic systems approaches to emotional Development* (pp. 349-372). Cambridge, UK: Cambridge University Press.

Ryan, R. M., & Deci, E. L. (2000a). Intrinsic and extrinsic motivations: Classic definitions and new directions. *Contemporary Educational Psychology, 25*, 54-67.

Ryan, R. M., & Deci, E. L. (2000b). Self-determination theory and the facilitation of intrinsic motivation, social development, and well-being. *American Psychologist, 55*(1), 68-78.

Ryan, R. M., & Deci, E. L. (2004). Autonomy is no illusion: Self-determination theory and the empirical study of authenticity, awareness, and will. In J. Greenberg, S. L. Koole, & T. A. Pyszczynski (Eds.), *Handbook of experimental existential psychology* (pp. 449-479). New York: Guilford Press.

Salovey, P., Caruso, D., & Mayer, J. D. (2012). Emotional intelligence in practice. In P. A. Linley, & S. Joseph (Eds.), *Positive psychology in practice* (pp. 447-463). Hoboken, NJ: John Wiley & Sons.

Sargent, M. C., Sotile, W., Sotile, M. O., Rubash, H., & Barrack, R. L. (2004). Stress and coping among orthopaedic surgery residents and faculty. *Journal of Bone and Joint Surgery American Volume, 86-A*(7), 1579-86.

Scheier, M. F., & Carver, C. S. (1992). Effects of optimism on psychological and physical well-being: Theoretical overview and empirical update. *Cognitive Therapy and Research, 16*(2), 201-228.

Schneider, S. L. (2001). In search of realistic optimism: Meaning, knowledge, and warm fuzziness. *American Psychologist, 56*(3), 250-263.

Schorr, Y. H., & Roemer, L. (2002). Posttraumatic meaning making: Toward a clearer definition. *Annual meeting of the International Society for Traumatic Stress Studies.* Baltimore, MD.

Schroevers, M. J., Helgeson, V. S., Sanderman, R., & Ranchor, A. V. (2010). Type of social support matters for prediction of posttraumatic growth among cancer survivors. *Psychooncology, 19*(1), 46-53.

Schwartz, B., & Sharpe, K. E. (2006). Practical wisdom: Aristotle meets positive psychology. *Journal of Happiness Studies, 7,* 377-395.

Schwartz, T., & McCarthy, C. (2010). *The way we're working isn't working: The four forgotten needs that energize great performance.* New York: Simon and Schuster.

Sears, R. W., Tirch, D. D., & Denton, R. B. (2011). *Mindfulness in clinical practice.* Sarasota, FL: Professional Resource Press.

Sears, W., Sears, M., Sears, J., & Sears, R. (2006). *The healthiest kid in the neighborhood: Ten ways to get your family on the right nutritional track.* New York: Little Brown.

Sedlmeier, P., Eberth, J., Schwartz, M., Zimmermann, D., Haarig, F., Jaeger, S., & Kunze, S. (2012). The psychological effects of meditation: A meta-analysis. *Psychological Bulletin, 138,* 1139-1171.

Segal, Z. V., Williams, J. M., & Teasdale, J. D. (2002). *Mindfulness-based cognitive therapy for depression: A new approach to preventing relapse.* New York: Guilford Press.

Segerstrom, S. C., Taylor, S. E., Kemeny, M. E., & Fahey, J. L. (1998). Optimism is associated with mood, coping, and immune change in response to stress. *Journal of Personality and Social Psychology, 74*(6), 1646-1655.

Seligman, M. E. (2008). Positive health. *Applied Psychology: An International Review, 57*(3), 3-18.

Seligman, M. E. (2010). The search for well-being. *Berliner Symposium der Positiven Psychologie.* Berlin.

Seligman, M. E. (2011). *Flourish: A visionary new understanding of happiness and well-being.* New York: Free Press.

Seligman, M. E., & Csikszentmihalyi, M. (2000). Positive psychology. An introduction. *American Psychologist, 55*(1), 5-14.

Seligman, M. E., Steen, T. A., Park, N., & Peterson, C. (2005). Positive psychology progress: Empirical validation of interventions. *American Psychologist, 60*(5), 410-421.

Selye, H. (1950). Stress and the general adaptation syndrome. *British Medical Journal*, 1383-1392.

Shakespeare-Finch, J. E., Smith, S. G., Gow, K. M., Embelton, G., & Baird, L. (2003). The prevalence of post-traumatic growth in emergency ambulance personnel. *Traumatology, 9*(1), 58-71.

Shanafelt, T. D., Sloan, J. A., & Habermann, T. M. (2003). The well-being of physicians. *American Journal of Medicine, 114*(6), 513-519.

Shanafelt, T. D., West, C. P., Sloan, J. A., Novotny, P. J., Poland, G. A., Menaker, R., . . . Dyrbye, L. N. (2009). Career fit and burnout among academic faculty. *Archives of Internal Medicine, 169*(10), 990-5.

Shapiro, S. L., & Carlson, L. E. (2009). *The art and science of mindfulness: Integrating mindfulness into psychology and the helping professions.* Washington, DC: American Psychological Association.

Shusterman, R. (2006). Thinking through the body, educating for the humanities: A plea for somaesthetics. *Journal of Aesthetic Education, 40*(1), 1-21.

Sibinga, E. M., & Wu, A. W. (2010). Clinician mindfulness and patient safety. *JAMA, 304*(22), 2532-2533.

Singer, T., Critchley, H. D., & Preuschoff, K. (2009). A common role of insula in feelings, empathy and uncertainty. *Trends in Cognitive Sciences, 13*(8), 334-340.

Slavin, L. A., O'Malley, J. E., Koocher, G. P., & Foster, D. J. (1982). Communication of the cancer diagnosis to pediatric patients: Impact on long-term adjustment. *American Journal of Psychiatry, 139*(2), 179-183.

Smallwood, J., Mrazek, M. D., & Schooler, J. W. (2011). Medicine for the wandering mind: Mind wandering in medical practice. *Medical Education, 45*(11), 1072-1080.

Sone, T., Nakaya, N., Ohmori, K., Shimazu, T., Higashiguchi, M., Kakazaki, M., . . . Tsuji, I. (2008). Sense of life worth living (ikigai) and mortality in Japan: Ohsaki Study. *Psychosomatic Medicine, 70*(6), 709-715.

Speca, M., Carlson, L. E., Goodey, E., & Angen, M. (2000). A randomized, wait-list controlled clinical trial: The effect of a mindfulness meditation-based stress reduction program on mood and symptoms of stress in cancer outpatients. *Psychosomatic Medicine, 62*(5), 613-622.

Stern, D. N. (2004). *The present moment in psychotherapy and everyday life.* New York: W. W. Norton & Company.

Sujiva. (1998). *Divine abodes: Meditation on loving kindness and other sublime states.* Sukhi Hotu.

Svensson, S., Kjellgren, K. I., Ahlner, J., & Säljö, R. (2000). Reasons for adherence with antihypertensive medication. *International Journal of Cardiology, 76*(2), 157-163.

Teasdale, J. D. (1999). Metacognition, mindfulness and the modification of mood disorders. *Clinical Psychology and Psychotherapy, 6,* 146-155.

Tedeschi, R. G., & Calhoun, L. G. (1996). The Posttraumatic Growth Inventory: Measuring the positive legacy of trauma. *Journal of Traumatic Stress, 9*(3), 455-471.

Tedeschi, R. G., & McNally, R. J. (2011). Can we facilitate posttraumatic growth in combat veterans? *American Psychologist, 66*(1), 19-24.

Thoen, M. A., & Robitschek, C. (2013). Intentional growth training: Developing an intervention to increase personal growth initiative. *Applied Psychology: Health and Well-being, 5*(2), 149-170.

Thomas, M. R., Dyrbye, L. N., Huntington, J. L., Lawson, K. L., Novotny, P. J., Sloan, J. A., & Shanafelt, T. D. (2007). How do distress and well-being relate to medical student empathy? A multicenter study. *Journal of General Internal Medicine, 22*(2), 177-83.

Timmons, K., & O'Leary, D. O. (2004). *Patient safety overview.* Amsterdam, NL: Joint Commission Patient Safety Initiatives. Retrieved from http://www.who.int/patientsafety/events/04/4_Timmons.pdf

Tribole, E., & Resch, E. (1995). *Intuitive eating.* New York: St. Martin's Press.

Tsuji, H., Larson, M. G., Venditti, F. J., Manders, E. S., Evans, J. C., Feldman, C. L., & Levy, D. (1996). Impact of reduced heart rate variability on risk for cardiac events. The Framingham Heart Study. *Circulation, 94*(11), 2850-2855.

Tugade, M. M., & Fredrickson, B. L. (2004). Resilient individuals use positive emotions to bounce back from negative emotional experiences. *Journal of Personality and Social Psychology, 86*(2), 320-333.

University of Essex GreenExercise Team. (2005-2014). *External Research.* Retrieved from Green Exercise: http://www.greenexercise.org/Research%20Publications%20Page.htm

Vaillant, G. E. (2008). *Spiritual evolution: A scientific defense of faith.* New York: Broadway.

Verrees, M. (1996). A piece of my mind. Touch me. *JAMA, 276*(16), 1285-6.

Vishnevsky, T., Cann, A., Calhoun, L. G., Tedeschi, R. G., & Demakis, G. J. (2010). Gender differences in self-reported posttraumatic growth: A meta-analysis. *Psychology of Women Quarterly, 34*(1), 110-120.

Watson, D., & Clark, L. A. (1994). *The PANAS-X: Manual for the positive and negative affect schedule-Expanded form.* Iowa City, IA: The University of Iowa.

Watson, D., & Naragon, K. (2011). Positive affectivity: The disposition to experience positive emotional states. In S. J. Lopez, & C. R. Snyder (Eds.), *Oxford handbook of positive psychology* (2nd ed., pp. 207-216). New York: Oxford University Press.

Watson, D., Clark, L. A., & Tellegen, A. (1988). Development and validation of brief measures of positive and negative affect: The PANAS scales. *Journal of Personality and Social Psychology, 54*(6), 1063-1070.

West, C. P., Shanafelt, T. D., & Kolars, J. C. (2011). Quality of life, burnout, educational debt, and medical knowledge among internal medicine residents. *JAMA, 306*(9), 952-960.

West, C. P., Tan, A. D., Habermann, T. M., Sloan, J. A., & Shanafelt, T. D. (2009). Association of resident fatigue and distress with perceived medical errors. *JAMA, 302*(12), 1294-1300.

Wheatley, M. J. (1992). *Leadership and the new science: Learning about organizations from an orderly universe.* San Francisco, CA: Berrett-Koehler.

Whitney, E., & Rolfes, S. R. (2005). *Understanding nutrition.* Belmont, CA: Wadsworth.

Williams, G. C., Minicucci, D. S., Kouides, R. W., Levesque, C. S., Chirkov, V. I., Ryan, R. M., & Deci, E. L. (2002). Self-determination, smoking, diet and health. *Health Education Research, 17*(5), 512-521.

Williams, G. C., Rodin, G. C., Ryan, R. M., Grolnick, W. S., & Deci, E. L. (1998). Autonomous regulation and long-term medication adherence in adult outpatients. *Health Psychology, 17*(3), 269-276.

Williams, J. M. (2006). *Applied sport psychology, personal growth to peak performance.* New York: McGraw-Hill.

Witte, F. M., Stratton, T. D., & Nora, L. M. (2006). Stories from the field: Students' descriptions of gender discrimination and sexual harassment during medical school. *Academic Medicine, 81*(7), 648-654.

World Health Organization. (1948). *Constitution of the World Health Organization.* Geneva, Switzerland: World Health Organization.

Young, A. (2013). Kaiser Permanente Study finds efforts to establish exercise as a vital sign prove valid. *Medicine & Science in Sports & Exercise, 45*(4). Retrieved from http://share.kaiserpermanente.org/article/kaiser-permanente-study-finds-efforts-to-establish-exercise-as-a-vital-sign-prove-valid/